P9-CRR-358

Pain Management

(PGPS – 136)

Pergamon Titles of Related Interest

Blanchard/Andrasik MANAGEMENT OF CHRONIC HEADACHES
DiMatteo/DiNicola ACHIEVING PATIENT COMPLIANCE: The
Psychology of the Medical Practitioner's Role
Karoly/Steffen/O'Grady CHILD HEALTH PSYCHOLOGY: Concepts
and Issues
Meichenbaum STRESS INOCULATION TRAINING
Varni CLINICAL BEHAVIORAL PEDIATRICS: An Interdisciplinary
Biobehavioral Approach
Weiss/Katzman/Wolchik TREATING BULIMIA: A Psychoeducational
Approach

Related Journals*

CLINICAL PSYCHOLOGY REVIEW
SOCIAL SCIENCE & MEDICINE

*Free sample copies available upon request

PERGAMON GENERAL PSYCHOLOGY SERIES
EDITORS
Arnold P. Goldstein, Syracuse University
Leonard Krasner, SUNY at Stony Brook

Pain Management
A Handbook of Psychological
Treatment Approaches

edited by

Arnold D. Holzman
Yale University School of Medicine and
West Haven Veterans Administration Medical Center

Dennis C. Turk
Center for Pain Evaluation and Treatment,
University of Pittsburgh School of Medicine

PERGAMON PRESS
New York   Oxford   Toronto   Sydney   Frankfurt

Pergamon Press Offices:

U.S.A.   Pergamon Press Inc., Maxwell House, Fairview Park,
                     Elmsford, New York 10523, U.S.A.

U.K.   Pergamon Press Ltd., Headington Hill Hall,
                     Oxford OX3 0BW, England

CANADA   Pergamon Press Canada Ltd., Suite 104, 150 Consumers Road,
                     Willowdale, Ontario M2J 1P9, Canada

AUSTRALIA   Pergamon Press (Aust.) Pty. Ltd., P.O. Box 544,
                     Potts Point, NSW 2011, Australia

FEDERAL REPUBLIC Pergamon Press GmbH, Hammerweg 6,
OF GERMANY   D-6242 Kronberg-Taunus, Federal Republic of Germany

BRAZIL   Pergamon Editora Ltda., Rua Eça de Queiros, 346,
                     CEP 04011, São Paulo, Brazil

JAPAN   Pergamon Press Ltd., 8th Floor, Matsuoka Central Building,
                     1-7-1 Nishishinjuku, Shinjuku, Tokyo 160, Japan

PEOPLE'S REPUBLIC Pergamon Press, Qianmen Hotel, Beijing,
OF CHINA   People's Republic of China

Copyright © 1986 Pergamon Press Inc.

Library of Congress Cataloging in Publication Data
Main entry under title:

Pain management.

   (Pergamon general psychology series ; 136)
   Bibliography: p.
   1. Pain--Treatment--Handbooks, manuals, etc.
2. Pain--Psychological aspects--Handbooks,
manuals, etc. I. Holzman, Arnold D. II. Turk,
Dennis C. III. Series. [DNLM: 1. Pain--therapy.
2. Psychotherapy: WL 704 P14655]
RB127.P3323   1985   616'.0472   85-12399
ISBN 0-08-031931-9

*All rights reserved. No part of this publication may be reproduced,
stored in a retrieval system or transmitted in any form or by any means:
electronic, electrostatic, magnetic tape, mechanical, photocopying,
recording or otherwise, without permission in writing from the
publishers.*

Printed in Great Britain by A. Wheaton & Co. Ltd., Exeter

To Susan for her limitless understanding, support and kindness.

A.D.H.

To Lorraine, Kenny, and Katy for all the times I was not there and without whose patience and understanding this book would not have been completed.

D.C.T.

CONTENTS

PREFACE

Perhaps the most universal form of stress encountered is pain. No medical symptom is more ubiquitous. Statistics on the magnitude of the problem are staggering. It has been estimated, for example, that there are 20 to 50 million arthritis sufferers in the United States with 600,000 new victims each year (American Arthritis Foundation, 1976). Chronic headaches, particularly migraine headaches, occur for approximately 25 million Americans (Paulley & Haskell, 1975). And low back pain, one of the most common pain complaints, accounts for over 8 million visits to physicians each year (Clark, Gosnell, & Shapiro, 1977).

Patients with chronic pain represent both an individual and societal problem in terms of their suffering, the impact on their families, time lost from employment, medical expenses, costs associated with litigation and disability compensation, and overutilization of health care resources. The first president of the International Association for the Study of Pain, Dr. J.J. Bonica, has gone so far as to call pain "one of the most pressing issues of our time" (Bonica, 1974).

Despite the prevalence of pain, the existence of pain since time immemorial, and medical advances, there is currently no treatment available that can consistently and permanently ameliorate pain for all patients. The recognition that many people experience persistent pain that is refractory to standard medical treatment and that their functional disability is often in excess of that expected on the basis of identified physical pathology has led clinical researchers to examine factors other than physiological ones that may contribute to the problem.

It has long been recognized that subjectively experienced pain is not solely dependent upon tissue damage or organic dysfunction. The intensity of pain reported and the amount of pain behavior displayed seem to be influenced by a wide range of factors, such as attention, anxiety, financial status, cultural background, and environmental contingencies. Thus, the role of psychological processes, especially dysfunctional ones, in the etiology, exacerbation, and maintenance of chronic pain has received increasing attention. The advent of a multidimensional perspective on pain in contrast to a view that is based largely on sensory–physiological factors has resulted in a proliferation of multidisciplinary pain clinics (over 1,200 in the United States) that focus on all aspects of the pain experience, both physical and psychological.

Interest in pain and pain treatments has grown rapidly over the past 15 years. International (the International Association for the Study of Pain) and national (American Pain Society) organizations have recently been founded. A journal (*Pain*) devoted exclusively to research on pain has been published since 1975, and a new journal devoted to clinically relevant topics in pain management (*The Clinical Journal of Pain*) has just begun publication. Moreover, many edited books and monographs on pain are published each year (e.g., Melzack & Wall, 1983; Smith, Merskey, & Gross, 1980; Stanton-Hicks & Boas, 1982; Turk, Meichenbaum, & Genest, 1983; Wall & Melzack, 1984).

Pain has become a major topic of interest within the developing fields of behavioral medicine and health psychology. Each new book in these areas includes a general summary chapter on pain and pain treatments (e.g., Doleys, Meredith, & Cimnero, 1982; Gatchel & Baum, 1983; Millon, Green, & Meagher, 1982). With two exceptions (Fordyce, 1976; Turk et al., 1983), none of the existing monographs or review chapters provide sufficient details of the various treatment approaches to enable a practitioner to apply them.

As leaders of workshops and participants in symposia, as well as consultants to pain clinics throughout the United States and Canada, we have been impressed by the growing number of professionals who are seeking information about the mechanics of treatment. Following presentations, we receive numerous requests from across the United States and around the world to visit our pain management program. Questions such as "How do you introduce your treatment to patients?", "How do you manage unmotivated patients?", "Do you involve spouses in your treatment?", and so forth, are typical. In short, they are asking "how to do it." The purpose of this book is to provide the reader with one source of sufficiently detailed and in-depth coverage of the mechanics of the major psychological approaches to treating pain.

Topics range from theoretical perspective (e.g., operant conditioning, cognitive-behavior therapy) to treatment modalities (e.g., biofeedback, hypnosis) to specific populations (e.g., children, cancer patients). The material presented in each chapter emphasizes the mechanics of the approach being described so that the reader will acquire a sense of the "nuts and bolts" of the interventions.

All contributors were asked to consider three aspects of their clinical work in preparing their chapter. The first was to include a brief overview of the theoretical rationale and supporting data for the particular approach. The second was to describe specific details of their treatment approach using case examples to illustrate important points. In this section, each author illustrates how the particular approach is actually applied.

The third aspect was to include a discussion of the case(s) that were described, emphasizing the application of treatment components. This discussion highlights clinical decision-making, how the clinical application followed from the particular theoretical rationale, and how particular or unexpected problems were addressed.

It is hoped that this book will serve as a valuable reference for students and practitioners in psychology, psychiatry, nursing, social work, occupational and physical therapy, and other disciplines utilizing nonmedical pain management approaches.

We would like to gratefully acknowledge the financial support of the Veterans Administration Merit Review Board during the production of this book.

Arnold D. Holzman
Dennis C. Turk
New Haven, Connecticut

April, 1985

REFERENCES

American Arthritis Foundation (1976). *Arthritis, the basic facts.* Atlanta, GA: Author.

Bonica, J.J. (1974). Preface. In J.J. Bonica (Ed.), *Advances in neurology* (Vol. 4). New York: Raven Press.

Clark, J.W., Gosnell, M., & Shapiro, D. (1977, April 25). The new war on pain. *Newsweek, 89,* 48–58.

Doleys, D.M., Meredith, R.L., & Ciminero, A.R. (1982). *Behavioral medicine: Assessment and treatment strategies.* New York: Plenum Publishing.

Fordyce, W.E. (1976). *Behavioral methods for chronic pain and illness.* St. Louis: C.V. Mosby.

Gatchel, R.J., & Baum, A. (1983). *An introduction to health psychology.* Reading, MA: Addison-Wesley.

Melzack, R., & Wall, P.D. (1983). *The challenge of pain*. New York: Basic Books.

Millon, T., Green, C., & Meagher, R. (Eds.). (1982). *Handbook of clinical health psychology*. New York: Plenum Press.

Paulley, J.W., & Haskell, D.J. (1975). Treatment of migraine without drugs. *Journal of Psychosomatic Research, 19*, 367–374.

Smith, W.L., Merskey, H., & Gross, S.C. (Eds.).

(1980). *Pain: Meaning and management*. New York: Sp-Medical & Scientific Books.

Stanton-Hicks, M., & Boas, R.A. (Eds.). (1982). *Chronic low back pain*. New York: Raven Press.

Turk, D.C., Meichenbaum, D., & Genest, M. (1983). *Pain and behavioral medicine*. New York: Guilford Press.

Wall, P.D., & Melzack, R. (Eds.). (1984). *Textbook of pain*. London: Churchill Livingstone.

1 CHRONIC PAIN: INTERFACES AMONG PHYSICAL, PSYCHOLOGICAL, AND SOCIAL PARAMETERS

Dennis C. Turk
Arnold D. Holzman

The quest to find means to control pain has probably existed since time immemorial. Historically, the majority of the attempts to alleviate pain have at least tacitly ascribed to a dualistic perspective formally promulgated by Descartes. That is, philosophers since the time of Aristotle have suggested that pain should be viewed as an emotion and consequently within the domain of the mind rather than the physical body. Thus, these philosophers suggested that pain was actually beyond the realm of physicians and surgeons. The Stoic philosophers further suggested that because pain was located within the mind it should be "overcome" through logic and "rational repudiation" rather than physical intervention. Religious leaders also viewed pain as beyond the scope of physical treatment. Some suggested that it was inappropriate for medical practitioners to treat pain because it was sent by God as punishment for the individual's sins or Original Sin (Fulop-Miller, 1938).

In contrast to those who viewed pain as a faculty of the mind were physicians, surgeons, and other healers who viewed pain as a sensory phenomenon associated with an organic cause. The history of medicine is replete with descriptions of diverse treatment modalities believed to be appropriate for treating pain, many of which are now known to have little therapeutic merit and some of which may actually have been harmful to the patient. For example, Haggard (1929, cited in Turk, Meichenbaum, & Genest, 1983) described the following treatment administered to King Charles II by the best physicians of his day:

> A pint of blood was extracted from his right arm and a half pint from his left shoulder. This was followed by an emetic, sneezing powder, bleedings, soothing potions, a plaster of pitch, and pidgeon dung was smeared on his feet. Potions containing ten different substances, chiefly herbs, as well as 40 drops of extract of human skull, were swallowed. Finally, application of the bezoar stone [gallstones from sheep or goats] was prescribed. Following the extensive treatment, the king died. (pp. 75–76)

1

Prior to the second half of the 19th century and the advent of research in sensory psychophysics and physiology, much of the pain treatment arsenal was composed of treatment modalities that had no direct mode of action upon organic mechanisms responsible for the symptoms. Yet, despite the absence of an adequate physiological basis, these treatments proved to have some therapeutic merit, at least for some patients. These effects have been disparagingly referred to as "placebo" effects or "psychological cures," with the implicit message being that the symptoms alleviated by such measures must be psychological (i.e., imaginary).

The same message has been applied to some more modern treatment modalities. Although some of these sophisticated treatment regimens are based on specific knowledge of physiology, the mode of action may be unrelated to modification of physiological processes. For example, in a recent study of headache patients treated by pharmacological means, Fitzpatrick, Hopkins, and Harvard-Watts (1983) concluded that although a large number of patients reported benefits from the drug treatment, most of the improvement appeared to be unrelated to the pharmacological action per se. Similarly, biofeedback has been reported to be of potential benefit for a wide range of pain disorders, from headaches to temporomandibular joint dysfunction syndrome to low back pain; the actual effect of biofeedback, however, may be unrelated to the modification of physiological activity (e.g., Denver et al., 1979; Dohrman & Laskin, 1978; Flor, Haag, Turk, & Koehler, 1983; Turk, Meichenbaum, & Berman, 1979).

Increased knowledge and advances in sensory physiology have resulted in the development of a contemporary treatment armamentarium that includes potent analgesic medications and sophisticated surgical procedures. This has served to reinforce the perspective of pain as a sensory phenomenon associated with tissue pathology. Even with such advances, however, pain remains very much a mystery, and *there is still no satisfactory set of treatments to consistently and permanently alleviate all sources of pain.*

On the other side of the coin, it can be noted that for some pain syndromes and for some patients, almost any treatment appears to have a beneficial effect. For example, Greene and Laskin (1974) followed 100 patients with temporomandibular joint myofascial pain syndrome from 6 months to 8 years following treatment by a host of modalities (i.e., analgesic medication, minor tranquilizers, exercises, splints, joint and muscle injections, physical therapy, psychological counseling, and placebo treatments ranging from inert drugs, nonoccluding bite plates, mock equilibration of the bite, and nonfunctional biofeedback) all "in combination with reassurance, explanation, advice for self-management, and a general attitude of sympathetic understanding" (p. 1366). These investigators reported that 92% of the patients had no or only minor recurrences of symptoms.

As an indication of how far we have *not* come, consider the host of current treatment alternatives available for a patient with chronic pain. Most experienced clinicians working in chronic pain management programs would not be surprised to come across a patient who is being treated simultaneously by multiple medical specialists and who may be receiving different interventions from each. Neurologists, neurosurgeons, orthopaedic surgeons, rheumatologists, radiologists, psychiatrists, osteopaths, among others, are medical specialists typically involved in the treatment of chronic pain. In addition to these medical specialties consider the nonmedical therapists that are available such as acupuncturists, chiropractors, masseuses, naturopaths, and so forth.

Modern day treatment at the hands of diverse specialists can be viewed as following the medical "dualistic" model; that is, disease is viewed as an abnormality in the function or structure of body organs and systems, and pain is a symptom of a biological process. Once the physical cause is identified and treated appropriately, the symptom — pain — will be eliminated. Physicians today search for a physiological cause and then offer a somatic treatment they believe to be appropriate for treating the physical cause. Often no consideration is given to the role of psychological or socioenvironmental parameters.

How far have we come in treating pain from the time of King Charles? Although the diagnostic and treatment procedures available today involve advanced technology, and are based on knowledge of anatomy and physiology that did not exist in the time of King Charles, the outcome is often similarly unsuccessful. Physicians are often unable to identify and treat a specific organic cause for pain.

Chronic pain remains a major problem for which we have no adequate solution. For example, it has been estimated that chronic pain afflicts as many as 50 to 75 million Americans (Bonica, 1974; National Institute of Neurological, Communicative Disorders and Stroke, 1979), with costs exceeding $50 billion per year (National Institute of Neurological, Communicative Disorders and Stroke, 1979). There are currently estimated to be 10 to 20 million migraine sufferers (Paulley & Haskel, 1975), 20 to 50 million arthritics (American Arthritis Foundation, 1976), and 8.5 million Americans permanently disabled by back pain (Vital and Health Statistics, 1974). There are over 1,200 pain clinics in the United States to deal with chronic pain problems.

To summarize the current status of pain treatment: Despite increased knowledge and sophistication, it is still unclear why patients with ostensibly the same medical diagnosis may respond differentially to identical treatments, and it is unclear why some treatments that have apparently no physiological basis for their action sometimes prove beneficial. From a dualistic perspective, one might be tempted to suggest that those patients who fail to respond to what is deemed to be an active and appropriate treatment, those who respond differentially to identical symptoms, and those who respond to "placebo" treatments have psychogenic pain, whereas those who respond appropriately have true somatic pain.

On the other hand, we might want to consider pain from what has come to be termed a biopsychosocial perspective (Engel, 1977). That is, pain is a complex phenomenon that is the product of the interaction of nociceptive sensory stimulation, psychological factors (i.e., cognitive, affective, and behavioral), and socioenvironmental factors (e.g., reinforcement from significant others and the health care system; ethno-cultural beliefs and societal norms). From the biopsychosocial perspective, each of these factors in combination contributes to the experience of pain and the response to treatment. Pain is neither solely somatic nor solely psychogenic, but is comprised of the interaction among all of these factors that produces the subjective experience of pain. In fact, we would expect that there would be a synergistic relationship whereby psychological and socioenvironmental factors can modulate nociceptive stimulation and the response to treatment. In turn, nociceptive stimulation can influence patients' appraisals of their situation and the treatment, their level of dysphoric mood, and the ways that they interact with significant others, including medical practitioners.

AN ILLUSTRATIVE BIOPSYCHOSOCIAL MODEL OF PAIN

Chronic low back pain (CLBP) is a significant medical problem that has been highly resistant to more than symptomatic treatment (Flor & Turk, 1984; Nachemson, 1979). Correlations between degenerative and structural abnormalities of the spine and reports of pain have consistently been low (e.g., Magora & Schwartz, 1980) suggesting that abnormal anatomical structure or physiology are not unique or significant causes or maintainers of CLBP. Psychological and socioenvironmental factors have been suggested as contributors to both the development and maintenance of CLBP (e.g., Dorpat & Holmes, 1962; Fordyce, 1976; Gentry & Bernal, 1977; Turk et al., 1983).

Recently, Turk and Flor (Turk & Flor, 1984; Flor, Turk, & Birbaumer, 1985) have proposed and provided a preliminary test of a biopsychosocial model of CLBP that they have labeled a "diathesis-stress" model. The central assumption of this model is that CLBP results from an interaction of environmental events with a predisposing organic or psychological condition or diathesis. The model states that the organic or psychological factors comprising the diathesis may vary for each individual. Factors contributing to this include physical build and health status, as well as psychological conditioning history. The specific physical or psychological events (e.g., injury, life events) interact with a predisposing diathesis resulting in the complaint of pain.

The occurrence of emotional and physical stressors with which the individual cannot adequately cope is thought to lead to an increase in muscular tension as a natural reaction in the fight–flight response to stress (e.g., Cannon, 1929). In a weak, already damaged, or otherwise unfavorably predisposed back (and if those stress experiences are of sufficient severity or are frequently recurring), a response stereotypy (Lacey & Lacey, 1959) may develop, consisting of an extreme and sustained muscular hyperreaction of the back muscles. The increase in muscular tension may lead to ischemia, which causes a reflex muscle spasm in the involved area. Thus, a vicious cycle of pain–muscle tension-pain may develop. Ischemia can also be induced by sympathetic arousal that leads to vasoconstriction and will subsequently cause reflex muscle spasm at the affected site. Both processes may interact (which is expected to be the case in a stress situation). Long-lasting ischemia leads to a release of pain-eliciting substances (e.g., bradykinen, substance P) that will cause the pain experience if the concentration is sufficiently high.

The pain that is felt may act as a new stressor contributing to an increase in the tension and thus more pain, especially if the individual possesses inadequate coping skills. Because movement often increases the pain further, an additional aggravating factor may be the increasing immobility of the spine that may develop out of a negative conditioned emotional response for movement. That is,

patients believe that if they engage in activity, they might exacerbate their pain or they might injure themselves even further. (One patient indicated that he did not engage in activity because he was afraid that he might "break my spinal fusion".) This may especially be the case when the original acute pain problem resulted from traumatic injury to the back, because inactivity helps avoid spasm-related movement pain.

Significant others may positively reinforce inactivity in an attempt to be sympathetic and to reduce the patient's suffering. Moreover, the system of pain-related compensation may discourage increased activity and return to work, leading to greater immobility, isolation, and preoccupation with pain. The state of heightened muscle tension and immobility may, in turn, have an additional complicating result of increasing the occurrence of muscle spasms. The entire process may eventually lead to oxygen depletion in the affected muscle tissue due to the sustained contractions and finally result in muscular degeneration and atrophy (e.g., de Vries, 1968).

A further complicating factor may be the occurrence of "protective muscle spasm" (de Vries, 1966, 1968) in reaction to spinal injury, which may make the paravertebral musculature (especially the erector spinae muscles) more susceptible to stress-related hypertension. On the other hand, habitual muscular overreaction with the back muscles to stressful stimuli may make the back more susceptible to injury.

Finally, dysphoric mood associated with perceptions of uncontrollable pain, limited control over life, and increased inability to engage in previously desired activities may exacerbate pain through muscle tension and reduced activity — a vicious cycle is thus perpetuated (Turk, Kerns, & Rudy, 1984). This relationship has to be considered as an interactive, biopsychosocial one.

The diathesis-stress model described illustrates the important interactions among physiological, psychological, and socioenvironmental factors and argues strongly for the need to consider psychological and socioenvironmental factors in the treatment of pain. It would hardly be surprising to find that treatments that focused on only one of these parameters were of limited success. Rather, more comprehensive, interdisciplinary approaches would appear to be required where the patient (within his or her social environment), and not the symptom, was being treated. The model also demonstrates that psychological and socioenvironmental factors need to be considered at two points. First, these factors may contribute to the etiology or development of various pain syndromes. Second, even if unrelated to the original cause of the pain, they may contribute to maintenance and exacerbation of the problem once a pathological process has been initiated.

The diathesis-stress model outlined noted the contribution of patients' appraisals and socioenvironmental parameters in the development and maintenance of symptoms. These factors are critical in considering how patients will respond to their plight and to treatments offered. In the next section, we will consider some of these parameters in more detail.

Psychological Parameters

People differ markedly in how frequently they complain about physical symptoms, in their propensity to visit a physician when experiencing identical symptoms, and in their response to the same treatments (Desroaches, Kamen, & Ballard, 1967; Zborowski, 1969; Zola, 1966). Often, the nature of patients' responses has little to do with their objective physical condition (Mechanic, 1962). For example, White, Williams, and Greenberg (1961) noted that less than one third of individuals with clinically significant symptoms consult a physician. There is increasing recognition that the presence of physiological perturbations are evaluated against some implicit or "common sense" representations of illness (Leventhal & Nerenz, 1982).

It may be useful to underscore the distinction between the medical concept of a *disease* that involves the malfunction or maladapta-

tion of biological processes and an *illness as construed by the patient* in his or her personal reaction to the disease and associated discomfort. Illness is a subjective experience that relates to the patient's unique perception of the symptoms, treatment, and appropriate responses. Patients will behave during illness in ways that are consistent with the conceptualizations they hold about their symptoms (Leventhal & Nerenz, 1982). Patients present their symptoms in ways that are related to their illness concerns, interpretation of symptoms, and personal beliefs.

Individuals are not passive responders to physical sensations, but rather, actively seek to make sense of their experience. They seem to appraise their condition and decide whether a particular sensation is a symptom of a physical disorder that requires attention by matching sensations to some preexisting implicit model. Thus, to some extent, each individual functions within a uniquely constructed reality. When information is ambiguous, he or she relies on general attitudes and beliefs based on his or her prior learning history. These beliefs determine the meaning and significance of the problem, as well as the perceptions of appropriate treatment.

When a patient experiences some form of intense nociceptive stimulation, he or she is likely to seek an explanation for the cause and try to determine the implications. What could be the cause of the nociceptive stimulation, was it something I did (e.g., "Did I hurt my back lifting a heavy object?"), and does this mean I might have a serious condition ("Maybe it's a sign of something really bad—cancer!")? The individual's response to such questions will affect his or her emotional and physiological arousal and his or her behavior. If the pain can be attributed to something that can be understood and that is familiar, then the patient may be less anxious and may decide whether and how to self-treat (e.g., take aspirins, lie down). If a patient interprets the sensations as serious, he or she may become tense and make an appointment to see a physician. The results of the selected action will also influence subsequent appraisals. For example, reduction in external stimulation by lying down in the bedroom may lead the patient to become preoccupied with his or her body and to focus on the sensations. If the symptoms do not follow the expected course, the patient may become more tense and distressed.

Most individuals have developed beliefs about illness that can be viewed as "acute illness" beliefs. That is, there is a specific cause for the symptoms, a specific treatment for the symptoms, and a definite time course (days or weeks). Moreover, socially sanctioned healers are expected to have available appropriate treatment modalities to alleviate the symptoms. This model is quite appropriate for many problems; however, for chronic medical syndromes, such as unremitting pain extending over many years, this model is inadequate and potentially detrimental. Often, the cause is unclear, the symptoms are unresponsive to all treatment efforts, and no end is foreseen for the problem. Physicians have not performed as expected. Given the discrepancy between the beliefs about acute illness and omnipotent physicians and the reality of chronic pain, it is hardly surprising that patients become despondent, perceive their plight as helpless and beyond their control, and become embittered and pessimistic about their future. These patients often reduce their activity levels, alter their social roles, and may come to view little contingency between their behavior and symptoms. All of these characteristics have been related to depression (e.g., Lewinsohn, 1974; Rehm, 1977; Seligman, 1975).

As patients become more and more demoralized, there is even less incentive to continue trying to cope with the situation. Thus, there is a spiraling downward from initial optimism, through repeated high expectancies for new treatments, followed by failures, eventually to giving up.

Socioenvironmental Parameters

Socioenvironmental factors affect the experience of pain in a number of ways. First, they may influence the beliefs of the patient regarding the meaning of symptoms and appropriate responses. Second, the beliefs and stereotypes of health care providers may influence the interactions between the patient and physician, the expectancies they have for each other, and the nature and type of treatment offered for the patient's symptoms. Finally, these factors may affect how significant others respond to the patient and, subsequently, the patient's behavior (e.g., Fordyce, 1976).

Common sense beliefs about illness and physicians are based on both prior experience and social and cultural transmission of beliefs and expectancies. Ethnic group membership influences how one perceives, labels, responds to, and communicates various symptoms, as well as from whom one elects to obtain care, when it is sought, and the types of treatments received (Mechanic, 1978). Several authors have specifically noted the importance of sociocultural factors in beliefs about and responses to pain (e.g., Wolff & Langley, 1968; Zborowski, 1969). Social factors influence how families and local groups respond to and interact with patients. Furthermore, ethnic expectations and sexual and age stereotypes may influence the practitioner–patient relationship (Chrisman & Kleinman, 1980).

Many chronic pain problems are extremely frustrating to physicians. Despite their best efforts, the patient continues to report the presence of pain. Furthermore, some patients complaining of pain do not demonstrate identifiable tissue pathology. The beliefs of the health care provider likely affect how patients are treated. For example, Pilowsky and Bond (1969) reported that older male cancer patients were less likely to be given potent narcotic analgesics than younger female patients. Additionally, Gillmore and Hill (1981) found that patients with ambiguous diagnoses were viewed as not having genuine pain. Moreover, these patients were viewed less favorably than patients for whom definite diagnoses were available. The frustration of physicians is, at least implicitly, conveyed to the patient.

Because pain is a subjective experience, we

have no "thermometer" that will enable us to assess the intensity of the pain the patient is experiencing. We are heavily dependent upon self-reports, which are likely to be highly idiosyncratic and affected by factors other than the extent of tissue damage or pathology. Because we do not have objective measures of pain intensity, the patient's manner of communicating becomes the sole basis for many decisions made by health care providers and significant others. And individual differences in symptom presentation affect the nature of the treatment and attention a patient receives. The more dramatic the presentation, the more seriously the patient's complaint might be taken ("You oil the wheel that squeaks"). If complaints lead to reduction in performance of undesirable activity and to positive reinforcement, then continued complaining may be fostered (Fordyce, 1976). If medication is taken when pain is most intense (prn), then medication may become a reinforcer of pain; and if aversive activities (e.g., job responsibilities) are reduced when pain increases, then pain is positively reinforced.

Sympathetic family members may unwittingly perpetuate pain by positively reinforcing what have been called pain behaviors (Fordyce, 1976). That is, if I grimace when I engage in an activity, my significant other may tell me to sit down and take it easy. The significant other has positively reinforced grimacing by giving the patient sympathetic attention and by encouraging inactivity and possibly some temporary reduction in pain perception. The social welfare system also reinforces continued pain and pain behavior by providing compensation based on *reported* pain.

CONCLUSIONS

An important point to consider is that the majority of knowledge of chronic pain is based on patients who attend our pain clinics. The psychological and sociocultural parameters mentioned, however, would lead us to expect that many patients with pain problems never appear at pain clinics (Lipton & Mar-

bach, 1984). We know very little about how representative the pain clinic sample is or how the majority of patients with pain problems cope with their plight. More research is required to understand how psychological and socioenvironmental parameters interact with somatic ones to determine which patients will be referred to pain clinics and which will not.

Another area for which little literature exists is the synergistic effects between psychological, socioenvironmental, and somatic parameters. For example, are there some somatic treatments that only prove effective when the patient and physician are optimistic about their potential or experience the right mental attitude (Melzack, 1973)? Some recent literature suggests that psychological factors may affect the production of endorphins (Chen, 1980), as well as the endocrine (e.g., Frankenhaeuser, 1980) and the immune systems (e.g., Rogers, Dubey, & Reich, 1979).

In summary, there are a growing number of reasons to consider a biopsychosocial model of chronic pain that incorporates psychological, socioenvironmental, and somatic parameters for understanding the development, maintenance, and exacerbation of pain, as well as response to pain and the nature of treatment. The first multidisciplinary pain management program that included a biopsychosocial perspective was developed by Bonica at the University of Washington School of Medicine only 15 years ago. The growth of such pain clinics to over 1,200 nationwide attests to the societal need.

It is important to realize that the biopsychosocial perspective is one that can serve as an umbrella for a diversity of specific treatment approaches. Careful examination of the treatment programs offered at various comprehensive pain centers reveals that no two programs are identical and a diversity of modalities are employed. In this volume, we have included chapters on the most widely used psychological modalities. To date, there is no satisfactory evidence to support the utility of one modality in contrast to any other. At the present time, no definitive statement can be made as to which modality should be employed with which patients, with what characteristics, and for which pain syndromes. Future research is required to answer such questions. At the present time, practitioners need to be aware of the range of options available and must rely largely on clinical judgment to decide on which modality(ies) to employ with different patients. The detailed description of treatment modalities, approaches, and case studies included in this volume will, we hope, assist practitioners in choosing among the range available. Further, it is our hope that the specific descriptions will permit investigators to evaluate systematically the different treatment strategies so that differential efficacy can be determined and future treatment decisions can be based on empirical research as well as clinical judgment.

REFERENCES

American Arthritis Foundation (1976). *Arthritis, the basic facts.* Atlanta, GA: Author.

Bonica, J J. (1974). Preface. In J.J. Bonica (Ed.), *Advances in neurology* (Vol. 4, pp. vii–x). New York: Raven Press.

Cannon, W.D. (1929). *Bodily changes in pain, hunger, fear and rage.* Boston: Charles T. Branford Co.

Chen, A.C.N. (1980, September). *Behavioral and brain evoked potential (BEP) evaluation of placebo effects: Contrast of cognitive mechanisms and endorphin mechanisms.* Paper presented at the second scientific meeting of the American Pain Society, New York.

Chrisman, N., & Kleinman, A. (1980). Health beliefs and practices. In S. Thernstrom (Ed.), *Harvard encyclopedia of American ethnic groups* (pp. 452–468). Cambridge, MA: Harvard University Press.

Denver, D.R., Laveault, D., Girard, F. et al. (1979). Behavioral medicine: Biobehavioral effects of short-term thermal biofeedback and relaxation in rheumatoid arthritis patients. *Biofeedback and Self-Regulation, 4,* 245–246.

Desroches, H.F., Kaiman, B.D., & Ballard, H.T. (1967). Factors influencing reporting of physical symptoms by the aged patient. *Geriatrics, 22,* 169–175.

de Vries, H.A. (1966). Quantitative electromyographic investigation of the spasm theory of ideopathic low back pain. *Journal of Physical Medicine, 45,* 119–134.

de Vries, H.A. (1968). EMG fatigue curves in postural muscles: A possible etiology of ideopathic low back pain. *Journal of Physical Medicine, 47,* 175–181.

Dohrmann, R.J., & Laskin, D.M. (1978). An evaluation of electromyographic biofeedback in the treatment of myofascial pain-dysfunction syndrome. *Journal of the American Dental Association, 96,* 656–662.

Dorpat, T.L., & Holmes, T.H. (1962). Backache of muscle tension origin. In W.S. Kroger (Ed.), *Psychosomatic obstetrics, gynecology and endocrinology* (pp. 302–321). Springfield, IL: Charles C. Thomas.

Engel, G.L. (1977). The need for a new medical model: A challenge for biomedicine. *Science, 196,* 129–136.

Fitzpatrick, R.M., Hopkins, A.P., & Harvard-Watts, O. (1983). Social dimensions of healing: A longitudinal study of outcomes of medical management of headaches. *Social Science & Medicine, 17,* 501–510.

Flor, H., Haag, G., Turk, D.C., & Koehler, G. (1983). Efficacy of EMG biofeedback, pseudotherapy, and conventional medical treatment for chronic rheumatic pain. *Pain, 17,* 21–32.

Flor, H., & Turk, D.C. (1984). Etiological theories and treatments for chronic back pain: I. Somatic factors. *Pain, 19,* 105–121.

Flor, H., Turk, D.C., & Birbaumer, N. (1985). Assessment of stress-related psychophysiological responses in chronic back pain patients. *Journal of Consulting and Clinical Psychology, 53,* 354–364.

Fordyce, W.E. (1976). *Behavioral methods for chronic pain and illness.* St. Louis, MO: C. V. Mosby.

Frankenhaeuser, M. (1980). Psychobiological aspects of life stress. In S. Levine & H. Ursin (Eds.), *Coping and health* (pp. 124–157). New York: Plenum Press.

Fulop-Miller, R. (1938). *Triumph over pain.* New York: Literary Guild of America.

Gentry, W.D., & Bernal, G.A.A. (1977). Chronic pain. In R.B. Williams & W.D. Gentry (Eds.), *Behavioral approaches to medical treatment* (pp. 173–182). Cambridge, MA: Ballinger.

Gillmore, M.R., & Hill, C.T. (1981). Reactions to patients who complain of pain: Effects of ambiguous diagnosis. *Journal of Applied Social Psychology, 11,* 14–22.

Greene, C.S., & Laskin, D.M. (1974). Long-term evaluation of conservative treatment for myofascial pain dysfunction syndrome. *Journal of the American Dental Association, 89,* 1365–1368.

Haggard, H. (1929). *Devils, drugs, and doctors.* New York: Harper.

Lacey, J.I., & Lacey, B.C. (1959). Verification and extension of the principle of autonomic response-stereotypy. *American Journal of Psychology, 71,* 51–73.

Leventhal, H., & Nerenz, D.R. (1982). Representations on threat and the control of stress. In

D. Meichenbaum & M. Jaremko (Eds.), *Stress management and prevention: A cognitive-behavioral approach* (pp. 5–38). New York: Plenum Press.

Lewinsohn, P.M. (1974). Clinical and theoretical aspects of depression. In K.S. Calhoun, H.E. Adams, & K.M. Mitchell (Eds.), *Innovative treatment methods of psychopathology* (pp.147–161). New York: John Wiley & Sons.

Lipton, J.A., & Marbach, J.J. (1984). Ethnicity and the pain experience. *Social Science and Medicine, 19*, 1279–1298.

Magora, A., & Schwartz, A. (1980). Relation between the low back pain syndrome and X-ray findings. *Scandinavian Journal of Rehabilitation Medicine, 12*, 9–15.

Mechanic, D. (1962). The concept of illness behavior. *Journal of Chronic Disease, 15*, 189–194.

Mechanic, D. (1978). *Medical sociology*. New York: Free Press.

Melzack, R. (1973). *The puzzle of pain*. Hammondsworth, England: Penguin.

Nachemson, A. (1979). A critical look at the treatment for low back pain. *Scandinavian Journal of Rehabilitation Medicine, 11*, 143–149.

National Institute of Neurological, Communicative Disorders and Stroke (1979). *Report of panel on pain to the National Advisory Council of National Institute of Neurological, Communicative Disorders and Stroke Council* (NIH Publication No. 81-1912). Rockville, MD: U.S. Public Health Service.

Paulley, J.W., & Haskell, D.J. (1975). Treatment of migraine without drugs. *Journal of Psychosomatic Research, 19*, 367–374.

Pilowsky, I., & Bond, M.R. (1969). Pain and its management in malignant disease. *Psychosomatic Medicine, 31*, 400–404.

Rehm, L.P. (1977). A self-control model of depression. *Behavior Therapy, 8*, 787–804.

Rogers, M.P., Dubey, D., & Reich, P. (1979). The influence of the psyche and the brain on immunity and disease susceptibility: A critical review. *Psychosomatic Medicine, 41*, 147–164.

Seligman, M.E.P. (1975). *Helplessness: On depression, development and death*. San Francisco, CA: Freeman.

Turk, D.C., & Flor, H. (1984). Etiological theories and treatments for chronic back pain. II. Psychological factors. *Pain, 19*, 209–233.

Turk, D.C., Kerns, R.D., & Rudy, T.E. (1984, August). *Identifying the links between chronic illness and depression*. Paper presented at the annual meeting of the American Psychological Association, Toronto, Canada.

Turk, D.C., Meichenbaum, D., & Berman, W.H. (1979). Biofeedback for the treatment of pain: A critical review. *Psychological Bulletin, 86*, 1322–1338.

Turk, D.C., Meichenbaum, D.C., & Genest, M. (1983). *Pain and behavioral medicine: A cognitive-behavioral perspective*. New York: Guilford Press.

Vital and Health Statistics. (1974). Washington, DC: Government Printing Office.

White, K.L., Williams, F., & Greenberg, B.G. (1961). The ecology of medical care. *New England Journal of Medicine, 265*, 885.

Wolff, B.B., & Langley, S. (1968). Cultural factors and the response to pain: A review. *American Anthropologist, 70*, 494–501.

Zborowski, M. (1969). *People in pain*. San Francisco, CA: Jossey-Bass.

Zola, I.K. (1966). Culture and symptoms—An analysis of patients' presenting complaints. *American Sociological Review, 31*, 615–630.

2 THE OPERANT APPROACH TO THE MANAGEMENT OF PAIN AND EXCESS DISABILITY

Alan H. Roberts

In 1968, Wilbert E. Fordyce published two reports describing the use of operant behavioral management techniques for treating problems associated with chronic pain (Fordyce, Fowler, & DeLateur, 1968; Fordyce, Fowler, Lehmann, & DeLateur, 1968). Following the publication of these papers, the use of operant methods to treat chronic pain increased rapidly. Rather than presuming an underlying medical or psychiatric cause for disability, the behavioral methods focused directly upon the actions or behaviors of patients and their families. Instead of treating the pain directly, behavioral techniques were applied to help patients change selected behaviors so as to improve function.

As published reports of these methods and the results of their applications have proliferated, they have been followed by critical articles and reviews (cf. Block, 1982; Latimer, 1982; Turk, Meichenbaum, & Genest, 1983; Turk & Flor, 1984; Turner & Chapman, 1982). In general, criticisms fall into two categories. The first questions the methodological adequacy of studies attempting to assess the efficacy of behavior management in the treatment of chronic pain. The second points out that operant methods do not treat "pain," but instead teach patients to live more effectively with the pain they may experience. I shall address both criticisms in turn.

Those who comment upon methodological inadequacies in the clinical studies of efficacy so far reported are, in general, accurate. The difficulties of designing prospective experimental studies in an area like this one are formidable and none have been reported to date. The consistency of positive clinical reports from a variety of settings over a long period of time does, however, argue for effectiveness (cf. Cairns, Thomas, Mooney, & Pace, 1976; Follick, Zitter, & Kulich, 1981; Fordyce, 1976; Roberts & Reinhardt, 1980; Seres & Newman, 1976; Sternbach, 1974).

This argument is strengthened when it is considered that these treatment methods are usually applied to patients who have not improved for long periods of time despite interventions by traditional medical and surgical treatment methods. When people remain disabled despite a variety of treatments and the disability diminishes when a new method is tried, the inference may be drawn that the new treatment is more effective than previous interventions. In a complex treatment program, however, it is difficult to determine just what the "active ingredients" might be.

A number of studies are available that provide data bearing upon the question of whether operant interventions are relevant to the expression and modification of pain behaviors. Four studies of the operant approach (Anderson, Cole, Gullickson, Hudgens, & Roberts, 1977; Cairns et al., 1976; Fordyce et al., 1973; Roberts & Reinhardt, 1980) all reported significant decreases in the amounts of medications used and increases in activity levels with follow-ups between 5 months and 7 years.

Cairns and Pasino (1977) compared the effects of graphic feedback alone, verbal reinforcement alone, and graphic feedback plus verbal reinforcement on increases in activity. They found that only the latter two interventions were effective. Dolcys, Crocker, and Patton (1982) compared the effects of verbal reinforcement, graphic feedback, and exercise quotas on activity for three pain patients. The exercise quotas and reinforcement resulted in a gradual increase in exercise behavior. Two studies by Fordyce, Caldwell, and Hongladarom (reported in Fordyce, 1979) demonstrated that the amount of exercise a chronic pain patient will do is influenced strongly by factors other than pain. Another study (Fordyce et al., 1981) found a negative correlation between exercise and pain complaints in chronic pain patients.

Fordyce, Shelton, and Dundore (1982) examined the relationships among patient communications about pain, associated impairment, and several other measures of patient reports about what they do. The data indicated a close relationship between patient ratings of pain and their ratings of how much pain interfered with their activities. These measures, however, had virtually no relationship to patients' reported accounts of health care utilization, pain-related medication consumption, hours spent sitting, standing, walking, or reclining, or frequency of engaging in a set of commonplace activities during the preceding week. These findings can be interpreted as questioning patient reports either of pain severity or of claimed impairment as an index of pain in chronic pain patients. Roberts

and Reinhardt (1980) reported similar findings. These studies demonstrate that pain behaviors may be little, if at all, related to inferences about underlying noxious stimulation.

Block, Kremer, and Gaylor (1980) classified a series of chronic pain patients into subgroups according to whether their spouses were supportive or nonsupportive of pain behaviors. Patients with supportive spouses rated their pain as higher when the spouse was present and lower when the spouse was absent. Patients with nonsupportive spouses did the opposite; they reported more pain when the spouse was absent and less pain when the spouse was present. Roberts and Reinhardt (1980) also demonstrated that spouse attributes have a systematic relationship to patient performance. They found that the spouses of successfully treated patients had lower scores on the hypochondriasis and hysteria scales of the Minnesota Multiphasic Personality Inventory (MMPI) than did the spouses of unsuccessfully treated patients. Their findings are consistent with the idea that spouse readiness to describe himself or herself as "sick" or to be concerned with physical symptoms, as reflected in higher scores on the hypochondriasis and hysteria scales of the MMPI, may predict spouse reinforcement or nonreinforcement of pain behaviors in patients.

Varni, Bessman, Russo, and Cataldo (1980) reported a case study using a sophisticated multiple-baseline design in which social contingencies to pain behavior were systematically manipulated in a young child with chronic pain. There was a striking effect on patient performance. This study again illustrates that therapist behavior has a marked effect upon expressions of suffering and patient efforts in therapy. Another case study by Redd (1982) describes the modification of social contingencies in order to help a suffering patient with terminal cancer to reduce screaming and crying. The results of Redd's efforts were very positive. Fordyce et al. (1981), also described a case study using a shifting-baseline single-subject experimental design. Working with a patient bound to a wheelchair because of pain and using rest as an exercise contingent reinforcer, they were able to help the patient achieve a brisk walking pace.

As a group, the studies and reports reviewed in this setting support the hypothesis that the pain behaviors of chronic pain patients are influenced in systematic ways by social reinforcement. Operant approaches to the management of chronic pain use methods derived from this hypothesis to reduce the disability of patients with chronic pain problems.

The second group of criticisms point out that operant methods do little to alleviate pain and instead teach chronic pain patients to be more stoical about their pain. These criticisms represent a misunderstanding of the goals of operant treatment. The misunderstanding arises when Fordyce's hypothesis that pain *behaviors* can be learned and unlearned is confused with the notion that *pain* can be learned and unlearned. Operant treatments for chronic pain are intended to reduce the disability associated with chronic pain problems. That large numbers of patients report decreasing pain following the application of these methods is not surprising, but decreased pain per se is not a primary goal for these rehabilitation methods.

I have found it useful to conceptualize operant treatment as treatment for *excess disability* instead of treatment for pain (Roberts, in press). The concept of excess disability highlights the major problem of people with chronic pain; namely, that they are more functionally disabled than is necessary.

The diagnosis of excess disability requires a clinical judgment that has a value judgment as a component. Contrast, for example, a quadriplegic who is unable to walk, with a paraplegic not otherwise physically impaired, who is unable to leave his or her bed and use a wheelchair. In most instances, the paraplegic would be judged to be suffering from disability in excess of physical limitations imposed upon him or her by a spinal cord injury, whereas the quadriplegic would not.

With chronic pain, the degree to which disability is excessive may not be as readily apparent. What judgment might be made about a 68-year-old woman who has had chronic low back pain for 7 years after twisting her back getting out of an automobile? Since that incident she has continued to have severe and debilitating pain. She spends most of her day reclining and is unable to perform more than minimal self-care chores and tasks. She has had many medical evaluations and there are no significant medical findings. She is severely physically disabled. Does the fact that there are no medical findings prove that there is no organic basis for her pain? If the judgment is made that she is not a malingerer, that she truly "experiences" the pain that she says she has, is she disabled by her pain or is she "excessively" disabled by her pain?

How would one judge a woman with polymyositis and pulmonary fibrosis, severe connective tissue disorders, that are still active after 13 years of treatment? She has an exogenous Cushing's syndrome and diabetic symptoms. Because of steroid treatments, she has osteoporosis with compression fractures of her spine that are generally considered to be very painful. For the past 3 months, she has been bedridden with muscle pain, back pain, and headaches. After dressing herself in the morning, she retires to the couch for the majority of the day and is unable even to sit for long periods of time. How much of her disability can be attributed to her medical problems? How much of it is excessive? With an appropriate program of rehabilitation, how much more is she capable of doing? Could her day-to-day functioning be improved enough to make a meaningful difference in the quality of her life?

Questions like these are not always easy to answer. They involve clinical judgments based upon experience with patients with similar medical problems combined with careful and extensive behavioral analyses of situational factors that may be influencing the patient's disability. These analyses require a combination of both medical and psychological expertise. Both physicians and psychologists involved in making these kinds of assessments must have knowledge of and experience with rehabilitation methods and their potential.

When a chronic pain patient is judged appropriate for an operant treatment program, the judgment is not that the pain is imaginary, feigned, or psychogenic. The clinical judgment that justifies this treatment recommendation is that the patient is excessively disabled by the pain syndrome and that he or she is capable of functioning at higher levels with less disability and, hopefully, less discomfort.

If the patient is seen only in the light of his or her presumed underlying problem (e.g., paraplegia, poor motivation, osteoporosis, pain of unknown origin, etc.), then the patient's potential for increased functioning may be overlooked or underestimated. In contrast, if the clinician attends to what the patient does or does not do, then it becomes possible to use learning technology to increase, decrease, or maintain selected behaviors to bring about improvements in function. These improvements may occur in the absence of changes in the underlying medical or psychological problems. The fact that many patients increase their function and quality of life without reporting concurrent decreases in pain is not a shortcoming of this treatment approach. For most of these patients, there is no alternative.

Case Study: A.B., A 68-Year-Old Man With Groin Pain

Mr. A.B. was first seen in our outpatient clinic complaining of pain in his scrotum and testicles. He lives in northern California and flew to the clinic with his wife because he was unable to drive a car or even sit in an automobile. The initial medical note by his internist stated that his pain developed following severe straining to have an erection. He had been sexually dysfunctional for the past 15 years. According to this evaluation, the patient went for a chiropractic treatment of his hips 3 days after the onset of pain

and felt that these treatments aggravated his pain.

He was also seen by a urologist and the patient also told him that the pain began after he strained himself in a prolonged fashion attempting to obtain an erection. Following this incident, he noted discomfort in his scrotum and both groins and, 3 days later, stiffness and discomfort in both hips. He saw a physician near his home who diagnosed epididymitis, which was treated with medication. In addition, he was seen by a chiropractor who treated his hips in some form of apparatus and the patient felt that this treatment aggravated the pain.

In discussing the onset of his groin pain with a consulting rheumatologist, Mr. B. did not mention the attempt to get an erection. He stated instead that he went to see the chiropractor for evaluation and manipulation because of neck pain. He had developed a "bad neck" several years ago following a game of golf. The chiropractor told him that he required a "realignment of his axis" and placed him in an apparatus to straighten his hips. This manipulation did not help his neck, but, according to Mr. B., he shortly thereafter developed the pain in his groin and scrotum.

Following these evaluations, he was diagnosed as having probable neuromuscular pelvic pain. Indocin and heat were prescribed. The rheumatologist specifically stated, "I would expect that he would improve somewhat by Thursday and progressively over the next 2 to 3 weeks." He was sent home to the care of his local physician.

One month later, Mr. B. returned to the clinic and was admitted to our hospital. He had now had his pain for over 2 months. The hospital admission reports now speak of the chiropractic evaluation and treatment as the cause of his groin pain. At the time of hospital admission, the patient said that he had been unable to sit in a chair or in a car for 2 months because of extreme burning discomfort deep in the groin near the scrotum. He is unable to walk or sit because of persistent pain. During his inpatient evaluation he was seen by the rheumatologist, an orthopedic surgeon, and a gastroenterologist. These evaluations were extensive and included repeated physical examinations that showed tenderness that was so severe that it prevented the patient from sitting upright or from walking.

Several different types of treatment were attempted in the hospital. These included injections of steroids, which provided approximately 2 days of relief: 1 week of high doses of phenalbutazone, which led to approximately 2 days of improvement, and prednisone, which also benefitted initially but only for a short time.

During hospitalization, he also received daily physical therapy treatments for what was now diagnosed as bilateral adductor tendonitis. He was seen twice a day for 12 days. The physical therapy examination indicated tight adductors, internal rotators, both hips and hamstrings. He was first treated with hot packs to both of his inner thighs and passive motion of the hips. The physical therapy notes indicated both increases and decreases in pain throughout the treatment program. On some days he would request ice as a treatment and other days he would prefer heat. Whatever he requested was provided. Ultrasound treatments were added, and the patient began to add or subtract that from his list of requested treatments. On the last day in the hospital, the physical therapist noted that none of these treatment modalities helped Mr. B.

Assessment

Mr. B. was discharged from the hospital. Two weeks later a behavioral medicine consultation was requested to evaluate his continuing problems with groin and leg pain. He was seen in the psychologist's office together with his wife. The psychologist introduced himself as follows:

P.: How do you do, Mr. and Mrs. B. I am Dr. Roberts, and I think I should begin by reminding you that I am a psychologist. I am not interested in mental illness or severe emotional problems, and I'm quite sure that that's

not the reason why Dr. D. asked you to come and see me. Nor does he think your problem is imaginary, because if he did he would have sent you to one of the psychiatrists down the hall. My job here at the clinic is to help patients change behaviors in ways that will improve their physical health, not their mental health. With that introduction, would you mind telling me why Dr. D. asked you to come and see me?

Mr. B.: Well, doctor, I really don't know.

P.: Well then, why don't you tell me about the problem that brought you to see your doctor.

It is extremely important to try to diffuse the patient's initial resistance to seeing a psychologist as early in the interview as possible. A majority of the patients who are seen by psychologists in a general medical setting do not think of themselves as having any kind of psychological problem. Their expectations about what psychologists do are frequently distorted by popular mental health stereotypes. Patients are often rejected and "dumped" into the mental health system after having experienced repeated failures in treatment (Roberts, 1981). Even when this is not the intention of the referring physician, patients make this inference. They may express their resistance by not making an appointment for a psychology consultation, or they make the appointment and fail to keep it. The problem is reduced when the psychologist's office is located in a traditional medical setting rather than in a setting identified as a mental health service.

Patients express their anger about having been sent to see a psychologist in many subtle and not so subtle ways. The problem is complicated and exacerbated by the fact that it is almost always true that a patient who has had severe pain for a long time will have developed significant emotional and behavioral problems. Even in a pain clinic, many, if not most, patients will interpret the psychological consultation as indicating that the referring clinician thinks that he or she is imagining his or her pain. This problem is most easily mitigated by the physician explaining to the patient why he or she is making the consultation request. Sometimes this is not done or, if it is done, the patient may distort what the physician has tried to communicate.

Mr. B. responded to the question concerning his reasons for seeing medical help by providing the previously described history. On this occasion he ascribed his pain to the chiropractic manipulations of his hips. He said that his pain was extreme and that he had never experienced anything like it before. He was unable to walk or to sit. He was no longer able to eat at the table and instead had to eat standing up. He said that he was unable to ride in a car for other than a short period of time. It was clear from his description, supported by his wife, that he was totally disabled and that he did little or nothing at home.

P.: Mr. B., what makes your pain worse?
Mr. B.: Walking, sitting up straight, driving, tension, and stress.
P.: Then you recognize that stress and tension play some part in making your pain worse?
Mrs. B.: My husband has always been high-strung.
Mr. B.: That's true, doctor.

This provides an early opportunity to make some connection between psychological factors and the experience of pain. If the patient does not volunteer stress or tension as a source of increased pain, I will ask about this.

P.: What makes your pain better?
Mr. B.: Nothing helps except the pain pills and sometimes smoking. I've tried everything, doctor, and nothing seems to help very much.
P.: Well what do you do to help him, Mrs. B.?
Mrs. B.: There's not very much that I can do. He lays around the house most of the time, and I get him things when he asks for them. Sometimes I rub his back and shoulders because of his neck pain, but there isn't very much I can do for the other pain except be sympathetic and listen to him when he talks about it. Sometimes he cries and that upsets me.
P.: Well, what do you folks talk about besides the pain and how he's feeling about it?
Mrs. B.: Not very much these days.
Mr. B.: Honey, you're exaggerating. We do talk about other things.

Mrs. B.: Well, you'll have to admit you're not very interested in many things besides how bad you feel.

A clear pattern of social reinforcement of pain behaviors has emerged from this part of the evaluation. His wife was both sympathetic and responsive to his pain complaints and behaviors. There were also indications that medications might be playing a role and this was evaluated.

At the time of evaluation, Mr. B. was taking 12 Ascriptin and 7 Tylenol with codeine each day as well as 30 mg of Elavil split morning and evening. He was smoking between one and a half and two packs of cigarettes a day and he had a 50-pack-a-year history of cigarette smoking. He used no alcohol whatsoever, and there was no family history of alcohol or drug abuse or of mental illness. He had been abusing pain medications, and this usually reinforces pain behaviors. There was, however, no indication of a primary drug problem; he was not abusing anything other than tobacco prior to the onset of his pain problem.

His appetite was good, and he had mild sleep onset problems and occasional early awakening. Mr. B. did not exercise on a regular basis even before the onset of his pain problem, and he readily admitted that he was physically deconditioned. Both depression and physical deconditioning were implicated as probable contributing problems. There was no evidence of a causal relationship, however.

Asked about the stress in his life, he spoke at length about his boredom since he retired. He had actively involved himself in business until he retired in order to move to California and live near his wife's relatives. He said that he regretted leaving his work and his friends and that he was unable to develop any new relationships because of his pain. Mr. B. also spoke spontaneously of concerns about his age and aging. This is not surprising, given the history he first provided of sexual discomfort and "straining to obtain an erection."

The only psychological test administered to Mr. B. was the MMPI. He produced a valid profile that, at the time of testing, indicated a distress syndrome of mild to moderate proportions including depression, nervousness, tension, and anxiety. The profile suggested that he relied heavily on repression and denial as defense mechanisms. He tested as strongly conscientious and as sensitive and easily hurt. The MMPI profile predicted that he would be particularly sensitive about performance. He would be seen by others as critical, overburdened, and feeling as though he were trapped in his current situation. The profile indicated that he was not psychologically minded and that he might resent any implications that psychological factors might be responsible for his problems.

At the time he was seen, there was no way to determine objectively what might have been the original cause of Mr. B.'s pain. He had clearly become a chronic pain patient, however, and was now almost totally disabled. He was obtaining considerable reinforcement for his pain problems and for his disability from his supportive wife, and possibly from medications. He was probably physically deconditioned even before the onset of his pain and had certainly become more so as his problem had begun to disable him more and more.

On the basis of this evaluation, an outpatient operant physical therapy program was recommended. Because Mr. B. lived so far from the clinic, a 2-week intensive program was prescribed during which he was to be seen twice a day in physical therapy and then he would be followed by another physical therapist near his home. During the 2 weeks of intensive operant treatment, I planned to see him and his wife on several occasions. I emphasized the importance of Mrs. B. participating in the treatment program. I did not attempt to explain the idea of social reinforcement to Mr. and Mrs. B. I did, however, point out that his extended disability must be having profound effects upon both of them. I asked her to involve herself in treatment so that she could learn ways of helping him improve. She seemed eager to cooperate.

Contingency Contract

Mr. and Mrs. B. signed a contingency contract which read, in part, as follows:

I, *A.B.*, agree to participate in and complete an outpatient treatment program for the management of excess disability at Scripps Clinic. I and others signing this understand that it is not a legally binding contract. It is, however, an understanding between me and members of the treatment team. It explains the purposes of the treatment program and what may be reasonably expected of me and the treatment team.

The purpose of the program is to help me learn to manage my pain and disability and to increase my level of functioning as much as possible. This will be done by providing me with a therapy program to help me increase and improve my strength, endurance, flexibility, posture, body mechanics, and ability to carry out day-to-day activities including work inside and outside the home. I understand that I am having particular problems with: *walking, sitting, standing, bending, lifting, and driving a car,* and the program will attempt to help me function better in these areas.

I understand that the program may or may not decrease my pain. The program is intended to promote relaxation, increase strength, increase range of motion, and generally to help me increase my level of function. When the treatment program is completed my goals include: *sitting for an hour or more, driving and riding in a car, being able to walk at least one hour, working at least part time outside my home.*

I understand that during the treatment program, members of the team will ignore any and all behaviors of mine indicating or communicating that I am experiencing pain. I give permission to significant others, including my spouse, to ignore my pains, complaints of pain, and behaviors related to pain in order to help me learn to pay less attention to them so I will be able to function better with less discomfort and suffering. In return, the members of the treatment team agree to respond positively to me as much as possible and assist and encourage me as I begin to increase my activities and level of functioning.

I am now taking the following medications which I agree to decrease and discontinue in the manner prescribed: *Tylenol with codeine*. I agree to follow the therapy program exactly as prescribed including attending all therapy sessions and doing all of the exercises and activities as scheduled at home as well as the clinic. I will keep up-to-date and accurate graphs showing my day-to-day progress. I understand that I alone am responsible for keeping these graphs. With help from the treatment team, I will keep them up-to-date and available for inspection at all times while I am in the clinic. I understand that my doctors will be interested in reviewing them with me.

If I miss two scheduled therapy sessions in a row or three altogether this program will terminate for me and I will be discharged. If I do not meet my scheduled goal on any single exercise or activity for 3 days in a row (as shown on the graphs) that exercise or activity will be lowered one step. In the event that I do not meet my goal at the lowered level for 3 days in a row, the program will terminate for me and I will be discharged.

The contingency contract also included sections that described follow-up visits and participation in follow-up research at 6 and 12 months following treatment. I signed the contract on behalf of the treatment team.

Treatment Program

The first 3 days of physical therapy were devoted to evaluation. He complained to the physical therapist of pain with sitting, standing, and walking, but not when lying down. He told the therapist that he was unable to walk for more than 100 feet at any time, and his tested walking tolerance in physical therapy was 10 minutes, whereas his sitting tolerance was 5 minutes.

On the 3rd day of physical therapy, a specific exercise program was prescribed for him as shown in Table 2.1.

The starting levels in each instance were well below his demonstrated tolerance levels observed during the 3-day evaluation. The rates of increase were also chosen to be well below his expected tolerance levels. The goals were judged to be reasonable for a 68-year-old man without physical problems.

Additional exercises were planned to be added to the program later. Mr. B. was asked to exercise to these criteria under the supervision of the physical therapist, who ignored any complaints of pain and all pain behaviors starting with the 3rd day. Brief rest periods were built in as a reinforcer at the end of each exercise. If the exercise were completed, Mr. B. could lie down for 2 minutes before going on to the next one.

At the time the exercises began, he had limited range of motion with respect to hip adduction, his hip strength was poor, and his hamstring flexibility was extremely limited. Mr. B. was very fearful that if he did these exercises he would have to "pay a price" later. This reaction is common in chronic pain patients who have restricted their movements to the point where even minor exercise or activity may cause pain. After the 4th day, however, he no longer mentioned this.

The physical therapist pointed out that Mr. B. complained of pain each time he was seen and that these complaints were ignored. She said that he complained more when his wife was present than when she was absent. The therapist instructed her to ignore his pain behaviors while Mr. B. listened and the therapist modeled this for her. Sometimes his complaints were so persistent that the physical therapist actually walked away from him and left the room. Mrs. B. would leave with her. Mr. B. found this to be amusing and he laughed when it happened. Nevertheless, the pain complaints decreased in frequency and intensity as the physical therapy program progressed.

He continued to do everything that was requested of him and began to walk not only further but faster. He stopped shuffling as he walked. The therapist called a physical therapist near Mr. B.'s home and discussed the

TABLE 2.1. EXERCISE PROGRAM FOR MR. B.

Exercise	Start	Increase	Goal
Modified sit-ups	3 repetitions	1 repetition every 3rd day	30 repetitions
Side-lying leg-lifts	2 repetitions	1 repetition every 3rd day	20 repetitions
Knee-to-chest	3 repetitions	1 repetition every 3rd day	20 repetitions
Stomach-lying leg-lifts	1 repetition	1 repetition every 3rd day	20 repetitions
Sitting	2 minutes	1 minute every 3rd day	60 minutes
Walking	2 minutes	1 minute every 3rd day	30 minutes
Bicycling	1 minute	1 minute every 3rd day	30 minutes

nature of the program with the new therapist. The new therapist seemed to understand what was required and agreed to follow Mr. B. 3 times a week initially and then gradually to reduce the frequency of physical therapy visits. Mr. B. was asked to do his exercises twice a day whether he was in physical therapy or not on that day.

Psychological Interventions

He returned to see me for his first revisit without his wife despite the fact that I had asked him to bring her each time. He did, however, carry with him a notebook full of physical therapy graphs, which I reviewed with him in great detail. I specifically praised him for what he was accomplishing. Dr. D., the rheumatologist, agreed to do the same thing when he saw him in revisit. During this interview, he was tearful and said that he felt his life was over, that he had no purpose, and that he was unneeded "like a fifth wheel." He said that he'd been unhappy since his retirement $2\frac{1}{2}$ years earlier and that he was disappointed about having moved to California. He felt that he would be happier if he moved again to a different location, but he felt that the pain must improve first. He volunteered that his pain seemed to be decreasing already. Although I listened to his concerns, I did not address them in any psychotherapeutic way.

A second meeting with the patient and his wife was devoted to going over all aspects of his program and encouraging him to follow the physical therapy program to the letter, neither doing more than was asked nor less.

During the second visit, he specifically asked for a whirlpool bath as a treatment and I agreed that he could do that after each exercise session, but if and only if he did all the exercises, thus turning what might have served as a reinforcer for pain into a reinforcer for exercise.

Follow-Up

One month later he returned to the clinic and he was reevaluated in physical therapy. He was doing the exercises at the levels indicated in Table 2.2.

Mr. B. was also continuing to do hamstring, hip adduction, and hip flexor stretches on a daily basis. They physical therapist told him that when he reached his goals in each exercise he was to decrease the frequency of that exercise from twice to once a day. This too served as a reinforcer. His gait was improved considerably and his hip muscles were stronger and more flexible. Mr. B. actually asked for some new exercises, but the

TABLE 2.2. EXERCISE LEVEL OF MR. B. AT ONE MONTH FOLLOW-UP

Exercise	Performance	Goal
Modified sit-ups	21 repetitions	30 repetitions
Knee-to-chest	20 repetitions	20 repetitions
Side-lying leg lifts	20 repetitions	20 repetitions
Hip extension	19 repetitions	20 repetitions
Sitting	43 minutes	60 minutes
Walking	30 minutes	30 minutes
Bicycling	28 minutes	30 minutes

physical therapist told him instead to concentrate on his current exercises and maintain them. She told him that she would see him again a month later, and at that time, if he continued to do as well as he was doing, she would be willing to assign additional exercises.

I saw him together with his wife and they were both proud that they had driven to the clinic instead of flying. He reported that he had some "discomfort" but that "the pain is almost nonexistent." He was using no medications other than the antidepressant medication that had been prescribed. He had been to visit relatives in a different state, and "they couldn't tell that there was anything wrong with me." His sleep and appetite were excellent, and he had been putting on weight, probably due, in part, to the fact that he had discontinued smoking cigarettes. He said that he was enjoying his exercises and that he had no intention of ever stopping. He was doing more things at home, but he said he still felt depressed when he was alone.

I spoke with him and his wife about the need for him to become involved in some gainful or voluntary activity outside the home as soon as possible. He agreed to do that. At no time during the treatment of his pain problem were his concerns with aging and sexual dysfunction addressed directly. Although these concerns might possibly have contributed directly or indirectly to the onset of his chronic pain problem, the disability was the focus of treatment. Contrary to conventional psychological wisdom, it is not always necessary to treat underlying psychological problems, even when they are presumed to contribute to etiology. From an operant perspective, that is an unnecessary step in resolving the disability that was the problem being treated.

His last visit to the clinic was 3 months later. At that time he had no groin pain or discomfort whatsoever. He was still not doing anything outside of his home, but he continued to think seriously of moving. His sleep and appetite were good, and he was using no medications other than the antidepressant

medication. The rheumatologist's final chart note stated in part, "I appreciated the opportunity of seeing the beneficial effects of behavioral therapy on Mr. B.'s illness. Impression: truly remarkable response — much appreciated by both the patient and me."

DISCUSSION

The case history illustrates the major aspects of evaluating and treating patients with chronic pain using an operant approach. These procedures and techniques are equally applicable to both inpatient and outpatient treatment programs. Inpatient programs allow greater control of the contingencies affecting the patient's behaviors. Outpatient programs are considerably less expensive and less demanding. The treatment team for the case described involved a physician, a psychologist, a physical therapist, and the patient's wife. Inpatient programs frequently have more extended treatment teams and may include nurses, vocational counselors, occupational therapists, work evaluators, or social workers. Descriptions of the functions of these health care professionals in operant treatment programs can be found in Fordyce (1976), Hudgens (1977), and Roberts (1977, 1981).

Assessment

The management of excess disability in chronic pain depends first of all upon its identification. For persons already in the health care system and suffering from severe chronic pain or illness, there is often reluctance to make a judgment that the person should be functioning at levels higher than current levels. It is necessary as a first step for a physician to identify the disability as excessive and to provide medical sanction and support for a program to decrease the disability. Medical involvement and sanction is a necessary requisite for both the initiation and maintenance of operant programs to manage most examples of excess disability.

Once the problem is identified and a person

is referred for evaluation and treatment, the next step is a functional behavioral analysis. The purpose of this analysis is to determine what social and environmental reinforcers are responsible for the development and maintenance of the disability. The medical diagnoses of these patients may range from physical deconditioning—with the patient complaining of such things as fatigue, weakness, tiredness, dizziness, or shortness of breath, as well as pain—to severe debilitating chronic disease.

The most common presenting complaint is that of pain. Sometimes the pain has a diagnosable but untreatable physiological etiology. At other times the origin of the pain is unknown. *It is important in assessment to focus not on the presumed medical problem responsible for the complaints and symptoms, but rather upon their behavioral consequences.* The common thread is inability to function at optimum levels.

The date gathered in the assessment provide the basis for making a decision about whether or not to treat a patient and also help to determine the appropriate components of an operant program. How disabled is the patient? How much time, effort, and expense is the patient and his or her family willing to put into a treatment program? Which components of a management program are necessary to increase function and which can be dispensed with? How long should a treatment program continue? How much follow-up is needed?

Will the patient need special treatment or attention for depression? In addition to the withdrawal of medications and focus on increasing activity and function, what special problems, such as alcohol, weight, or marital problems, need to be addressed? If the patient has a weight problem that is medically significant, will diet need to be a component of the program or can it be managed by exercise alone? What are the marital and family relationships contributing to the disability? Can intervention change these sufficiently to assure reasonably that the patient will not only increase his or her activity but also maintain these changes? If marital stress is involved, are interventions possible or appropriate to reduce these stresses? The answers to these questions generally flow from the assessment and determine not only whether or not the patient will be treated, but also the outlines of specific programs for individual patients.

Correcting Misperceptions

Many patients do not perceive their disability to be excessive. To be effective, the evaluation must often include an element of confrontation and education. A bedridden, medication-dependent person suffering from severe and intractable pain has great difficulty in accepting the notion that he or she can learn to live a more normal life even though pain might continue. A program that is presented inaccurately as intending to cure or alleviate the presenting complaint might persuade the patient to participate in a treatment program, but the program is almost certain to fail when the presenting symptom persists.

During the course of chronic illness the patient has acquired misinformation and misperceptions. These must be corrected. Some of these incorrect beliefs directly support disability and may be an underlying cause of some of the patient's problems. An example is the medical advice commonly provided to patients with musculoskeletal pain: "If it hurts, don't do it." Such advice, if taken literally for other than brief periods of time, may lead to progressive physical deconditioning. A common misperception is that the best treatment for pain is rest. Although this may be good advice for short periods of time, decreased activity frequently causes more pain as time passes. As muscles become weak and tight from misuse or disuse, there is increasing pain and, frequently, muscle spasm when these muscle groups are activated.

Further preparation of patients for treatment requires education concerning the idea that pain behaviors can be learned and unlearned. This assumption underlies many of the behavioral techniques used in an operant treatment program. If patients understand this, they may understand partly why some of these techniques are used in their treatment. Even if they don't accept the assumption, the knowledge provides some rationale for the seemingly odd things that are done during treatment, such as ignoring their complaints or other pain behaviors.

It is not necessary that patients believe or agree with any of the underlying assumptions about the treatment program. Patients do, however, need to have some understanding about why these methods are being used if they are to behave in ways consistent with that program. Even if informed patients and families are skeptical, many will go along with the rationale. Most often they have few other options.

Family Involvement

The participation of the family in both the assessment and treatment of excess disability problems is in most cases mandatory. It is increasingly evident that family members are primary reinforcers of disability and of activity. Treatment programs are much more likely to be successful when family members are involved and cooperative (Hudgens, 1977; Roberts, 1983; Roberts & Reinhardt, 1980). When operant programs fail, it is most often because significant operant contingencies have not been fully controlled. Involvement of the family at all levels of assessment and treatment increases the likelihood that these contingencies can be managed more effectively and more broadly. A treatment program that is primarily an outpatient program must be supported at home as well as in the clinic both during and after the treatment program. Families who subvert the program, who will not withhold reinforcement for disability, or who will not provide reinforcement for activity make it extremely unlikely that the patient can be treated successfully (Hudgens, 1977).

Psychological Tests

Usually an MMPI is administered to both the patient and his or her spouse prior to the evaluation. This allows for the screening of psychopathology, levels of depression and anxiety, the degree to which the patient and his or her spouse are focusing on somatic concerns, perceived energy levels, ego strength, addiction proneness, dependency, and similar variables. It is possible, in comparing the MMPI of a patient and spouse, to make some predictions about the way the two will interact. There are data suggesting that elevations on certain MMPI scales of the spouses of patients may be better predictors of treatment outcome than the MMPI scores of the patients themselves (Roberts & Reinhardt, 1980).

A common use of the MMPI is to evaluate whether or not the patient's complaint is organic or functional. This is misleading and ill-advised (Roberts, 1983). People with acute organic pain frequently have many of the same psychological symptoms found in people with chronic pain (e.g., dysphoria, anxiety, autonomic arousal, or cognitive impairment). Similarly the psychological problems of patients with chronic pain (e.g., depression, anxiety, sleeplessness, the excessive use of repression and denial, somatic overconcern, or passive-aggressive behaviors, to name only the more prominent ones) are no different in kind or degree from those of many patients with any chronic disabling disease or of people who become dependent upon drugs or medications obtained from either the street or the pharmacy. Thus, attempts to use the MMPI or other psychological tests to try to determine whether the patient's presenting problem is "real" are bound to mislead and ultimately fail.

Drugs and Medication

The misuse or abuse of medications, alcohol, or recreational drugs frequently contributes to excess disability. Medications, particularly analgesics, tranquilizers, and muscle relaxants, have been amply documented as reinforcers for pain and disability (Fordyce, 1976; Roberts, 1981; Roberts, 1983). A primary goal in the management of excess disability is to have patients discontinue all unnecessary medications.

Among the most prevalent of these are prescription analgesics, anti-anxiety or muscle relaxing medications, and sedative hypnotics. These medications may increase dysphoria, as well as reinforce pain behaviors. In either case, they contribute to the increasing disability. The inappropriate use of medications is both a cause and a consequence of excess disability.

An evaluation of drug and alcohol use requires the participation of family members because those who are abusing substances frequently deny that they are to themselves and others. We frequently find patients who are surprised when told that they are abusing a particular medication or group of medications. After all, their doctors prescribed the drugs. An appropriate evaluation should include data about past as well as current use of alcohol, family histories for alcohol abuse, and past and current use of medications or drugs.

Reinforcers for Disability

The assessment must cover the degree of disability and dysfunction, with the reinforcers for disability being the primary foci of attention. Inquiry is directed at how long the person has been having problems, how many health care professionals have been consulted, the number of hospitalizations, and the particular kinds of treatments that have been tried and failed.

Many leads concerning reinforcement for pain and disability may be obtained by asking the patient what kinds of things help the pain and what things seem to make it worse. A question such as "If your pain were gone, what would you do that you're not able to do now?" provides data about the areas and amount of disability. For example, the patient might reply that he or she would do his or her homemaking chores, drive a car, travel more, or return to employment outside the home if the pain were gone.

Predicting Outcome

The decision to treat a disabled patient is based on the judgment that the patient will improve functionally if treated. If a major complaint is pain, one must decide if the patient will maintain improvements even if the pain continues after treatment. Although many patients are willing to "live with pain" as long as they can improve function, a few insist that the pain must be alleviated by the treatment program. We generally decide not to treat patients who insist on a "cure" for their pain, because they are very likely to regress once treatment is completed and their expectations are not met.

Other variables that predict poor outcome include severe mental illness, pending litigation, relatively high levels of compensation that will be lost if the patient improves, or families unwilling to participate in and cooperate with the treatment program and its goals (Roberts & Reinhardt, 1980). Each of these variables must be weighed before embarking upon a treatment program.

Severe mental illness makes it more difficult to treat patients. Sometimes a severe emotional disturbance (e.g., agitation, paranoia, hostility) makes it more difficult for the staff to work with the patients, and the staff may undermine the program. The limitation of mental illness or disturbed behavior may not be a limitation of the operant method; it may instead be a limitation of staff tolerance. Some clinical judgment must always be made concerning whether or not to proceed. We have, however, worked successfully with patients retarded by depression and with a few who have had brief, intermittent psychotic episodes while they were being treated. Inability to focus or concentrate, or severe memory loss, makes it more difficult to work with the patient and increases the likelihood that the program will not be maintained following treatment.

Pending litigation, the outcome of which may be influenced by the results of treatment, is a serious limiting factor. We have worked successfully with patients whose litigation is still pending, but this tends to be effective only when the outcome of litigation is independent of the outcome of the treatment program. One way to assess this is to ask the patient to have his or her attorney send a letter stating that a positive treatment outcome will not change significantly the outcome of litigation. If the attorney is unwilling to make a statement to that effect in writing, our decision has usually been to defer treatment until the litigation is settled. When we have not done this, we have most often been disappointed.

TREATMENT PROCEDURES

The components of a program to decrease excess disability include: (a) medical sanction and support from a physician; (b) discontinuing all unnecessary medications; (c) increasing physical activity; and (d) involving family members in reinforcing physical activity and withholding reinforcements of disability. Other components and goals may become relevant based upon the assessment, but these four are those most generally applicable to patients with chronic pain.

Informed Consent

It goes without saying that the informed consent of the patient is needed. If patients or their families are unwilling to participate in a treatment program, then I know of no other way to involve them. The issue of informed consent can be addressed through the contingency contract. A treatment program should include a treatment contract signed by the patient, the spouse, and a key member of the treatment staff. The contract, properly written and executed, serves to set appropriate levels of expectations for the patient and his or her family, specifies the contributions of the patient, the family, and the treatment team, and provides contingencies for failure to perform. A well-written treatment contract should meet all requirements for fully informed consent.

Selecting Reinforcers

All members of the treatment team are concerned with issues of reinforcement throughout the treatment program. A wide variety of positive reinforcements are used for behaviors that we wish to strengthen. A conscious attempt is made to avoid using reinforcers that are not fully under the control of the treatment team. Cigarettes and television watching, for example, are avoided because the patient clearly has access to these from sources other than those controlled by the staff. Most often, reinforcers are kept as simple as possible.

The most common reinforcer is praise and attention from members of the health care team and family. Because patients have had a long history of using the health care system, health care professionals frequently acquire reinforcing properties.

Additional reinforcers may be chosen, such as soft drinks following the completion of exercises in the therapeutic area, if the patient finds this reinforcing. Activities that the patient likes to do are often used by an occupational therapist to reinforce the patient, especially during another activity that, in itself, may not be pleasurable but requires positive reinforcement. An example of this might be requiring the patient to sit for progressively longer periods each day; the therapist might provide a task that the patient enjoys for the period when he or she is sitting.

Because the patient is disabled and thus inactive, easily fatigued, and in pain, rest is commonly used as a reinforcement to reward the completion of activities. In this instance, rest is used as a reinforcement for exercise, allowing the patient to perform the activity we want to decrease (rest) as a reinforcement for the behaviors we wish to increase (activity).

The withdrawal of reinforcements for behaviors that we wish to decrease is also important. At the same time, we begin reinforcing behaviors that are incompatible with those that are to be decreased. During the treatment program, all identifiable pain behaviors are ignored by all members of the treatment team. During exercise if the patient winces, complains, screams, or talks about pain, the therapist ignores these behaviors, acting as if he or she had not heard. Therapists will change the subject or, if absolutely necessary, walk away from the patient. The treatment team members should be made aware of the fact that ignoring a well-established response will tend to increase that response initially rather than decrease it. Only later will it decrease.

Shaping and Modeling

Shaping is an integral part of the strategy of treatment. The desired behaviors are divided into successive gradual steps that are taught sequentially. Each of these steps is rewarded, and the patient moves on to the next step after he or she has completed the previous one. In this way, a new behavior is learned slowly as the patient comes closer and closer to approximating normal levels of activity.

Modeling is used both consciously and unconsciously by the treatment team. Therapists participate in exercises and activities with the patients. Sometimes, treatment team members who are not usually present during therapy attend therapy sessions and participate in the exercise programs with the patients at those times. Family members are encouraged to attend therapy and exercise with the patients. They are also asked to do so at home.

Medication Withdrawal

In the majority of outpatient programs, patients need only be told of the necessity of withdrawing from medications after pointing out to them how they have become dependent upon them. Many patients are genuinely surprised when told that they are dependent upon the drugs. They are even more surprised when it is explained to them that these medications, when used for more than brief periods of time, tend to make the pain worse rather than better. Most often patients will adhere to a progressive withdrawal schedule

for these medications, if the schedule is slow enough to minimize withdrawal symptoms. Patients unable or unwilling to withdraw from their unnecessary medications are typically candidates for an inpatient treatment program and use of a "pain cocktail" (Fordyce, 1976; Roberts, 1981).

Alternatives to prescription analgesics, tranquilizers, and muscle relaxants are primarily plain aspirin or plain acetominophen. The patient is told that these medications are the most effective analgesics that can be used on a long-term basis without increasing pain. As the other medications are gradually withdrawn, plain aspirin or plain acetominophen is gradually added to the regimen on a *time-contingent* rather than a pain-contingent basis; the medication is administered according to prearranged time intervals, not according to the patient's perception of pain.

Physical and Occupational Therapy

Physical and occupational therapy programs to increase activity levels and exercise are primary components of an operant program for excess disability. The program must be designed so as to promote adherence during treatment, as well as to generalize after the program has been formally completed.

It is important that therapists working with patients in programs like this make continuous efforts to discriminate between what the person says about his or her pain and disability and what the patient actually does. The focus of the program is entirely upon behavior change. The amount of pain or fatigue that is described by the patient may change very little during the course of a treatment program, but what the patient does in terms of increasing activity level and reducing disability will change significantly. Patients' verbal complaints are not themselves measures of success or failure in a treatment program like this. It is the objective measures of decreasing disability and increasing function that are the criteria for success.

A typical program for outpatients lasts from 6 to 8 weeks and includes from 10 to 12 exercises and activities designed to promote strength, endurance, stretching, posture, body mechanics, and Aids to Daily Living (ADL) activities. A 6- to 8-week program seems to provide enough time to evaluate a patient, prescribe a program, and reinforce significant progress in that program to the point where the patient should be able to continue it on his or her own and maintain the program when specific goals have been reached. Usually, the patient is expected to do the prescribed exercises and activities twice a day, every day, whether seen that day in therapy or not. This is later reduced to once a day for maintenance as each exercise goal is reached.

Aerobic exercises are included to promote endurance as well as to assist patients in the management of stress and tension and to relieve fatigue and tiredness. Therapists are specifically asked to focus on exercises and activities that the patient has particular difficulty performing. If patients are unable to stand, for example, exercises designed to increase standing are included in the program. If they are unable to bend, then stretching and bending exercises are given special attention. Patients who state that they are unable to sit for long periods of time because of pain are provided with "sitting exercises."

The first 3 to 5 days of therapy are spent evaluating the patient. The patient is asked to do a large variety of exercises covering the areas previously noted, doing each of these exercises and activities to tolerance. For example, the patient might be asked to do as many partial sit-ups as possible each day for 3 to 5 days in a row or to do a particular stretching or strengthening exercise as many times as possible. He or she may be asked to ride an exercise bicycle for as many minutes as can be tolerated. The patient will walk with the therapist, and minutes of walking and heart rate are recorded. He or she may be asked to sit in a "standard" chair for as long as possible.

If homemaking tasks are a problem, the patient will be evaluated by an occupational therapist in the same way. Tolerance of the usual homemaking responsibilities will be evaluated by asking the persons to actually sweep, do dishes, launder, make beds, get up and down from low places, and similar tasks. Homemaking is promoted only when this area of activity is a problem for the patient, and he or she wants or needs to be able to do these tasks. Activities outside the home are always encouraged regardless of sex or need for gainful employment. The patient is clearly informed that it is perfectly all right for a spouse to do these tasks or share them after treatment is concluded, but for reasons other than the patient's pain or fatigue. Sharing of responsibilities within the family is encouraged, but not in ways that reinforce inactivity or disability.

After a few days of performing each exercise to tolerance, a baseline is obtained that tells the therapist precisely how much of each exercise the patient is capable of doing. This baseline provides a database for prescribing exercise and activity to carefully chosen criteria levels instead of performing to tolerance.

Once the database has been compiled, a number of exercises and activities are chosen. The patient will then be expected to do these chosen exercises twice a day at a slowly increasing rate throughout the program. It is important that repetition levels start at no greater than one third to one half of the average baseline level obtained during the evaluation period.

Both the beginning level and the rate of increase are chosen to ensure that the patient never fails an assignment throughout the program. It is more important that the patient do the exercise at a low level and succeed each time than it is that he or she do it at a higher level and sometimes fail. *Failure is never reinforcing.* The most common error made by therapists is to set required levels too high or to raise them too rapidly. Whenever there is a question about this, therapists are encouraged to be extremely conservative. Each time the patient reaches his or her quota of exercise, the therapist provides rest, praise, attention, and other selected reinforcers.

Failure to do an exercise must be managed so as to minimize reinforcement from the failure experience. Patients sometimes refuse to come to therapy or else come to therapy and refuse to do one or more of the prescribed exercises or activities. The contingencies for managing this should be specified in the treatment contract.

If the patient does not meet his or her performance criterion for any particular exercise on any given day, the therapist simply ignores this and goes on to the next exercise. If the patient fails a particular exercise for 3 days in a row, however, the criterion is dropped one level. If the patient is unable to meet the criterion after it has been lowered for an additional 3 days in a row, the patient is discharged from the treatment program.

Only rarely, if at all, will renegotiating the contract improve the situation. There are few ways to coerce a patient. If the patient cannot meet exercise criteria that have been selected to insure that he or she will not fail, then it is obvious that we are unable to help that particular patient.

Graphs and Charts

All exercises and activities required of the patient are graphed. These include regular exercises and activities or special prescribed activities, such as increasing standing or sitting time. The patient is asked to carry all the graphs in a folder whenever in the clinic. These graphs may be self-reinforcing; when the patient plots the required data, he or she sees immediately that progress has been made. The graphs also provide a basis for reinforcement from other team members. When physicians, psychologists, or others who are not present when the exercises are being done visit with the patient, the team member can look at the graphs and provide verbal reinforcement for what has been occurring.

Family Intervention

In the outpatient program, a member of the team, usually a psychologist or social worker, meets with the patient and spouse at least once or twice a week. The details of the kinds of work that are done with the family members have been described by Hudgens (1977). In general, the family members of chronic pain patients either enable the disability through various forms of reinforcement or fail to reward healthier kinds of behavior. The team member working with the family helps the family become aware of and change this pattern of reinforcement. Family members are taught to identify pain behaviors, and these observations are discussed. Spouses are also asked to observe and record their own behaviors in the presence of the patient and to become alert to ways in which they have been responding when the patient complains of pain or acts in other ways communicating illness or disability.

The professional working with the patient and spouse teaches the spouse and others to behave appropriately by modeling and role-playing ways in which spouses can ignore sick behavior and reward healthy behavior. Family members are taught that "negative attention," such as fussing, nagging, complaining, threatening, coercing, and similar behaviors, is a form of attention that may reinforce pain behavior and disability. It is also critical that spouses learn that ignoring sick behavior is not enough; healthy, active behaviors must be attended to and reinforced systematically.

Working with the families is essential to ensure the generalization of newly learned healthy behaviors. If the patient returns home to the same setting with the same reinforcements for sick behavior, the learning that is achieved during the clinic visits will invariably deteriorate. The family is always taught to allow the patient to assume full responsibility for the management of his or her own body, medical problems, medications, and treatment program.

An operant program that does not generalize from the treatment setting to the home and work situation is worthless. An outpatient treatment program has an advantage over inpatient treatment in that patients in outpatient programs spend more time at home than they spend in the clinic. Therefore, there is a built-in opportunity for generalization. Exercises and activities are done where they will continue to be done after treatment. Requiring exercises to be done twice a day insures that the exercises will be done at least once at home even on days they visit the clinic.

Outside Physicians

Sometimes the patient will return for primary care to a physician who is not associated with the clinic where the treatment program is located. It is necessary to explain to the referring or primary physician what has occurred and the need for a different kind of patient–physician relationship. This must be done in ways that will enhance understanding, cooperation, and support. Health care professionals have often reinforced disability unwittingly with high levels of caring, concern, sympathy, and medication prescription. Many physicians are unfamiliar with the operant model, and they conceptualize the patient's problems entirely as a disease. It may be difficult for a physician who has been treating a chronically disabled patient for a long period of time to refrain from represcribing medications when a patient asks for them.

A verbal or written contingency contract can be negotiated between the patient and the referring physician that defines more appropriately their future relationship. For some patients it is helpful if the primary physician agrees to visits by the patient at regular intervals, contingent upon the patient not using pain or sickness as an excuse for these visits. This can be agreed upon in writing through the use of a brief contingency contract signed by both the patient and the physician.

SUMMARY AND CONCLUSIONS

There is an incredible amount and variety of pain in the world. There are also an enor-

mous number of perspectives and treatment approaches for pain, depending not only on the etiology, location, and intensity of the pain, but also the training and orientation of the person prescribing the treatment. Pain is not a disease; it is a symptom. *Chronic* pain is not a disease either, but over the years it has assumed the status of a pseudodisease because it appears to have a "natural history" that is different from acute pains of similar location and intensity.

Acute pain is assumed initially to have an organic etiology. If a pain problem persists for weeks or months, if the degree of pain appears to exceed normative expectations for a particular organic pathology, or if the pain disables the person more than might generally be expected, the hypothesis may be changed and the person accused of having some form of "psychogenic" pain.

The diagnosis and treatment of a particular pain problem often depends upon the perspective of the person responsible for diagnosis and treatment. A close companion of mine recently developed severe pain in the vicinity of her left hip and thigh that was extremely sensitive to touch. In a relatively short period of time, she was evaluated by a large number of doctors including a general practitioner, two radiologists, a rheumatologist, and an orthopedic surgeon. The general practitioner diagnosed hip dysplasia and spondylosis. Two radiologists and the rheumatologist decided independently that she did not have hip dysplasia and instead diagnosed disseminated idiopathic skeletal hyperostosis, which is a benign form of osteoarthritis with a generally favorable prognosis. The orthopedic surgeon said that she was in imminent danger of a prolapsed disk with impending paralysis and recommended surgery to prevent disaster. Treatment recommendations thus ranged from rest and aspirin to immediate spinal surgery. The fact that my companion is a dog does not alter the point being made, namely, that the diagnosis and treatment of pain problems are very much dependent on the perspective of the specialist.

The observation that a dog cannot speak is

not critical. Humans speak of pain in many tongues. Many years ago I attempted to treat a depressed woman by means of traditional psychotherapy. Once or twice a week for months she came to my office and spoke with me of her pain, suffering, and anguish. I, in turn, tried to understand, to empathize, to console, and to reassure. One day she brought me an artistic gift, a beautifully constructed, handmade poster for my office that read "Pain Hurts." We laughed a little together, and I communicated as best I could that I understood how much she had been suffering. She seemed to accept my reassurance, but that weekend she went into her garage after her family was asleep, turned on the engine of her automobile, and asphyxiated herself. One of the many things I learned from that experience was how closely the language of depression can mirror the language of physical pain.

We understand very little about pain from a neurophysiological point of view and even less about the interactions between the somatosensory aspects of pain and the psychological aspects of it. The Melzack and Wall (1965) gate control theory of pain does little more than point out the complex interaction among sensory–discriminative, affective–motivational, and cognitive–evaluative systems that determine both the perceptions of pain and their expressions in behavior. The overall lack of understanding and the complexity combine to evoke a multitude of sometimes incompatible treatment strategies from medical, surgical, and psychological perspectives. For these and other reasons, it seems highly unlikely that any of the current treatment or management approaches for chronic pain — medical, surgical, or psychological — will provide the ultimate answer to what both Melzack (1973) and Hilgard (1969) described as the "puzzle of pain."

Usually, judgments are made about whether or not to attempt to use psychological approaches on the basis of a belief about whether or not the pain is "organic" or "psychogenic." If the patient is behaving as if he or she is experiencing significant pain and

there is an absence of physical findings that might account for this pain, the pain behaviors of the patient are presumed to stem from some kind of personality, emotional, or motivational difficulty. The patient doesn't have a sick body; he or she has a sick mind. When that assumption is made, the clinician often thinks of the patient's pain as not real, as imaginary, or malingered. The implication is that the patient is not really suffering, just as one might assume that a depressed person is not "really" experiencing pain. Overall, the effect of this approach is to blame the victim.

A variety of formal and informal diagnoses are available to convey these judgments in subtle and not so subtle ways: hysteric, hypochondriac, conversion reaction, secondary pain, psychogenic pain, imaginary pain, and, in the absence of the patient, "crock," "turkey," or "difficult" (all nouns). All too often the patient with a chronic pain syndrome will indeed be found to have concurrent emotional or personality disturbances. This does not, however, establish a causal relationship between the psychological problems and the pain, although the assumption of causality is made frequently.

The operant approach to the management of chronic pain also hypothesizes psychological factors. The psychological factors hypothesized, however, are not derived from psychopathology but instead from learning theory. Learning theory hypothesizes that a prominent source of the behaviors that indicate pain is the contingent reinforcement of pain behaviors. Pain behaviors may lead to consequences in the environment that are directly reinforcing of these behaviors.

The operant perspective, then, differs from most other approaches by declining to treat a presumed underlying etiology, whether organic or psychiatric. This may be seen as a shortcoming by some, but others might consider this a positive attribute. Its successful application is well documented. If an operant approach has any merit, then the next application should be in the area of the prevention of chronicity, which would include the reduction of iatrogenic and social interventions and the elimination of financial incentives that reinforce disability. The operant approach demonstrates that pain behaviors may be learned and unlearned. From this it follows that learned pain behaviors can be prevented (Roberts, 1983).

REFERENCES

Anderson, T.P., Cole, T.M., Gullickson, G., Hudgens, A., & Roberts, A.H. (1977). Behavior modification of chronic pain: A treatment program by a multidisciplinary team. *Clinical Orthopedics and Related Research*, *129*, 96–100.

Block, A.R. (1982). Multidisciplinary treatment of chronic low back pain: A review. *Rehabilitation Psychology*, *27*, 51–63.

Block, A., Kremer, E., & Gaylor, M. (1980). Behavioral treatment of chronic pain: The spouse as a discriminative cue for pain behavior. *Pain*, *9*, 243–252.

Cairns, D., & Pasino, J. (1977). Comparison of verbal reinforcement and feedback in operant treatment of disability due to chronic low back pain. *Behavior Therapy*, *8*, 621–630.

Cairns, D., Thomas, L., Mooney, V., & Pace, J.B. (1976). A comprehensive treatment approach to chronic low back pain. *Pain*, *2*, 301–308.

Doleys, D., Crocker, M., & Patton, D. (1982). Responses of patients with chronic pain to exercise quotas. *Journal of the American Physical Therapy Association*, *62*, 1111–1114.

Follick, M.J., Zitter, R.F., & Kulich, R.J. (1981). Outpatient management of chronic pain. In T.J. Coates (Ed.), *Behavioral medicine: A practical handbook*. Champaign, IL: Research Press.

Fordyce, W.E. (1976). *Behavioral methods for chronic pain and illness*. St. Louis: C.V. Mosby.

Fordyce, W.E. (1979). Environmental factors in the genesis of low back pain. In J. Bonica, J. Liebeskind, & D. Alba-Fessard (Eds.), *Advances in pain research and therapy* (Vol. 3, pp. 659–666). New York: Raven Press.

Fordyce, W.E. (1983). *Chronic pain and social contingencies*. Unpublished manuscript, University of Washington, School of Medicine, Seattle.

Fordyce, W.E., Fowler, R.S., & DeLateur, B. (1968). An application of behavior modification technique to a problem of chronic pain. *Behaviour Research and Therapy*, *6*, 105–107.

Fordyce, W.E., Fowler, R.S., Lehmann, J.F., & DeLateur, B.J. (1968). Some implications of learning in problems in chronic pain. *Journal of Chronic Disease*, *21*, 179–190.

Fordyce, W.E., Fowler, E., Lehmann, J.,

DeLateur, B., Sand, P., & Treischman, R. (1973). Operant conditioning in the treatment of chronic pain. *Archives of Physical Medicine and Rehabilitation*, *54*, 399–408.

Fordyce, W., McMahon, R., Rainwater, G., Jackins, S., Questad, K., Murphy, T., & DeLateur, B. (1981). Pain complaints — exercise performance relationship in chronic pain. *Pain*, *10*, 311–321.

Fordyce, W., Shelton, J., & Dundore, D. (1982). The modification of avoidance learning in pain behaviors. *Journal of Behavioral Medicine*, *5*, 405–414.

Hilgard, E.R. (1969). Pain as a puzzle for psychology and physiology. *American Psychologist*, *24*, 103–113.

Hudgens, A.J. (1977). The role of the social worker in a behavioral management approach to chronic pain. *Social Work in Health Care*, *3*, 77–85.

Latimer, P.R. (1982). External contingency management for chronic pain: Critical review of the evidence. *American Journal of Psychiatry*, *139*, 1308–1312.

Melzak, R. (1973). *The puzzle of pain*. Harmondsworth, England: Penguin.

Melzack, R., & Wall, P.D. (1965). Pain mechanisms: A new theory. *Science*, *50*, 971–979.

Redd, W.H. (1982). Treatment of excessive crying in a terminal cancer patient: A time-series analysis. *Journal of Behavioral Medicine*, *5*, 225–236.

Roberts, A.H. (1977). *The pain clinic and pain treatment program procedure manual* (2nd ed.). Minneapolis, MN: Department of Physical Medicine and Rehabilitation, University of Minnesota.

Roberts, A.H. (1981). The behavioral treatment of pain. In J.M. Ferguson & C.B. Taylor (Eds.), *The comprehensive handbook of behavioral medicine: Vol. 2. Syndromes and special areas* (pp. 171–189). Jamaica, NY: Spectrum Publications.

Roberts, A.H. (1983). Contingency management methods in the treatment of chronic pain. In J.J. Bonica, U. Lindholm, & A. Iggo (Eds.), *Advances in pain research and therapy* (Vol. 5, pp. 789–794) New York: Raven Press.

Roberts, A.H. (in press). Exercise for the elderly: The behavioral management of excess disability. In L. Teri & P.M. Lewisohn (Eds.), *Clinical assessment and treatment of older adults*. New York: Springer.

Roberts, A.H., & Reinhardt, L. (1980). The behavioral management of chronic pain: Long term follow-up with comparison groups. *Pain*, *8*, 151–162.

Seres, J.L., & Newman, R.I. (1976). Results of treatment of chronic low back pain at the Portland Pain Center. *Journal of Neurosurgery*, *45*, 32–36.

Sternbach, R.A. (1974). *Pain patients: Traits and treatment*. New York: Academic Press.

Turk, D.C., & Flor, H. (1984). Etiological theories and treatment for chronic back pain. II. Psychological models and interventions. *Pain*, *19*, 209–233.

Turk, D.C., Meichenbaum, D., & Genest, M. (1983). *Pain and behavioral medicine: A cognitive-behavioral perspective*. New York: Guilford.

Turner, J.A., & Chapman, C.R. (1982). Operant conditioning, hypnosis and cognitive behavioral therapy. *Pain*, *12*, 22–46.

Varni, J., Bessman, C., Russo, D., & Cataldo, M. (1980). Behavioral management of chronic pain in children: A case study. *Archives of Physical Medicine and Rehabilitation*, *61*, 375–379.

3 THE COGNITIVE-BEHAVIORAL APPROACH TO THE MANAGEMENT OF CHRONIC PAIN

Arnold D. Holzman
Dennis C. Turk
Robert D. Kerns

The cognitive–behavioral treatment for chronic pain evolved and grew simultaneously with the application of cognitive–behavioral theory and procedures to more traditional psychological problems (e.g., Meichenbaum, 1974). Similar to the growth of cognitive-behavioral procedures for traditional behavioral disorders, the rationale for the application of cognitive–behavioral procedures to pain included enhanced breadth of treatment effects and improved generalization beyond the treatment environment (Kerns, Turk, & Holzman, 1983).

It was the hope of the early cognitive-behavioral therapists that the utilization of cognitive constructs would enhance generalization beyond the treatment environment, but, possibly more importantly, also tap aspects of certain disorders not otherwise directly affected by purely behavioral approaches (e.g., Beck, Rush, Shaw, & Emery, 1979; Meichenbaum, 1977). The cognitive-behavioral approach to the treatment of chronic

pain has similar foundations. First, this approach grew out of the frustrations in generalizing the effects of operant treatments beyond the treatment unit or with the limited focus of biofeedback. Second, the cognitive-behavioral approach, and its conception of the multidimensional aspects of chronic pain, was found to be theoretically compatible with Melzack and Wall's (1965) gate-control theory of pain. Melzack and Wall's neurophysiological explanation of a multicomponent pain construct provided converging scientific evidence of not only the sensory but also the cognitive and affective aspects of pain and, thus, the need for a multidimensional treatment approach (Turk & Kerns, 1983).

In this chapter, we will describe the major components of the cognitive–behavioral approach that we have developed. Many of the features of the operant approach and biofeedback-assisted-relaxation are incorporated as part of our multidimensional treatment.

A number of recent studies have examined

the efficacy of the cognitive–behavioral approach with different pain populations, such as those who suffer with headaches (Holroyd, Andrasik, & Westbrook, 1977; Bakal, Demjen, & Kaganov, 1981); arthritis (Randich, 1982); temporomandibular joint pain (Stenn, Mothersill, & Brooke, 1977); low back pain (Turner, 1982). There have also been a number of comprehensive reviews of this body of research (Tan, 1982; Turk, Meichenbaum, & Genest, 1983; Turner & Chapman, 1982). In general, the results have been promising, although many of the studies cited are preliminary and include many methodological problems. The interested reader should examine these studies, as we will not review this body of literature in this chapter. Out intent is to describe the components of the cognitive–behavioral treatment in sufficient detail so that readers who are not familiar with this approach can decide whether they would like to learn more and perhaps to try this with their own patients. A much more thorough presentation appears in the 1983 text by Turk et al., entitled *Pain and Behavioral Medicine: A Cognitive-Behavioral Perspective.*

STRUCTURE OF THE PROGRAM

The cognitive–behavioral treatment program can be broadly outlined into four interrelated phases: screening, assessment, intervention, and follow-up. In the rest of this chapter, we will discuss each of these phases, using clinical examples to illustrate our approach.

Screening

The majority of patients referred for pain management have been given little or no information about our program and often have developed distorted conceptions about what participation may entail. Some patients referred to us have indicated they expected that we would provide the "best pain medicine." Others have indicated that they expected an extensive medical evaluation that

would be followed by some unspecified medical procedure. Many patients who are aware that the pain management program is headed by psychologists suspect that the referring physician considers them to be a "crock" or a malingerer — believes that their pain was "all in their head."

Anticipation of possible misconceptions about the program and active attempts to reassure the patient and provide an accurate perception of what the program can offer are critical goals of the initial contact with the staff member responsible for the screening interview. Successful engagement of appropriate referrals often hinges on an initial brief contact with a clinician who skillfully acknowledges the patient's concerns, fears, or anger while beginning to develop a collaborative problem-solving style of interaction.

Few patients are excluded from the program at this phase of treatment, as there is essentially no consistent literature indicating the demographic characteristics of successful versus nonsuccessful candidates for pain management (Holzman et al., in press). We find it nearly impossible to confidently differentiate appropriate and inappropriate candidates or to predict success in our program.

Our exclusionary criteria are minimal and include: (a) plans for alternative medical or surgical procedures; (b) pain of less than 4 months duration; (c) acute need of psychiatric services (e.g., actively psychotic, suicidal); and (d) pain related to terminal illness.

A typical screening interview begins:

> My name is Dr._____ of the Pain Management Program. You were referred to this program by Dr._____. I'd like to begin by asking you to tell me what he (she) told you about the program. Did Dr._____ describe our program to you? . . . What I would like to do today is briefly learn about your pain problem and then describe to you what our program is all about.

The interview proceeds by eliciting from the patient basic information about his or her pain, the pain's duration and perceived intensity, a brief medical history and plans, and a brief mental status evaluation. If the patient meets none of the exclusionary criteria, the purpose and procedures of the program are explained:

> Your doctor has referred you to this program because he (she) has determined that there is nothing that he (she) can do medically or surgically to alleviate your pain. This program is specially designed to treat people just like you — people suffering from chronic pain that has not been controlled satisfactorily. You may be surprised to learn that you are not alone. There are many people who suffer from chronic pain that medical treatments cannot successfully control. The purpose of our program is not to give you more medication or to perform other medical or surgical procedures on you. Rather, what we will attempt to do in this program is to work with you and to teach you more effective ways to cope with and to control your pain by means of a number of strategies you can learn. We call these self-management or self-control strategies, and you may be surprised to learn just how much of your pain, and its effect on your lifestyle, you can learn to control. Are there any questions? . . .

> Some patients are skeptical about this approach. They think that we don't think their pain is real. To the contrary, we know your pain is real, and we have confidence that the procedures that we use in our program will be beneficial to you if you give them a try. We are not asking you to believe us on faith, but rather we encourage you to work with us. If you are willing to give it a try, we believe you will be surprised to learn how much control you can have over your suffering.

> The strategies we will teach you include what we call progressive relaxation and cognitive and behavioral pain-coping techniques. They are difficult to describe in detail now, but will become more clear to you as you progress through the program. Do you have any questions? . . . What I would like to do now is to have your first evaluation appointment scheduled. If any questions or concerns occur to you between now and your next appointment, please jot them down so that we can talk about them.

Several points need to be made about this explanation. First, the explanation of the program is made within a positive framework and with an expectancy for success. As we have already mentioned and will discuss in more detail in the following sections, many chronic pain patients are defensive and demoralized and thus have little belief that the program will succeed. Although many patients may feel as if they are the "special case" that cannot be cured, it is important to let them know the pain program personnel are experienced and have been successful with other patients "just like them."

It is critical to solicit questions. Many patients tend to be nonassertive in doctors' offices. For patients who do not ask questions, it is often worthwhile to say something such as, "Although it may not have occurred to you yet, many patients are often concerned about . . . . ." These concerns may focus on the belief that because we are psychologists only people with imaginary pain get referred, or that we are going to take away all of their pain medication and they will be left with more pain following this program, and so forth. It is imperative to address these points. It is likely the patient is thinking about these things; and, if not addressed, these fears and concerns may interfere with their participation in the program.

Initial patient attitude and incentives for changing their behavior are very important issues and need to be directly addressed. One patient attending a screening interview came wearing a cervical collar despite the fact that it had not been prescribed for him and he had not worn it since the original injury 5 years earlier. This patient was giving a strong nonverbal message that his pain was real and "not in his head." The clinician's response to this patient was not to address the collar directly but to overemphasize our treatment of patients only with "real pain," stressing that people whose pain was "all in their head" would not have been referred to our program. This overemphasis allowed the patient to develop a belief in the credibility of our services, without feeling as if his pain was not being taken seriously.

In summary, the screening phase serves several functions. It is our first contact with the patient and thus allows us to address any misconceptions and provide him or her with appropriate and positive expectations for treatment. It is the initial point at which we inform patients that our program is different from previous treatments for their pain, that they will be active participants in the treatment process, and that, although no guarantees for success are made, they are provided with a positive expectancy of treatment success.

Most of the points made during the screening phase are repeated many times in treatment. Therefore, none of these issues are critical for the patient to recall. What is most important is that the patient leaves with a positive attitude toward the program (and the individuals on the treatment team), a general willingness to participate, and an expectation for treatment success.

Assessment

A complete discussion of the cognitive–behavioral assessment of the chronic pain patient is beyond our purposes here. The interested reader is referred to Turk and Meichenbaum (1984) and Turk et al. (1983).

The first goal of the assessment phase is data collection. Typical of any cognitive-behavioral assessment, date are collected through multiple modalities (e.g., interview, questionnaire, psychophysiology, behavioral observation) and sources (e.g., patient, significant others).

Data collection is performed: (a) to determine appropriateness for treatment; (b) to provide a baseline against which treatment progress can be evaluated; (c) to develop working hypotheses and a treatment plan; (d) to provide the therapist with examples of problems and situations that can be employed later in treatment as illustrations; and (e) to establish a basis for developing goals and homework assignments. The following case will illustrate cognitive–behavioral assessment of the chronic pain patient.

Case Study: Assessment

Mr. M., a 48-year-old divorced male, was referred to us by a psychiatrist working in a substance abuse clinic. The patient had a 5-year history of chronic neck and shoulder pain and secondary problems of narcotic (Percocet) medication addiction and depression. He came to our office complaining of "horrible and constant" pain that was moderately relieved only by excessive use of narcotics. In the screening interview conducted 2 weeks prior to beginning the assessment phase, the patient had stated that his physician had explained that treatment in the pain management program would help him to learn to control some of his pain on his own and thus hopefully reduce his dependence on narcotics. The patient revealed that he expected no help from our program and feared that the result would be forced medication reduction with no other means to control his pain. These concerns had been directly addressed in the screening interview; however, not surprisingly, the patient continued to express this fear at the first assessment session. The purposes and procedures of the pain management program were explained to the patient again, and he was reassured that our goals and his goals were the same and that gradual medication reduction would not be initiated until other pain management techniques were effectively learned.

We believe that a comprehensive assessment of all aspects of a patient's life (cognitive, emotional, marital, recreational, social, sexual, vocational) are essential in individualizing components of our treatment (Turk & Kerns, 1985). The results of the assessment were as follows.

Continuous hourly self-monitoring of pain over a 2-week period (Turk et al., 1983) indicated that Mr. M. acknowledged relatively high pain levels (3,4, and 5 on our 0–5 scale), with little variability across days or within any given day. Careful scrutiny of the data revealed that Mr. M.'s pain experience worsened in the evening and at bedtime.

Mr. M. acknowledged several factors occasionally associated with changes in his experience of pain, including the weather, time of day (consistent with his self-monitoring of pain), and stress. He considered exacerbations of his pain to be largely unpredictable and uncontrollable.

Mr. M. was taking 8 to 10 Percocet tablets per day on an as needed (PRN) basis having gradually increased to this level over the 5 years of his pain problem. He stated strongly that the narcotic medication was his only effective pain reliever and that he considered the drug dependence to be "worth the price of the pain relief." In addition to the drug dependence, this patient met the criteria for a Diagnostic and Statistical Manual (DSM) III diagnosis of Major Affective Disorder, Depressive type.

A psychosocial history revealed that Mr. M. had been self-employed, owning a small machinery company until the time of his accident. He had been a college scholarship athlete and until the time of the injury participated actively in sports. He had been divorced for 2 years. By his report, his wife had divorced him due to his mood and activity changes subsequent to the pain. We were unable to interview his former wife for corroboration.

A medical history indicated that Mr. M.'s pain problem began following a fall from a ladder while changing a light bulb at his business. The fall resulted in a broken collarbone and other structural damage to his shoulder. Two surgeries had been performed. The patient reported that his pain was unaffected by either surgery and had gradually increased the first several years following the injury until it reached an asymptote at the current level. Mr. M. had also pursued treatment with physical therapists and a chiropractor without benefit.

At the time of the assessment, Mr. M. acknowledged almost no vocational, social, or recreational activities. He was unemployed and had returned to living in his mother's house due to financial limitations. Mr. M. described his typical day as lying in bed or on the couch in his house and, on good days, taking his dog for a walk.

His Beck Depression Inventory score was 26 and his Depression Adjective Check List score was 22. These results were consistent with the diagnosis of depression and his report of dysphoric mood and behavior. No preaccident mental status data were available. However, his report of his preaccident successful vocational and marital functioning compared with his postaccident status suggested that his depression was most likely secondary to his pain and its ramifications. It was our hypothesis at the completion of the assessment that Mr. M.'s depression was probably a result of the degree of interference, perceived lack of control, and subsequent loss of multiple sources of reinforcement, for example, marital, vocational, recreational (Kerns & Turk, 1984). With the presence of depression, it was difficult to attribute his low activity levels to either pain or depression, as both have been noted to result in decreased activity.

Two questionnaires developed by our research group, the Pain Experience Scale (PES) (Turk, 1982) and the West Haven–Yale Multidimensional Pain Inventory (WHYMPI; Kerns, Turk, & Rudy, in press) were administered. Space does not permit us to discuss these instruments in detail. They are, however, available upon request. The primary purpose of the PES is to assess cognitive and affective responses to pain exacerbations. The WHYMPI is designed to evaluate the adjustment to and effect of pain on various aspects of the patient's lifestyle as well as the responses of significant others.

The PES results indicated that Mr. M's typical response to pain included self-statements of worry ("I wonder when it will end") and negative affect (i.e., "I feel overwhelmed"). His responses were significantly higher than most chronic pain patients referred for treatment in our program. These results suggested that Mr. M.'s cognitive and affective responding to pain exacerbations possibly resulted in increased arousal, anxiety, and depressed mood, and fewer coping behaviors.

The results of the WHYMPI were consistent with the PES and indicated the perception of a large degree of interference in most aspects of his lifestyle. Mr. M. reported substantial vocational, social, and familial disruptions attributed to pain that he felt relatively helpless to control.

A psychophysiological evaluation was also performed (Flor, Turk, & Birbaumer, 1985). Generalized (galvanic skin response, GSR, heart rate, HR, frontalis electromyogram, EMG) as well as site-specific (trapezius EMG) recordings were taken during baseline conditions and in response to neutral imagery, personally relevant stress imagery, and pain imagery. One secondary benefit of this assessment is that it has face validity and supports our message that we accept the patient's pain as real.

The trapezius EMG results of the psychophysiological assessment indicated that Mr. M. responded with heightened and sustained levels of muscle tension to thoughts of previous pain and stressful episodes. Minimal evidence of reactivity was observed for the neutral imagery (control) trial. The results were consistent with the interview and questionnaire assessment, suggesting extremely ineffectual coping skills. It was our hypothesis following these results that this patient's poor cognitive and affective coping were associated with heightened muscular arousal at the site of his pain. This heightened muscular arousal reciprocally appeared to be causing increased pain perception, expectations of future pain episodes, and avoidance of activity.

The results of a naturalistic pain behavior observation procedure corroborated the rest of the assessment results. Mr. M. was found to score high on both verbal (i.e., complaining) as well as nonverbal (i.e., protective posture) pain behaviors across several interviews.

With the comprehensive cognitive–behavioral assessment protocol, we were able to develop a useful working hypothesis with which to develop a treatment plan. It was our hypothesis that Mr. M. perceived a high degree of interference with various aspects of his lifestyle due to the pain. Further, it was our hypothesis that his affective disorder was due, not to the pain directly, but to the perceived interference of the pain, perceived loss

of control, and subsequent loss of significant reinforcement in his environment. The affective disorder and ineffectual coping were considered to be reciprocally exacerbating each other.

In sum, the cognitive–behavioral assessment utilizes multiple methods of data collection and is concerned not only with the pain per se, but with the patient's current ability to cope and with the effects of the pain on the patient's lifestyle. The cognitive–behavioral clinician is also interested in the specific ramifications of the pain (e.g., psychophysiology, mood changes) as possible targets for intervention.

The cognitive–behaviorally oriented clinician assumes that the assessment, by itself, will have therapeutic value. For example, patients may be asked questions about their pain that they have never been asked before by a health professional. Many patients have never considered these questions themselves. Previously, health professionals may have only evaluated such issues as how much does it hurt, where, and so forth. Assuming that people are active processors of their environment, cognitive–behavioral therapists expect that consideration of a broader perspective of their pain will lead patients to reevaluate their behavior and attitudes and contribute to subsequent behavior change.

Besides the information-gathering function of the assessment process, this phase begins the collaborative process that will be critical in the intervention phase. Inherent in all the data-gathering activities of the assessment is the notion that the patient is the "expert" related to his or her own situation. Questions are phrased in a manner requiring judgment on the part of the patient and respect for his or her beliefs. The therapist does not generally assume the role of the expert, but rather assumes the role of the facilitator. This approach to the assessment establishes the collaborative relationship that is central to the cognitive-behavioral intervention (cf. Turk et al., 1983; Turk, Holzman, & Kerns, in press).

An example of the collaborative process is

the process of goal-setting. Goal-setting typically completes the assessment phase. Similar to the therapy contract in any therapeutic relationship, we feel that the formal establishment of observable, measurable, and *mutually agreed upon* goals is essential for treatment progress and for avoiding missed communications and inappropriate expectations. Therapy goals are individually negotiated and thus are unique for each patient. They are developed in consideration of the individual's current status, of his or her particular limitations or disabilities, and of the more general goals for treatment. The result of the negotiation process must be the establishment of goals that the individual feels are obtainable as well as personally relevant to his or her particular needs. Thus, treatment goals cannot be dictated to the patient. They must be individually considered and must emanate from the patient's needs, albeit guided by the therapist.

An example of goal-setting comes from a session with Mr. R., whose general treatment goal was to return to a computer programming course from which he had dropped out due to pain. It was pointed out that returning to school was a worthwhile and objective goal; however, it was important to determine what was now preventing him from returning and ultimately to work on these specific behavioral problems.

Mr. R: With all this pain I just can't go to school.
Therapist (T): I understand that going to school is difficult and also very important for you. But what exactly does school involve that you can't do?
Mr. R: I just can't do anything.
T.: Such as?
Mr. R.: Well, for one, I can't sit. They expect me to sit in front of those terminals for 2 hours at a time. Like I told you last week, I can't sit for more than 20 minutes without the pain becoming unbearable.
T.: So increasing your sitting tolerance should be one goal?
Mr. R.: Yeah, that sounds like a good idea, but I can't sit for long.
T.: What do you think your goal should be?
Mr. R: Well I need to sit for 2 hours in class. So I guess I have to make it 2 hours.

T.: Do you think that's feasible for you?
Mr. R: To be honest, I don't see how.
T.: Gee, you can only sit now for 20 minutes and you don't think you can ever reach 2 hours. Do you think there's a way around this?
Mr. R: I don't see how? What do you mean?
T.: Well, I'm wondering if you really have to sit for 2 hours straight or if there are other things you can do?
Mr. R: You mean like getting up and stretching or walking around the room for a minute.
T.: Great ideas!
Mr. R: Yeah, I guess I can sit for a while and then take little breaks.
T.: Great idea. How long do you want to sit for, before you take your break?
Mr. R: Forty minutes sounds like a good goal to me. I can take a break every 40 minutes.
T.: Great, so you've come up with the goal of sitting for 2 hours with a break every 40 minutes. What else interferes with your ability to go to school?

Notice that the therapist attempts to orchestrate the intervention so that the patient suggests those goals that the therapist has in mind. The therapist does not dictate what the goals are, but encourages the patient to generate realistic and appropriate solutions. This approach has the additional advantage of reinforcing the patient's sense of competence and problem-solving.

The therapist and Mr. R. went on to identify poor concentration due to excessive medication use and difficulty falling asleep. Thus, in a similar collaborative manner, decreasing medication and improved sleeping became other goals. These goals were developed in a collaborative process and were personally relevant to this patient. The process allowed Mr. R. to attribute the development of each goal as his idea. We know that when individuals consider an idea as theirs, they are more likely to carry out that behavior (Kopel & Arkowitz, 1975).

Intervention

The general goal of a cognitive–behavioral pain treatment program is to develop on the part of the patient a reconceptualization of his or her pain. This reconceptualization should be from a view of the pain as a medical symptom that is all encompassing and uncontrollable, to a belief that the pain is (at least partially) subject to the patient's control. The purpose of all of the cognitive–behavioral procedures and treatment strategies is to develop these reconceptualized beliefs about self-control of pain.

The cognitive–behavioral approach to intervention is designed to be optimistic, emphasizing the patient's ability to alleviate much of his or her pain and suffering. Throughout the intervention, pain is reconceptualized so that the patient comes to view his or her situation as amenable to change by means of a combined psychologically and physically based approach. The treatment teaches the patient a range of coping skills to assist him or her in dealing with maladaptive thoughts and feelings as well as noxious sensations that may facilitate or exacerbate suffering. The cognitive–behavioral treatment relies heavily on active patient participation and emphasizes a collaborative problem-solving approach between the patient and the therapist (and at times family members), whereby the therapist remains focused on the idiosyncratic thoughts of patients and attempts to engage them in a socratic dialogue. In this manner, problems, concerns, and misunderstandings, in short, anything that can undermine successful treatment, are openly addressed throughout the intervention.

Kanfer and Karoly (1982) suggest that for self-management to operate there must be a shift in the patient's repertoire from well-established, habitual, and automatic but ineffective responses toward systematic problem-solving and planning, long-term control of affect, and behavioral persistence. Cognitive–behavioral techniques are employed to teach the patient to recognize and alter the association between thoughts, feelings, behaviors, environmental stimuli, and pain. From the cognitive–behavioral perspective, therapeutic gain is enhanced when the patient is actively involved and accepts responsibility for change (e.g., Schorr & Rodin, 1982). Improvement is thus a function of both therapist and patient efforts. An implicit assumption of the cognitive–behavioral perspective is that when a patient believes that he or she has the responsibility for some action, that a successful outcome is due to personal competence, that his or her behavior is voluntary and not controlled by external events, and that he or she has chosen voluntarily among alternative courses of action, then the patient will tend to learn more easily, be more highly motivated, report more positive feelings, and demonstrate greater behavioral change.

To summarize, the cognitive–behavioral treatment approach can be viewed as having four major objectives. These are: (a) reconceptualize the patient's view of his or her plight from helplessness and hopelessness to resourcefulness and hopefulness; (b) ensure that patients learn to monitor their thoughts, feelings, and behaviors during activities to identify relationships between thoughts, feelings, behaviors, the environment, and symptoms; (c) ensure that patients can execute necessary behaviors for dealing effectively with problems; and (d) develop and implement increasingly more effective and adaptive ways of thinking, feeling, and responding.

Given the assumptions of the cognitive–behavioral perspective, it is expected that the assessment phase will have some therapeutic value. Although no specific pain-coping strategies are taught, the nature of the questions asked and the overall collaborative approach assumed by the therapist encourage patients to think differently about their pain; thus, many patients on their own begin to develop alternative pain-coping strategies. This reactive property of the assessment phase clearly serves as the initial therapeutic aspect of the treatment program. However, it is the goal of the intervention phase specifically to develop this reconceptualization.

The treatment we will be describing can be applied to inpatient or outpatient programs. We consider an outpatient program to be the treatment of choice for the less severely affected patients for several reasons, including: (a) It is less invasive; (b) it enhances the probability of generalization of treatment gains because treatment and generalization environments are identical; (c) problems that arise in the natural environment can be dealt with more easily; and (d) cost of treatment is decreased. For some patients, such as those who live a great distance from the medical center, those whose medication reduction needs to be closely monitored, those with severe secondary affective problems, or those whose initial level of motivation is low, an inpatient program or at least an initial inpatient phase is desirable. For patients initially seen on an inpatient basis, we encourage continued outpatient follow-up treatment after discharge.

The intervention phase can be subdivided into four components: (a) education, (b) skills acquisition, (c) cognitive and behavioral rehearsal, and (d) generalization and maintenance. For the most part, these four components are not presented sequentially, but rather are presented simultaneously and in interaction with one another.

Educational Component

This component consists of a collaborative presentation of the cognitive–behavioral perspective of coping with and control of chronic pain (i.e., the role of cognitions, affect, and behavior). During the screening and assessment phases, the cognitive–behavioral perspective has already been explained to the patient. Nevertheless, we find it useful to present it once more upon initiating the intervention phase. The presentation should be individualized to the specific situation, goals, and competencies of the patient. It should include didactic as well as socratic learning aspects. At this point, we also find it useful to review assessment data as a way of demonstrating to the patient how this perspective relates specifically to his or her situation.

The gate-control theory of Melzack and Wall (1965) is also presented during one of the initial intervention sessions. The gate-control theory is presented, not as a complex scientific theory, but rather to demonstrate to the patient the multidimensional aspects of pain (sensory, affective, cognitive). It is presented in a way the patient can understand using personally relevant examples.

There have been scientific challenges to the Melzack and Wall (1965) gate-control theory. By presenting this theory, we are not suggesting that it is "the gospel," rather we are acknowledging, and attempting to communicate to the patient, the multidimensional aspect of pain and the role of other than purely sensory–physiological processes in its control.

Skills Acquisition

We cannot emphasize too strongly the distinction between the cognitive–behavioral perspective (described previously) and cognitive–behavioral treatment techniques or strategies (Turk et al., in press). The cognitive–behavioral perspective assumes that individuals are active processors of their environment. When they confront situations that are not consistent with their cognitive schemata (expectations, appraisals, beliefs), they attempt to alter the situation or accommodate their cognitions to be consistent with their environment. Cognitions can elicit or alter affect and can also serve as an impetus for behavior. Conversely, affect and behavior can facilitate or inhibit the production of cognitions. Thus, from a cognitive–behavioral perspective, behavior is reciprocally determined by both the individual and his or her environment.

Cognitive–behavioral treatment techniques consist of a whole range of strategies and procedures, both cognitive and behavioral, designed to bring about alterations in patients' perceptions of their situation and thus their ability to control their condition. The rationale for the cognitive–behavioral strategies assumes that individuals can learn new ways of thinking and behaving through experience.

The cognitive–behavioral therapist serves as a teacher, coach, collaborator, and at times "cheerleader" helping patients learn new ways of behaving, feeling, and thinking. The therapist encourages the patient to feel like an active contributor to his or her experience and not a victim. The responsibility for carrying out the program and maintaining any treatment gains rests ultimately with the patient.

Various strategies and techniques are available to the cognitive–behavioral therapist. *We have found no one treatment technique that is essential for all patients.* This highlights the need to individualize the treatment program to the specific patient. Although two individuals both participate in a cognitive–behavioral pain management program, the specifics of their treatment, or the treatment techniques that are employed, may be very different. Therefore, commonalities among treatments may be obscured if only the techniques utilized are considered. Rather, the rationale for the techniques used and the overall plan of treatment are most important in this approach. We will describe some of the different treatment strategies that are available and discuss and illustrate with case examples the decision criteria for each strategy as well as how they are applied in the following sections.

Relaxation Training. Although no one treatment technique is employed for all patients, relaxation training, in one of its various forms, is clearly the most often used technique. A type of relaxation training is typically employed because of the multiple roles relaxation can serve in pain management. Relaxation can be utilized for its direct muscular relaxation effects (e.g., Keefe, Block, Williams, & Surwit, 1981), for its reduction of generalized arousal (e.g., Linton & Melin, 1983), for its cognitive effects (i.e., as a distraction or attention diversion strategy, or for its initial placebo value.

Muscular and Generalized Autonomic Arousal. The heterogeneity of chronic pain patients precludes generalized statements about common psychological or psychophysiological processes. Our research, as well as that of others, has suggested that patients with specific-site pain syndromes often demonstrate specific psychophysiological processes (e.g., Flor et al., 1985; Laskin, 1969). A commonality among the findings of these studies

was specific EMG reactivity at the pain site in response to the presentation of a stressful stimulus. Theoretically, muscular hyperarousal, developing coincident with, or subsequent to the injury or other etiological factor, serves to maintain or increase the pain experience. Therefore, one rationale for relaxation training is a method of decreasing muscular hyperreactivity and thus decreasing the exacerbation and maintenance of pain.

Orthodox biofeedback approaches for chronic pain are based on a rationale assuming resting level or stress-related muscular hyperarousal. Our concern with this type of approach is the unidimensional view taken of the problem. Muscular arousal is not isomorphic with pain perception. The multidimensional nature of pain presumes that it has multiple response components — sensory, affective, cognitive, and behavioral. Thus, we consider biofeedback or relaxation-only treatment approaches to be incomplete in their focus on this one response channel. Nevertheless, relaxation training for reduction of muscular activity or reactivity is an important component of the multidimensional cognitive–behavioral treatment program.

Muscular hyperarousal is thought to be initiated as a reflexive response to acute pain (unconditioned response). In the chronic pain patient, however, this response is often observed to function as a conditioned response, occurring in the presence of particular stimuli and possibly leading to avoidance responses or overt pain behaviors (Gentry & Bernal, 1977; Linton, Melin, & Gotesman, 1984). The discriminative stimuli eliciting these responses may be situational or internal in the form of beliefs, expectations, or feelings. Direct techniques for the alteration of cognitions and emotions are employed in addition to relaxation procedures. Thus, from the cognitive–behavioral perspective, relaxation procedures for reduction of muscular arousal are utilized as one in a set of strategies, focusing on both stimulus- and response-based aspects of pain perception and behavior.

In addition to site-specific muscular activity, generalized autonomic arousal or anxiety may occur and, via more central processes, contribute to pain perception and overt expressions of pain behaviors. Relaxation procedures are utilized here similarly to specific-site arousal as one component in a treatment program focusing on the amelioration of generalized arousal.

Relaxation procedures cannot be effectively utilized without a simultaneous focus on cognitive procedures. The cognitive-behavioral therapist presumes the interactive and reciprocally determining role of cognitions, behavior, and emotion. The therapist must identify the cognitive components of both the antecedent stimulus complex as well as the response. If the muscular or generalized psychophysiological response is a function of a complex set of antecedent and concurrent cognitions, then focusing on only the psychophysiological response will not be successful. The unaltered cognitions will continue to reinforce the problematic psychophysiological response.

Cognitive Effects of Relaxation. The most commonly considered role for relaxation is reduction of specific muscular or generalized arousal. Relaxation training procedures, however, have clear cognitive components and effects. Therapist or self-directed imagery, autogenic self-statements, controlled attentional focus, or fantasy are all cognitive strategies incorporated in different relaxation techniques and have been reported to elicit or enhance the effects of relaxation. Such strategies in pain management may also serve to distract or to directly alter the focus of attention away from the location of pain.

The results of the assessment frequently suggest that patients are hypervigilant regarding their health status and pain. Examples include patients for whom slight and otherwise innocuous aches and pains signal a turn for the worse. There are also patients who constantly focus on the pain site and whose anticipations of pain exacerbations become self-fulfilling prophecies. Attention diversion strategies, taught via relaxation, can allow these patients to learn other than internally directed, symptom-focused attention.

Relaxation-based attention diversion strategies can work very effectively in specific situations, as well. Sleep disorders, particularly sleep-onset insomnia, are common to the vast majority of chronic pain patients. In fact, virtually every pain patient referred to our program complains of significant sleep difficulties. During assessment, many of these patients report increased pain perception at hours of sleep, thereby causing sleep difficulty. Also at this time, however, most patients report that most external stimuli are removed (i.e., lights, TV, radio are turned off), thereby increasing internal focusing of attention that may exacerbate the experience of pain. Relaxation, alone and combined with other strategies, with the goal of attention diversion or distraction, can serve to reduce pain perception and enhance sleep.

Relaxation as Placebo. An important aspect of nonmedical treatment for pain is the patient's belief that the clinician (a) views the patient's pain as "real" or "legitimate," and (b) can prescribe treatment techniques that are conceptually understandable by the patient (i.e., they make sense given his or her understanding of the problem). Likewise, placebo interventions require the patient's acceptance of the rationale and efficacy of treatment and expectation of treatment success. Relaxation training meets these requirements. The manner in which relaxation training is presented and the manner in which initial training sessions are carried out are all geared to heighten the potential placebo benefits of treatment.

The rationale that is presented to the patient for relaxation training follows the same principles as the presentation of the treatment rationale. The goal is to develop or enhance motivation and participation. The way the rationale is presented depends on the patient's particular way of thinking about his or her pain problem and life situation. The rationale is presented within a framework that sets a high expectation for success, that indicates that this treatment is clinically indicated, and that is within the patient's own competencies to accomplish.

Furthermore, the relaxation procedure can be presented in a manner that is highly "face-valid," by providing the patient with a demonstration of self-control of pain (both increases and decreases in pain intensity). We choose to initially use muscle tension-reduction procedures (Bernstein & Borkovec, 1973). Slight pain exacerbations that often accompany muscle tensing clearly demonstrate to the patient the role of muscle activity in chronic pain. If muscle tension results in increased pain, we can reason that the converse, muscle relaxation, leads to pain reduction. Furthermore, the results of even the first relaxation training session are often inherently reinforcing by reducing generalized arousal. The therapist can build on this to predict the potential beneficial treatment effects with extended practice.

Throughout the practice of relaxation, the therapist continues to take the collaborator's role. This is very important for developing the conceptualization of relaxation as a self-management skill, thereby facilitating self-control of pain. The therapist should also assume a role that fosters the patient's perception of success. The perception of failure, especially at the initial stages of treatment, should be avoided. The patient is frequently encouraged with statements about his or her progress. Likewise, all possible indications and reports of success by the patient should be highly reinforced.

In summary, the placebo value of relaxation training is enhanced by presentation of a rationale that is logical, that includes physiological aspects that are face-valid and acceptable to the patient, that includes a high expectation for success, that demonstrates to the patient the potential for self-control of pain, and that is perceived as immediately reinforcing. With these considerations, the perception of success is insured, the patient continues to believe in the efficacy of treatment, and, most importantly, will continue to participate in treatment.

Case Study: Relaxation Training

Mr. C. was a 51-year-old married male referred for pain management for chronic leg and arm pain due to diabetic peripheral neuropathy. This patient had a medical history that included coronary artery disease, cancer in remission, and an episode of major depression 10 years earlier, coincident with the diagnosis of coronary artery disease. The results of the assessment indicated that Mr. C. was experiencing constant pain in his legs, which increased in intensity during physical activity and when under stress. Avoidance of activities in order to reduce his suffering had resulted in his spending most of his day in bed or otherwise reclining. Due to pain exacerbation, he required a wheelchair to ambulate more than a few steps. Mr. C. was a retired military officer. The main areas of interference due to the pain included vocational (the pain and disability caused him to retire) and domestic activities. He reported frustration at not being "an adequate father" to his two teenage sons. He described his preferred parenting style as being a strong disciplinarian. He considered his pain an indication that he was getting "old and more feeble." Thus, when pain exacerbations occurred, he became increasingly depressed and less likely to leave the house and perceived himself as helpless to cope with the pain. At the initiation of treatment, he was taking 6 to 8 Percocet tablets per day.

During screening, this patient had reported that he had little belief in the efficacy of "mental health treatment" for his pain. He was unhappy with previous psychotherapy for depression 10 years earlier.

Relaxation was considered appropriate for Mr. C. for several reasons. First, he reported that generalized stress resulted in increased pain. The mechanisms of the pain exacerbation may have been muscular or psychological in the form of increased vigilance to the unpleasant sensation and/or poorer affective and cognitive coping during stress. Second, the interview and questionnaire evaluation suggested that Mr. C. rarely attempted distraction or attention diversion activities.

Rather, he was found to be overly vigilant to his symptoms.

Finally, Mr. C. had little confidence in psychological pain treatment. The relaxation technique could be presented to him in a manner that suggested its scientific validity and described its physiological mechanisms of action. Using this type of rationale, the placebo value of relaxation could be strategically employed to insure initial motivation and participation.

Relaxation training was introduced and implemented with this patient as follows:

As I mentioned during the assessment, what I am going to do is teach you various techniques to help you cope with and control your pain. The first of these techniques is called progressive relaxation training. Progressive relaxation training is a technique that has helped many of the patients I see control their pain.

Relaxation training is a technique that once learned will allow you to: (a) discriminate tense versus relaxed muscles and (b) decrease the amount of tension in your muscles, thus possibly resulting in less pain. When I use the term "relaxed," I don't mean relaxed as in not-active or calm and quiet. Rather, I am referring to a state of physiological relaxation associated with decreased electrical activity of muscles. This type of relaxation may be somewhat of a new sensation for you, but may eventually allow you more effective control of your pain.

Many people who experience chronic pain also experience effects on their muscles — chronic tension and deterioration due to lack of activity. While increased muscle tension is a natural and adaptive response to acute pain, it is not adaptive for chronic pain. Rather, chronically aroused muscle tension often makes the muscles susceptible to spasm and thus more pain. The fact that your muscles have deteriorated due to lack of use does not allow you to control your muscles as you would like. And, as I learned during the assessment, not only is muscle spasm extremely painful for you, but the fear of spasm or pain exacerbation due to spasm has caused you to significantly decrease your activity, thereby enabling

your muscles to deteriorate further, resulting in a cycle of pain resulting in fear of activity leading to a greater susceptibility to pain and thus greater fear of movement.

Relaxation training is a complex skill that will take you some time to learn. Don't expect immediate results, but in a few weeks or so expect to see some positive effects of the relaxation. Because it's a relatively complex skill it requires practice. As a rule of thumb, the more you practice, the better you will get. We will talk more about this later, but now I would like to go through the exercise with you.

A muscle tension-reduction relaxation training procedure (e.g., Bernstein & Borkovec, 1973) was selected because: (a) It has face validity; (b) it is a relatively concrete procedure and thus easy to recall and practice at home; and (c) it is therefore less prone to failure due to distraction by pain or cognitive intrusions.

Following the initial exercise in the office, Mr. C. reported some pain relief. This information was reframed by the therapist as a very positive sign and indicating a good prognosis with practice. Social reinforcement is required during early stages to enhance the likelihood of continued practice until the effects of relaxation training become more obvious.

As treatment progressed, Mr. C. became more skilled in the application of the relaxation exercise and the ability to discriminate pain- and/or anxiety-producing situations. He became more able to interrupt or reduce pain exacerbations. As this skill became more effective at reducing pain, other cognitive and behavioral strategies were able to be introduced with a shared expectation of treatment efficacy.

Cognitive Techniques

Cognitive techniques consist of several different types of procedures, including cognitive distraction or attention diversion techniques, and cognitive coping-strategy training or restructuring.

Distraction Training. Patients are often found to be overly preoccupied with their pain and bodily symptoms in general. Every new sensation is seen as an indication of deteriorating status or a new health problem. Also, many patients describe being unable to focus externally. Rather, their focus of attention is always on their body (i.e., their pain or other symptoms). When asked how they distract themselves from pain, many patients describe being unable or unwilling to do so. This latter group often needs to understand that it is "OK" to disattend from their pain sensations. Cognitive distraction techniques are often best utilized during discrete, low- to moderate-intensity pain episodes, where the pain may be predictable and can be prepared for.

Case Study: Distraction Training

Mr. A. was referred for pain management due to a 6-year history of upper back and neck pain. During the first assessment session, an immediate problem became apparent. He could not sit in his car a sufficiently long time to reach the hospital without substantial pain exacerbation. A brief assessment indicated that Mr. A. typically focused on his pain, waiting for it to reach his tolerance level as he grew more and more tense. The anticipation appeared to result in muscle tension that exacerbated his pain.

The therapist made two basic suggestions. First, Mr. A. was to consider changing the radio station in his car from music to a news or talk show. While doing this, Mr. A. found topics he was interested in, thus easily keeping his attention focused externally. Second, Mr. A. always drove 55 miles per hour on the highway. He decided to count the number of cars that passed him each day on the way to the hospital and keep a record by month. These two cognitive activities allowed Mr. A. to direct his attention away from his pain, prevented subtle increased tension levels, and thus led to decreased pain perception and ability to do the required task (drive to the hospital).

Cognitive distraction tasks, like all procedures in cognitive–behavioral treatment programs, are individualized. There are a large number of potential distraction strategies. They have been categorized by Turk (1977).

Cognitive Restructuring. The cognitive–behavioral perspective assumes that the way an individual perceives his or her situation determines behavior and affect. Likewise, affect and behavior reciprocally affect cognition. For example, the thoughts of patients during pain episodes can clearly influence the intensity and duration of the episodes and the degree to which the pain disrupts instrumental activities and coping efforts. Lefebvre (1981) provided indirect support for this notion by demonstrating that depressed pain patients acknowledged more frequent negative and distorted cognitions than did nondepressed pain patients or depressed patients without pain. Research by Turk, Kerns, and Rudy (1984) further demonstrated that perceptions of a high degree of behavioral interference and low self-control are important links between the experience of pain and the development of depression. As noted previously, Mr. C. interpreted his pain episodes as indications of "becoming more feeble." Consistent with this belief, Mr. C. viewed himself as weak, helpless, and ineffectual, resulting in feelings of overwhelming sadness and a greatly restricted lifestyle.

The ability to develop alternative cognitive responses to the experience of pain is, at the same time, a process and a goal of the cognitive–behavioral perspective. Cognitive restructuring refers generally to the process of reconceptualization that has been emphasized throughout this chapter as well as to a more formal phase of intervention. In this phase, the therapist directly attempts to elicit the patient's idiosyncratic thoughts and feelings associated with the pain experience and collaborates with the patient in an effort to alter those thoughts and feelings that may have negative effects on the pain experience.

From the first contact with the patient, the phrasing of the therapist's questions and the explanation of the treatment rationale is geared to providing an alternative view of his or her pain experience. Questions such as "What do you do to relieve your pain?" and

"What factors have you identified that affect your pain?" intuitively imply an aspect of controllability and predictability. Other aspects of the intervention phase (e.g., discussion of the gate-control theory, relaxation training) reinforce this conceptualization. This process sets the stage for more direct attempts by the therapist to focus specifically on the patient's maladaptive thoughts regarding his or her pain experience.

Cognitive restructuring requires active collaboration between the patient and therapist. Skillful probing by the therapist is required in order to elicit specific high-frequency thoughts of the patient, especially those associated with periods of exacerbation. The Pain Experience Scale (described previously) may be a useful tool in this regard. Once negative or distorted thoughts are acknowledged by the patient, it is usually intuitively obvious to the patient that these thoughts may have a negative influence on his or her pain experience, as well as mood and behavior.

Much more difficult for most patients to appreciate is the notion that thoughts can be altered. Our clinical tactics during this aspect of treatment remain very much consultative and within a problem-solving framework. Patients are not told what to do! Our clinical experience and research data both support the belief that people are more likely to accept and participate in behaviors they consider to be of their own volition (e.g., Kopel & Arkowitz, 1975). Thus, the therapist's goal is to assist the patient to learn experientially and in a framework that allows the learning of new cognitive coping strategies.

Rather than simply tell the patient to stop negative thinking, the therapist encourages the patient to consider how his or her particular thoughts may be untrue and distorted. For example, it is not uncommon for patients with a several-year history of pain with no evidence of progressive deterioration in physical status to continue to worry that their pain is indicative of some gross pathology, perhaps even terminal illness. The therapist must acknowledge this concern but work with the patient to appreciate that the fear is most likely unfounded and illogical. The patient is encouraged to acknowledge alternative positive thoughts that may compete with the maladaptive thought. This process typically requires frequent repetition and practice, with emphasis placed on the adaptive consequences of more positive and accurate thinking. An example may help describe this process.

Mrs. D. was a 56-year-old woman with a 12-year history of episodic head pain. Repeated neurological evaluations had failed to reveal significant findings. The following is an excerpt of the seventh treatment session.

T.: What thoughts come to mind as you notice your pain beginning to increase?

Mrs. D.: I immediately worry about having a tumor or something. I think that this time the pain is not going to go away and that I'm going to end up in a hospital again and that I'll never see my children grow up. I imagine myself in the hospital and my family is there worrying about me, but there's nothing anybody can do.

T.: So you get extremely worried that there's something terribly wrong and you feel helpless to do anything about it. Let's examine those thoughts for a minute.

Mrs. D. (interrupting): Yes, I know they're not true but I cannot help it.

T.: You don't think you have control over your thoughts?

Mrs. D.: Yes, they just come to me.

T.: Well, let's come back to the idea that your thoughts are automatic. First, let's break down your flood of negative thoughts and look at each part separately. Do you really think that you have a tumor?

Mrs. D.: I don't know. I guess not (pause) but it's hard not to worry about it. My head hurts so bad.

T.: Yes, I know. So how do you convince yourself that you don't have a tumor or something else seriously wrong?

Mrs. D.: Well, as you know I've been examined many times by the best neurologists around. They say I'm OK. Also, my pain always goes away and I've never had any other neurological problems. My only problem is the pain. But, it's hard to remember these facts when my pain is so awful.

T.: It's much easier to be positive about your condition when you're not suffering. Nevertheless, rationally, you really are convinced that there's nothing seriously wrong.

Mrs. D.: I guess so. If only I could remember that when my pain starts coming on.

T.: So the goal of our work today could be to figure out a strategy to increase the likelihood that you'll remember the positive thoughts during a pain episode.

Mrs. D.: Yes, that sounds good.

T.: Let's start by generating a list of accurate statements about your pain. Then we can talk about ways you can cue yourself to remember the list when you begin to feel pain. You already mentioned a couple of beliefs about your pain; that is, that there's nothing seriously wrong, that the pain always goes away, and that, other than the pain, you feel pretty healthy. Can you think of other accurate and positive thoughts?

This excerpt exemplifies the collaborative process in which the therapist carefully elicits the troublesome thoughts and concerns of the patient, acknowledges their bothersome nature, and then constructs an atmosphere in which the patient can safely challenge the validity of his or her own beliefs. Rather than suggesting alternative thoughts, the therapist always attempts to elicit competing thoughts from the patient and then emphasizes their adaptive nature. In this excerpt, the patient continues to acknowledge a degree of uncertainty about the etiology of her problem by stating "I guess so" in response to questions about her belief that nothing serious is wrong. In this case, it was critical that this belief remained a focus of cognitive restructuring exercises during the last sessions of treatment. Only after numerous repetitions and practice in the cueing of competing positive statements during rehearsal in therapy sessions (see the next section) and in vivo practice during pain episodes did Mrs. D. decrease the frequency of her negative thoughts. As these thoughts decreased, her pain episodes significantly diminished, further reinforcing her positive beliefs about her problem.

Cognitive and Behavioral Rehearsal

The next stage of treatment is the rehearsal phase. In this phase, the patient practices and further consolidates the skills he or she has learned during skills acquisition and learns to apply them to natural situations. The techniques often used during the rehearsal stage include rehearsal during mental imagery, role-playing, and various homework activities. These are standard behavior therapy procedures and do not differ substantially in their application in the treatment of pain.

One means of providing patients with an opportunity to rehearse coping skills is to use imagery rehearsal. As in the procedure of systematic desensitization (Wolpe, 1959), the patient is asked, while relaxed, to imagine himself or herself in various situations in which the intensity of pain and stress varies.

In systematic desensitization, the patient is asked to imagine scenes from a graded hierarchy. If the patient experiences any stress (anxiety, pain), he or she signals the therapist, who then instructs the patient to terminate the image and continue relaxing. The procedural steps follow from the concept of counter-conditioning as outlined by Wolpe (1959). In recent years, however, the explanation of desensitization has been subjected to much theoretical and empirical criticism (cf. Davison & Wilson, 1972). An alternative view of the desensitization process suggests that imagery rehearsal is a useful way to teach the patient a set of coping skills or to foster self-control (Goldfried & Davison, 1976).

Our view of imagery rehearsal presumes that when patients are instructed to imagine hierarchy scenes, they are providing themselves with a model for their own behavior (e.g., Goldfried & Davison, 1977). The closer the imagery comes to representing real experiences, the greater the likelihood of generalization. Through imagery, patients may mentally rehearse the specific thoughts, feelings, and behaviors they will use to cope with stress and pain.

To maximize the similarity between the images used in desensitization and real-life experiences, a cognitive-behavioral approach to desensitization adds coping images (e.g., Meichenbaum, 1971) to the mastery images that have been commonly used. Mastery imagery involves patients' viewing themselves successfully handling the problem situation. Coping imagery, in contrast, involves patients' imagining themselves becoming anxious, beginning to experience pain, or having maladaptive thoughts, and then coping with these difficulties using approaches they have already developed to deal with the situation. Several authors (Kazdin, 1973; Meichenbaum, 1971; Sarason, 1975) have provided evidence of the therapeutic value of coping over mastery modeling in the change process.

We utilize mental imagery within a stress-inoculation paradigm such as that described by Meichenbaum & Turk (1976). Patients are taught to view coping as a four-stage event: (a) preparing for a pain episode, (b) confronting and handling the pain, (c) coping with feelings at critical moments, and (d) utilizing self-reinforcement for successful coping.

Case Study: Coping Strategy

Ms. C. was a 29-year-old female suffering from upper back and shoulder pain following a fall 1 year earlier. She was employed as a typist in a large corporation. Among other findings, assessment results indicated increased pain at work due to extended sitting at her desk or when she felt pressured to complete a task.

Relaxation was successfully learned, but Ms. C. reported it to be ameliorative only under optimal circumstances (i.e., in the clinic, at home) and without effectiveness beyond the actual exercises. Imagery procedures were employed to enhance generalization.

An imagery hierarchy was developed that ranged from lying in her own bed to the final scene of working overtime feeling pressured to complete a report. These scenes were paired with relaxation while gradually progressing through the hierarchy. The general instructions for each scene were:

> Now that you are relaxed, I would like you to imagine the following scene that we discussed previously. I would like you to try to imagine that scene as vividly as possible — as if you were right there. As you will be imagining this scene, you may feel some tension or pain. Do not stop imagining, but rather try to see yourself coping with the situation as successfully as you can. By coping, I mean providing yourself with coping self-statements as we have practiced before and/or doing brief relaxation exercises. You may not be successful at first, but keep trying in your imagination, and you may eventually experience some success.

The therapist then went on to present the scene and through each stage of the hierarchy directed the patient through the most appropriate coping strategy as determined prior to the exercise.

Role-playing. Role-playing is another method used to rehearse and consolidate the skills learned during the acquisition phase. We find role-playing useful not only in the rehearsal of new skills but also in the identification of potential problem areas that may require special attention. Most typically, the patient is asked to identify and participate in a role-playing situation indicative of a particular problem area. As treatment progresses, the patient is able to practice and demonstrate gradually improved abilities over time. For example, the patient may learn the ability to assertively request that significant others refrain from being overly solicitous and frequently drawing attention to the patient's pain. Also in role-playing situations, the patient may learn that methods of communication that do not consist of pain complaints would still result in satisfactory outcomes.

Reverse role-playing is also beneficial. This procedure is employed because we know from research on attitude change that when people are placed in adversary positions, they generate exactly the kinds of arguments they regard as most personally appealing (Janis & King, 1954). Also, dissonance theory tells us that once an individual has expressed a particular point of view for no or little extrinsic reinforcement, he or she is more likely to subsequently uphold that view (e.g., Festinger, 1954).

Homework

An essential component of our approach to pain management is the active involvement of the patient and significant others outside of the therapy sessions. Tasks to be carried out between sessions begin during the assessment phase and continue throughout the therapy process. Homework assignments fulfill a number of purposes:

    1. To assess various areas of the patient's and significant others' lives and how these influence and are affected by the pain problem.

    2. To assess the typical responses of significant others and the patient to pain and pain behavior.

    3. To make the patient and significant others more aware of factors that exacerbate and alleviate suffering.

    4. To help the patient and significant others identify maladaptive responses to pain and pain behavior.

    5. To consolidate the use of coping procedures discussed during therapy sessions.

    6. To increase physical activity.

    7. To illustrate to the patient and significant others that progress can be made in living with pain.

    8. To serve as reinforcers and as enhancers of self-efficacy as the patient achieves goals.

    9. To assist the therapist and patient in assessing progress and in modifying goals and treatment strategies. (Turk et al., 1983)

Homework assignments are determined within the same consultative framework that all therapy is practiced. Each homework assignment is geared toward observable and manageable tasks, starting with those that are most readily achievable and progressing to more difficult ones. The purpose of such graded tasks is to enhance the patient's sense of competence and to reinforce his or her continued efforts. The therapist uses the assessment results to establish short-, medium-, and long-term goals, and the accompanying tasks are designed to achieve these goals. Goals and assignments are individually tailored to the particular condition and lifestyle of each patient.

Generalization and Maintenance

We have described previously how Marlatt and Gordon's (1980) approach to relapse prevention in addictive behaviors may also be appropriate for chronic pain patients (Turk, Holzman & Kerns, in press). Briefly, their approach is to help patients, prior to completion of treatment, learn to identify and successfully cope with factors that may otherwise lead to relapse. They help the patient identify high-risk situations and the types of cognitive and behavioral responses that may be necessary for successful coping.

In the final stage of treatment, discussion is focused on possible ways of predicting and avoiding or dealing with pain following treatment termination. Discussion of relapse must be done in a delicate manner. On the one hand, the therapist does not wish to convey an expectancy of treatment failure, but, on the other hand, the therapist wishes to anticipate and assist the patient to learn how to deal with potential recurrences or problematic situations.

We have found this process to be most successful by assisting the patient to anticipate future stress or pain-producing events and to plan coping strategies before they occur. Actual, planned, possible, as well as unlikely, events should be considered and strategies developed for use when needed. For example, one patient was anticipating a car ride from Connecticut to Florida soon after termination. Utilizing a future-oriented problem-solving approach, the patient was able to identify both expected and possible pain-eliciting situations (e.g., extended time sitting, possible interpersonal stressors due to car breakdown and poor repair service in an unfamiliar area). In this case, the patient was able to develop a plan to cope with a range of situations and thereby decrease the likelihood of relapse. It is important to encourage the patient to use the problem-solving approach, with as little guidance from the therapist as needed, in order to foster a sense of self-efficacy. Greater perceived self-efficacy should enhance persistence in any problem situations that arise (Bandura, 1977).

It is important to note that all possible situations cannot be anticipated. Rather, our goal during this phase, like the rest of the treatment, is to enable the patients to develop a problem-solving approach to coping with their pain. In this manner, the patient will learn to try to anticipate future problems, to develop plans for coping, and to adjust his or her behavior accordingly.

The relapse prevention phase serves at least two purposes. First, it allows the patient to anticipate and plan for future events. Second, and possibly more important for long-term success, it provides the patient with the expectation that minor setbacks may in fact occur, but that these setbacks *do not* signal complete failure and in fact should be considered cues to utilize the coping skills already learned in a more effective manner. It is important for the patient not to think of his or her work as ending, but rather as switching into a different phase.

During the final session, all aspects of the training are reviewed. A review with the patients of what they have learned and how they have changed from the assessment phase can encourage recognition of how *the patient's own efforts contributed to this change.* Discussion can enhance the patient's sense of competence and mastery. The goal is to help patients to realize they have plans and abilities to cope with these events. By this type of discourse, the therapist conveys the expectation and conviction that the changes that have been achieved will be maintained.

SUMMARY

It should be obvious that the cognitive–behavioral approach is complex and requires considerable therapeutic skills. More important than any specific technique is the general perspective that fosters patient responsibility, resourcefulness, and control; in short, this is a reconceptualization of the pain problem that is diametrically opposed to the typical view of pain as overwhelming and uncontrollable with the patient a passive and helpless victim. The success of the cognitive–behav-

ioral treatment is based on the therapist's ability to combat demoralization and to assist in the reconceptualization process. The diversity of procedures described here are geared toward this end.

REFERENCES

Bandura, A. (1977). Self-efficacy: Toward an unifying theory of behavioral change. *Psychological Review, 84,* 191–215.

Bakal, D.A., Demjen, S., & Kaganov, J.A. (1981). Cognitive behavioral treatment of chronic headache. *Headache, 21,* 81–86.

Beck, A.T., Rush, A.J., Shaw, B.F., & Emery, G. (1979). *Cognitive therapy of depression.* New York: Guilford.

Bernstein, D.A., & Borkovec, T.D. (1973). *Progression relaxation training.* Champaign, IL: Research Press.

Davison, G.C., & Wilson, G.T. (1972). Critique of "Desensitization: Social and cognitive factors underlying the effectiveness of Wolpe's procedure." *Psychological Bulletin, 78,* 28–31.

Festinger, L. (1954). A theory of social comparison processes. *Human Relations, 7,* 117–140.

Flor, H., Turk, D.C., & Birbaumer, N. (1985). Assessment of stress-related psychophysiological reactions in chronic back pain patients. *Journal of Consulting and Clinical Psychology, 53,* 354–364.

Gentry, W.D., & Bernal, G.A.A. (1977). Chronic pain. In R.B. Williams & W.D. Gentry (Eds.), *Behavioral Approaches to Medical Treatment* (pp. 173–182). Cambridge, MA: Ballinger.

Goldfried, M.R., & Davison, G. (1976). *Clinical behavior therapy.* New York: Holt, Rinehart, & Winston.

Holroyd, K.A., Andrasik, F., & Westbrook, T. (1977). Cognitive control of tension headache. *Cognitive Therapy and Research, 1,* 121–133.

Holzman, A.D., Turk, D.C., Rudy, T.E., Sanders, S.H., Gerber, K.E., Zimmerman, J., & Kerns, R.D. (in press). Chronic pain: A multiple setting comparison of patient characteristics. *Journal of Behavioral Medicine.*

Janis. I.L., & King, B. (1954). The influence of role-playing on opinion change. *Journal of Abnormal and Social Psychology, 49,* 211–218.

Kanfer, F.H., & Karoly, P. (1982). The psychology of self-management: Abiding issues and tentative directions. In P. Karoly & F.H. Kanfer (Eds.), *Self-management and behavior change.* Elmsford, NY: Pergamon.

Kazdin, A.E. (1973). Covert modeling and the reduction of avoidance behavior. *Journal of Abnormal Psychology, 81,* 87–95.

Keefe, F.J., Block, A.R., Williams, R.B., Jr., & Surwit, R.S. (1981). Behavioral treatment of chronic low back pain: Clinical outcome and individual difference in pain relief. *Pain*, *11*, 221–231.

Kerns, R.D., & Turk, D.C. (1984). Depression and chronic pain: The mediating role of the spouse. *Journal of Marriage and the Family*, 845–852.

Kerns, R.D., Turk, D.C., & Holzman, A.D. (1983). Psychological treatment for chronic pain: A selective review. *Clinical Psychology Review*, *3*, 15–26.

Kerns, R.D., Turk, D.C., & Rudy, T.E. (in press). *The West Haven-Yale multidimensional pain inventory. Pain.*

Kopel, S., & Arkowitz, H. (1975). The role of attribution and self-perception in behavior change: Implications for behavior therapy. *Genetic Psychology Monographs*, *92*, 175–212.

Laskin, D.M. (1969). Etiology of the pain-dysfunction syndrome. *Journal of American Dental Association*, *79*, 147–153.

Lefebvre, M.F. (1981). Cognitive distortion and cognitive errors in depressed psychiatric and low back pain patients. *Journal of Consulting and Clinical Psychology*, *49*, 517–525.

Linton, S.J., & Melin, L. (1983). Applied relaxation in the management of chronic pain. *Behavioral Psychotherapy*, *11*, 337–350.

Linton, S.J., Melin, L., & Gotesam, K.G. (1984). Behavioral analysis of chronic pain and its management. *Progress in Behavior Modification*, *18*, 1–42.

Marlatt, G.A., & Gordon, J.R. (1980). Determinants of relapse: Implications for the maintenance of behavior change. In P.O. Davidson & S.M. Davidson (Eds.), *Behavior medicine: Changing health life styles.* New York: Mazel.

Meichenbaum, D.H. (1971). Examination of model characteristics in reducing avoidance behavior. *Journal of Personality and Social Psychology*, *17*, 298–307.

Meichenbaum, D.H. (1974). *Cognitive behavior modification.* Morristown, NJ: General Learning Press.

Meichenbaum, D.H. (1977). *Cognitive behavior modification.* New York: Plenum Press.

Meichenbaum, D.H., & Turk, D.C. (1976). The cognitive behavioral management of anxiety, anger, and pain. In P.O. Davidson (Ed.), *The behavioral management of anxiety, depression, and pain.* New York: Brunner/Mazel.

Melzack, R., & Wall, P.D. (1965). Pain mechanisms: A new theory. *Science*, *50*, 971–979.

Randich, S.R. (1982). Evaluation of a pain management program for rheumatoid arthritis patients. (abstract). *Arthritis and Rheumatism*, *25*, 11.

Sarason, I.G. (1975). Anxiety and self-preoccupation. In I.G. Sarason & C.D. Spielberger (Eds.), *Stress and anxiety* (Vol. 2). Washington, DC: Hemisphere.

Schorr, D., & Rodin, J. (1982). The role of perceived control in practitioner-patient relationships. In T.A. Wills (Ed.), *Basic processes in helping relationships.* New York: Academic Press.

Stenn, P.G., Mothersill, K.J., & Brooke, R.I. (1979). Biofeedback and a cognitive-behavioral approach to treatment of myofacial pain dysfunction syndrome. *Behavior Therapy*, *10*, 29–36.

Tan, S-Y. (1982). Cognitive and cognitive-behavioral methods for pain control: A selective review. *Pain*, *12*, 201–228.

Turk, D.C. (1977). A coping skills-training approach for the control of experimentally produced pain. Unpublished doctoral dissertation, University of Waterloo, Waterloo, Ontario, Canada.

Turk, D.C. (1982). *The pain experience scale.* Unpublished Manuscript, Yale University, New Haven, CT.

Turk, D.C., Holzman, A.D., & Kerns, R.D. (in press). Chronic pain: Emphasis on self-management. In Kenneth A. Holroyd and Tom Creer (Eds.), *Self-management in health psychology and behavioral medicine.* New York: Academic Press.

Turk, D.C., & Kerns, R.D. (1983). Conceptual issues in the assessment of clinical pain. *International Journal of Psychiatry in Medicine*, *13*, 15–26.

Turk, D.C., & Kerns, R.D. (1985). Assessment in health psychology: A cognitive-behavioral perspective. In P. Karoly (Ed.), *Measurement strategies in health psychology*, (pp. 335–372). New York: John Wiley & Sons.

Turk, D.C., Kerns, R.D., & Rudy, T.E. (1984). *Identifying the links between chronic illness and depression: Cognitive-behavioral mediators.* Paper presented at the annual meeting of the American Psychological Association, Toronto, Canada.

Turk, D.C., & Meichenbaum, D. (1984). A cognitive-behavioral approach to pain management. In P.D. Wall & R. Melzack (Eds.), *Textbook of pain.* London: Churchill Livingstone.

Turk, D.C., Meichenbaum, D.H., & Genest, M. (1983). *Pain and behavioral medicine: A cognitive-behavioral perspective.* New York: Guilford Press.

Turner, J.A. (1982). Comparison of group progressive relaxation training and cognitive-behavioral group therapy for chronic low back pain. *Journal of Consulting and Clinical Psychology*, *50*, 757–765.

Turner, J.A., & Chapman, C.R. (1982). Psychological interventions for chronic pain: A critical review. *Pain*, *12*, 23–46.

Wolpe, J. (1959). *Psychotherapy by reciprocal inhibition.* Stanford, CA: Stanford University Press.

4 TRADITIONAL INDIVIDUAL PSYCHOTHERAPY AND PSYCHOPHARMACOTHERAPY

Harold Merskey

In this chapter, I aim to describe the theory and application to pain of the types of individual psychotherapy that are traditionally identified with medical and psychological practice. These extend from psychoanalysis on the one hand to the overt use of suggestion or placebos on the other. Sometimes, active medication is also employed and, besides its physiological effects, provides an additional placebo benefit. In between the extremes lie exploratory psychotherapy, insight-oriented therapy, transactional analysis, existential therapy, client-centered therapy, and supportive therapy. Most of the theoretical differences between the above approaches are not appropriate topics for discussion here, nor are they my field. Fortunately, there is an abundance of works that deal with the principles of psychotherapy in general and the differences between the particular approaches. These are readily available for reference.

The main psychological approaches among the above themes can largely be reduced to five principal headings: (a) psychoanalysis; (b) dynamically oriented insight therapy; (c) abreactive experimental treatments, on which little has yet been published in rela-

tion to pain; (d) supportive therapy; and (e) suggestion.

THE EMERGENCE OF PSYCHOTHERAPY FOR PAIN

By Hill 60 . . . everything I could see seemed to be made of jelly. I bit the end of my tongue, and then shot over the debris of no man's land like a clockwork man. My feet seemed to be six inches off the ground most of the way. The spike of a barbed wire strand stuck in the back of my knee and I pulled it out with the flesh hanging to it. But couldn't feel any pain. It seemed like someone else's leg. (Newspaper account of a man's experiences in the First World War)

Whoever has read Hippocrates or Dr. James Mackenzie, and has considered well the effects which the passions and affections of the mind have upon the digestion (why not of a wound as much as a dinner?) may easily conceive what sharp paroxysms and exacerbations of his wound my Uncle Toby must have undergone upon that score alone. (*Life and Opinions of Tristram Shandy, Gentleman*, by Laurence Sterne, 1940)

To those who have not encountered the

proposition previously, it is prima facie surprising that any psychological techniques should be held to be important in the management of pain. Workers in the field are acquainted, however, with plentiful evidence about the significance of psychological and behavioral topics on these themes. It is worth noting how these concepts emerged and developed towards present practice.

Historically, there has long been some awareness that the emotions were important in the experience of pain. Jeremiah, Aristotle, Montaigne, Shakespeare, and Sterne provide a ready quintet of illustrations (Merskey, 1980b). At the same time, pain was traditionally classed by physicians as one of the symptoms that could be hysterical. So far as I can determine, the management of hysterical pain was not a specific separate topic prior to the 20th century. It was part of the general treatment of hysteria and did not achieve separate consideration. Perhaps quite a few hysterical pains were treated as neuralgias, gastralgias, and so forth; and there are many references to the management of relatively chronic pains in the 19th century with the help of opiates. Even when Freud (Breuer & Freud, 1893–5) first noted the relationship between a psychological cause and its solution with a hysterical pain, he did not focus on pain specifically. His psychodynamic explanation of the origin of hysterical pain has, however, had obvious fruit since then.

Graven (1924) was one of the earliest psychoanalytically oriented writers to make therapeutic comments on pain, and Schilder (1931) provided some specific psychoanalytic ideas about the relationship between humiliation in childhood and the need for pain in adult life. These psychoanalytic themes were reviewed by Hart (1947), then by Engel (1951, 1959), and by Szasz (1957). Jelliffe (1933), Engel (1959), and others also documented a tendency on the part of some patients to seek excessive operations.

Through this literature, the view developed that psychotherapy of an analytic type was valuable in removing pain in patients who either had headache or an affliction in some other part of the body. I have counted over 30 such contributions to the literature between 1924 and 1959. Most of them were single, uncontrolled observations. Theories about the mechanism of the pain tended not to be well defined except in terms of repression and hysteria. Scattered comments and suggestions of this nature persist throughout the literature to the present time. One of the most recent papers in this field is by Lakoff (1983).

In company with the development from the traditional idea of hysterical pain to the view that pain might be treated psychoanalytically, there also emerged a recognition by internists that pain was frequently emotional in origin. One of the most important conditions in this connection is DaCosta's syndrome or "irritable heart" or "effort syndrome," which was commonly marked by precordial pains and often occurred in soldiers. DaCosta himself does not appear to have recognized its psychological significance. Indeed, his first case (DaCosta, 1871) was a man who developed an aphonia that was labelled catarrhal, but which one must presume to be hysterical because the patient recovered without any other treatment 10 months subsequent to onset. Internists like Sir Thomas Lewis (1917) had trouble recognizing the psychological aspects of this condition. By 1918 others (e.g., Oppenheimer & Rothschild, 1918) related the condition to psychological causes and to a premorbid predisposition to psychological illness.

Physicians from the time of the First World War increasingly emphasized the importance of psychological factors in patients with pain, particularly those with gastrointestinal complaints or "rheumatic" or musculoskeletal complaints. Merskey and Spear (1967) reviewed a good deal of this information. It became natural to accept or suppose that if psychological factors were important in the production of these pains, the psychological approach to treatment would be relevant. Engel (1951, 1959) was especially influential in encouraging psychiatrists and psychoanalysts to assume that it was thoroughly justified to attempt to treat patients with chronic pain

by means of psychoanalytic and deep exploratory psychotherapy techniques. Other reports
about the influence of motive on pain
(Beecher, 1956) and theories of chronic pain
(Barber, 1959) readily fostered a climate of
ideas in which such approaches were favored.

THEORETICAL EXPLANATIONS

As the editors make clear at the beginning of
this volume, chronic pain is a problem of
enormous dimensions. There are six different
ways of accounting for the frequency of pain
reported in psychiatric populations, and they
will be taken in order. The first three ways of
explaining the phenomenon are essentially
traditional medical ones that argue that pain
can result from an emotional state. They are
complementary to each other and they are as
follows.

First, it is possible that pain may arise as
an hallucination. This can happen, for example, in schizophrenia and might happen also
in endogenous depression (Merskey & Spear,
1967). No one really disputes this. Most
accept also, as has been claimed (Watson,
Chandarana, & Merskey, 1981), that a
schizophrenic hallucination of pain is very
rare, and depressive hallucinations are certainly not very common.

Second, pain may arise as a hysterical conversion symptom. This is a traditional view,
amplified by Freud's notions, illustrated from
time to time in different articles (e.g., Merskey, 1980a), and supported to some extent
by the profusion of hysterical and hypochondriacal features in patients who are to be
found in pain clinics. There may be some
reservations about the frequency with which
hysterical features represent a psychodynamic
explanation for the production of pain, but no
one seems to reject specifically the idea that
such pain can occur. Some writers, who prefer other formulations, however, do not use
the terminology (e.g., Roberts, Chapter 2 of
this volume).

The third classical mechanism by which
pain has been attributed to mental processes

is that of muscle tension giving rise to pain.
The muscle tension may follow from overuse
or overactivity of some part and particularly
from anxiety giving rise to excessive muscular
contractions. When it is present, it is held
that waste metabolites are not adequately
removed from nerve endings, which are then
stimulated leading to the subjective experience of pain. There is readily available experimental evidence in support of this idea:
Active contraction of muscles in a limb to
which circulation has been interrupted by a
tourniquet quickly leads to pain that is abol-
ished on restoring the circulation. Further, a
series of studies by Wolff and his colleagues
(1948) demonstrated a relationship between
pain and muscle overuse. Although all these
mechanisms can be understood as causing
chronic pain, their exact importance in individual populations has never been well determined, except that in recent years many of
the so-called tension headache patients have
been shown *not to have* as much muscle contraction as would be expected. (See Merskey,
1981, for a discussion of this topic.)

A fourth approach treats pain as arising by
operant conditioning. The types of patient
who seem to fit the operant concept are
apparently all those in whom an organic
cause is no longer applicable, or never has
been applicable. This means that the one
word covers a rather broad range of individuals who may be separated out by the different
mechanisms and associated diagnoses
(schizophrenia, depression, hysteria, anxiety)
that follow from the first three mechanisms
previously outlined. It may also apply
wrongly to the patients in the next group to
be considered, in whom emotional changes,
such as reactive depression and anxiety, follow the physical cause. Thus, the operant
term tends to be rather unselective and may
mask differences between groups that can be
usefully discriminated if the classical psychiatric diagnostic approach is employed,
despite the limitations of the latter.

Fifth, another of the ways in which pain
may be related to the emotions is that chronic
painful illness will produce psychological

PM-C

change. The general medical and psychiatric literature of the past few decades has neglected this idea in favor of the notion that it is the emotional state that produces the pain. These ideas are not, of course, necessarily in conflict, except in their application to any particular case, and even then it is possible to assume both that the emotional cause engenders some pain and that a physical cause then makes the emotional state worse. The best example — in theory — would be of a person who was anxious after developing a peptic ulcer and then became somewhat depressed because of the pain of the ulcer.

For practical purposes, it is important to recognize that there are indeed many patients who have troublesome pain that gives rise to emotional change. One of the early controlled (or comparative) reports on this theme was by Woodforde and Merskey (1972) who observed that patients without lesions (organic) but with pain were in fact slightly less depressed, anxious, and obsessive than patients who had lesions to which their pain could be attributed. The organic group also tended to score rather high on the Lie scale of the Maudsley Personality Inventory. These findings were interpreted as indicating that those who scored high on the Lie scale were actually reporting events correctly as, prior to their illness, and unlike the usual trend with psychiatric patients, they were more likely to have been relatively well adjusted in their social relationships and premorbid personality.

One way to explore this topic further has been to look at the childhood of different groups with pain (Merskey & Boyd, 1978; Salter, Brooke, Merskey, Fichter, & Kapusianyk, 1983). Another source of support for the view that secondary emotional changes may arise from pain could be found in the frequent observation of elevated scores on the hypochondriasis and hysteria scales of the Minnesota Multiphasic Personality Inventory (MMPI) in patients with chronic pain. If those patients have primary lesions that give rise to their pain, then the emotional changes implied by the MMPI elevations in the clas-

sical conversion V triad might well be attributed to the psychological effects of the chronic painful lesions. Relief of the pain could then be followed by a reduction of scores on those scales as has been shown by Sternbach, Wolf, Murphy, and Akeson (1973). One fallacy that has gone little noticed, however, is that the hypochondriasis and hysteria scales in the MMPI rely upon complaints of bodily symptoms to produce their scores. Although this is valid for patients who do not have physical illness, it hardly seems correct in patients who do have physical illness and who might be erroneously scaled as having a psychological disorder merely because they acknowledge the presence of organic symptoms. Be that as it may, there is an accumulating recognition in the literature that anxiety and depression, and to some extent hysterical complaints, may result from chronically troublesome or painful disease.

In connection with the foregoing mechanisms, it is also worth recognizing that one of the most common situations is to find somebody who has a modest physical lesion but whose pain is out of proportion to that lesion. This has been repeatedly noted and was particularly emphasized by Walters (1961) in his survey of 430 psychiatric patients with pain. A substantial minority of chronic pain patients probably present this situation, that is, they have both emotional and physical problems, which combine to produce severe pain. When the emotional state is treated successfully — and it is often more easy to treat than the physical state — the pain usually becomes of minor importance. A typical example is a patient who has had a previous coronary infraction or may have modest angina, gets depressed, and then has severe chest pain. Another instance would be of someone who has definite lesions of post-herpetic neuralgia that, when he is not depressed, present only a mild intermittent buzzing or tingling sensation, but who has severe pain in that area when depressed. Most clinicians have seen cases of this sort.

The sixth consideration that may determine the psychological importance of pain has to do with the attitudes of the patient toward chronic suffering and the selection process that develops from that. All patients seen in professional practice will have undergone a process of selection. Merely having a headache is not enough to bring a patient to a health professional. The practitioner must also be aware that only some patients will take the next step after recognizing a symptom and go and seek professional assistance. Many others dose themselves with over-the-counter preparations, rest, relaxation, a day off work, or distract themselves from the symptom altogether and continue to go about their usual activities. Others may seek consultation on one occasion and rest content with that. The result is that there is a steady progression of forces operating to select for specialist clinics those patients who have the most concern and the most psychological disturbance.

The recognition of this phenomenon has been somewhat belated. The literature of the years prior to 1970 seems to take almost no account of it except for one report (Pond & Bidwell, 1959). Subsequently (Banks, Baresford, Morrell, Waller, & Watkins, 1975; Merskey, 1975; Merskey, 1980a), increasing emphasis has been laid upon this phenomenon. Some of the findings that have been demonstrated are: (a) Patients take to general practitioners only 3% of the symptoms they experience in any given period (Banks et al., 1975); (b) compared to patients without psychological problems, patients with psychological problems are referred to neurologists twice as often for *epilepsy*; and (c) the closer migraine patients come to being drawn from a representative sample of the general population, the more normal they tend to be (Crisp, Kalucy, McGuinness, Ralph, & Harris, 1977; Merskey, 1975; Rees & Henryk-Gutt, 1973).

With the recognition of this regular pattern of events, whereby those who are more concerned present more often with nonfatal or nonprogressive conditions, we have one final and alternative explanation for every case of chronic pain in which psychological factors seem to be important. It is that people may have modest or unimportant physical illnesses that give rise to a modicum of pain by their own account, but that such pain becomes much more significant because of the attitudes and emotional state of the person in whom it is present. This has already been accepted in looking at the clinical cases where it is recognized that a transitory emotional illness makes pain from an established lesion worse. It can now be emphasized that, in patients with chronic pain, the characteristics of the personality may be a persistent factor in exacerbating the complaint of pain.

A number of inferences and conclusions will follow from the foregoing in regard to ways in which pain should be treated. Clearly, all persistent pain must be thoroughly assessed physically and psychologically. Then, appropriate measures will be introduced according to either the physical, psychiatric, or psychological diagnosis. Everyone who practices in this field is aware that the thorough review of the patient's complaints may itself be therapeutic. Often enough, patients who have had examination and investigation at one center or another may be left "up in the air," or feel that they are so left, because no one person has thoroughly put together the physical and psychological possibilities and discussed them with them.

In my personal practice, at least some patients attend for perhaps two or three occasions so that I can complete history-taking and collection of data and hold an extended discussion with them. Following that, a number are content to accept the physical or psychological situation as it is—if I think no more can be done for it—and to maintain their lives at an appropriate level of activity. This effect is sometimes known as "reassurance." It is no doubt a good deal more. It may involve a fundamental supportive relationship. It certainly involves a commitment to what all professionals should provide, which is a clear investigation and exposition of the situation to the patient or client, and it sometimes also involves new thoughts which the individual reviews and uses for a change of attitude. For example, one patient who had been asked to complete some routine questions and brief psychological tests in relation to her feelings (the Wakefield Irritability, Depression and Anxiety Questionnaire [Snaith, Constantopoulos, Jardine, & McGuffin, 1978]; the Hysteroid Obsessional Questionnaire [Caine & Hope, 1967]; the General Health Questionnaire [Goldberg, 1972]; and the Parental Bonding Instrument [Parker, Tupling, & Brown, 1979]) added the following note at the end, "I found this form very difficult to complete . . . it made me think very hard. I realize there are a lot of things I have to work through."

CRITERIA FOR ACCEPTANCE OF PATIENTS FOR PSYCHOTHERAPY

I do not personally accept for treatment, or recommend psychiatric treatment for, anybody who does not in my view have a psychological condition that can be demonstrated to be in need of attention. This is obviously common sense, and one might suppose that everyone would follow it. Occasionally, however, one is expected to treat someone for whom one cannot demonstrate a psychological disorder. In those cases, it should never be assumed that the situation can be explained psychologically. Evidently, what has happened is that a chronic pain state has not been explained by physical examination, but it also has not been explained by psychological examination.

When this occurs, I state the situation as I see it very firmly to the patient. I then proceed to point out that I might have missed something, or other specialists might have missed something, and that the long duration of the pain makes it probable that the condition is not dangerous. The best we can then do is suspend judgment or else make further inquiries along particular lines. Some of those lines may include additional tests, the opinion

of another colleague, and so forth. If steps of that nature have been fully taken, all that can be done is to explore further psychologically, if it seems justified, but without forming a firm diagnosis. This may be undertaken — and is undertaken by me if the patient and I both agree — for perhaps two or three occasions of 30 to 60 minutes each, with family interviews in addition to everything else that should have been done. Minor analgesics may also be tried or, alternatively on an empirical basis, psychotropic medication that is analgesic (Amitriptyline, Methotrimeprazine) but without the physician prejudging the particular diagnosis.

It is important for the psychologist and psychiatrist to remember that organic causes can be missed, often because the particular diagnosis is not well known or is clouded by other considerations, and that the hapless psychologist or psychiatrist might find himself vainly struggling to drum out of the patient some symptom that is organically founded. It would be unreasonable to suggest that psychologists and psychiatrists could become expert at diagnosing all cases of obscure organic disease that their colleagues missed. What they have to do, however, is treat only psychological conditions that they are satisfied are present.

This last comment states the first general criterion for accepting patients for psychotherapy or psychiatric treatment or any other psychological approach. It is that there should be a defined psychiatric condition or psychological state for which treatment is appropriate. For the psychiatrist, this may be an anxiety state, depressive illness, or even hysteria (albeit rarely as the latter alone). For some other health professionals, it may be "operant pain" or, perhaps more likely, "pain behavior." In any case, the practitioner must be satisfied that there is something to deal with on psychological grounds and not just a failure to explain organic illness.

The second general criterion is that the pain might be amenable to psychological maneuvers even though its cause is primarily, or perhaps principally, physical. Thus, a patient with overt physical lesions might be referred for training in cognitive techniques of management. Supportive psychotherapy can be appropriate in such cases as an alternative or adjunct to cognitive measures. For example, in a patient with chronic severe back pain following a fusion operation, I also offered advice about tactical maneuvers that would enable him to distract himself from pain when it was most troublesome. As it happens, he had already developed a number of these himself.

Once I accept a patient for psychotherapy or drug therapy, it is virtually automatic that the minimum treatment offered will be support and advice. A new patient, seen the day before writing these lines, represents the minimum case. He was 57 years old and unemployed because of rheumatoid arthritis. He was referred because his family doctor was concerned about the extent to which his disability might be psychological in origin. I decided he was not depressed or otherwise psychologically ill but was frustrated by his inability to work as a foundry foreman. Thus, the primary function of the consultation, diagnosis and evaluation, was completed quite quickly. Inquiry had shown, however, that he was fluently bilingual in English and French and had always stood high in his class at school, but had come from a large family with little interest in further education. He was referred, optimistically, despite his age, for vocational advice and retraining. This was clearly a second purpose of the consultation, when found to be relevant.

As a problem-solving activity the consultation had produced a statement about his condition, had defined an explanation for his distress (not for his pain), and had offered a tentative solution. None of that was a specific treatment, and none more might appear necessary. Nevertheless, the interview also endowed the patient with the feeling that his ability and motivation were recognized and appreciated.

Other cases, of course, will require different pragmatic strategies and psychological messages, but all are liable to involve direct practical aid and psychological encouragement. This is obviously something that arises most efficiently from the fact of contact with the patient and review of his or her problems. Because it is largely an automatic consequence of almost any specialist psychiatric consultation, the question of whom one chooses for these approaches mainly devolves back upon the family doctor, other referring agent, or person who refers himself or herself. It seems likely that anyone who is concerned over a failure to resolve a persistent pain, or distressed by disability and its consequences, may be helped by such measures. Certainly once the patient is referred to me, it is routine that I attempt to assist him at least in this fashion.

To whom is continuing supportive psychotherapy offered? The answer is anyone who feels it is beneficial, requests more treatment (overtly or by implication), and appears to be benefiting. The benefit may be better adaptation to an unchanged pain, or relief of other concomitant distress (e.g., depression, feelings of frustration), as well as, of course, actual relief of pain. Most often, the continuing psychological support develops out of a series of attempts to ensure thorough investigation and treatment of a noninvasive nature. For example, physiotherapy, arrangements for Transcutaneous Electrical Nerve Stimulation (TENS), family interviews, advice about work, advice about cognitive maneuvers, and drug adjustments may all be undertaken, and during this process the patient is being supported psychologically as well.

Specific indications are employed to determine if patients should be selected for other psychological treatments such as exploratory psychotherapy or antidepressant medication. Thus, typically the patient chosen for more exploratory work will have a recognizable problem in human relations, will want to change at least part of it, and will undertake this approach. Patients may be given antidepressants for depression whether it is categorized as reactive depression, endogenous depression, or major affective disorder. Amitriptyline will also be prescribed empirically, as it is believed to be analgesic (Monks & Merskey, 1984; Watson et al., 1982).

Decisions about these diagnoses are reached by conventional clinical practice and, for me, in accordance with the diagnostic categories of the Ninth Revision of the International Classification of Diseases (ICD-9). My goals, besides relief of pain, are relief of any other defined problem, whether it be depression, unemployment, family disputes, or intrapsychic conflicts. The conclusion that the treatment has been successful rests upon mutual discussion, symptomatic relief, increased activity, occupational change or return to employment, and similar alterations in the activities of daily living. For research purposes, of course, these would have to be scaled and categorized more systematically and definitively. For day to day clinical practice, it is sufficient that the parties concerned recognize the presence of the change or reject the notion that one has occurred.

PLACEBOS

Beecher (1955) showed that a placebo response was obtained in 35% of patients with pain. His evidence related largely to acute experiments or comparisons in anesthesia and analgesia. Although the placebo response was known before that, Beecher established its importance in all studies of pain. The meaning of a placebo effect, however, requires further attention. In its literal sense, the term implies that, because of pleasure or satisfaction with the treatment offered, the patient feels better even though the treatment has had no direct physical action in relieving the condition that produced the symptom.

When a patient is given a treatment that may have a placebo effect, alternative explanations for a recovery may also exist. One is that the illness could be evolving spontaneously and undergo a natural remission. That is common, for example, with some cases of migraine, rheumatoid arthritis, and mechanical back pain. Hence, a response by a patient may reflect not only psychological improvement from faith in the treatment but also con-

comitant spontaneous physical change. There is yet another possibility. This particularly applies to conditions that have a psychological basis. A change in the environment may result in an alleviation of the factors that were causing the symptom. For example, a man with chronic headaches who retires from a job that he does not like, or gets a change of supervisor, may have a remission of symptoms for the latter reason. It is customary to control for the benefits of a treatment by having a group that receives placebo treatment. The conclusion is usually then drawn that any improvement in this group was due to placebo. However, it can be seen from the above that alternative explanations for improvements in a control group must always be considered.

The relevance of these effects to treatment of pain is immediately obvious. Because pain is a subjective symptom, the response of patients with pain is hard to measure, and it may in any case be affected by any of the three processes outlined. Accordingly, all systematic studies of treatment require evaluation of appropriate control groups. There is reason to suppose, however, that patients with chronic pain do not respond readily to placebos. One factor in this is the basic definition of their symptom as chronic. Acute conditions of anxiety and readily remitting illnesses often show improvements that may be true placebo responses or spontaneous environmentally induced recovery. The opportunities for these changes to occur in patients whose pain is already chronic are fewer. In my personal observation, a pure placebo response or significant remission is uncommon in the typical chronic pain patient who is so often studied in the literature. For research purposes it is thus legitimate, initially, to study groups of patients whose pain is of long standing, without controls. This can only be for pilot purposes, however, as many studies are now available indicating the benefits of various treatments by comparison with each other. Thus, even though the expectation of major improvement in chronic pain without treatment is low, no new treatment can readily come forward without undergoing controlled investigations.

PATIENTS AND PROCEDURES

In this section, illustrative cases are chosen from my personal practice that reflect the following situations: (a) purely psychiatric illness giving rise to persistent pain; (b) the treatment of a patient with a definite neurological lesion causing pain and emotional disturbance; (c) problems of motor vehicle accidents with particular reference to the so-called whiplash syndrome (this case is also a good example of how both physical and psychological problems play a part).

Case Study:
An Essentially Psychiatric Problem

Mr. A. illustrates some of the problems associated with the diagnosis and treatment of hypochondriacal depression. In fact, the major measure that in the end produced worthwhile improvement was the use of an antidepressant. His case is presented mainly to illustrate how plausible psychological observations could lead to a wrong emphasis in treatment. Yet, psychological or psychiatric skills were needed in order to reach the most appropriate diagnosis and to maintain a relationship with the patient and his wife so as to permit effective treatment.

Mr. A., a skilled workman, was born in 1938. I saw him first, with his wife, in May 1983. He said, "For a long time I have had pains and no one believes me." Every morning he woke with a stiff neck "as if a tugging match had gone on," and it only wore off gradually. He also noted a "surge of blood to the head," felt very depressed and down, and had "a give-up type of feeling," which he disliked. Symptoms had appeared about 4 years previously with back pain in which pain went onto the inside of the left leg, and had become worse in the past year. He had been concerned about a "white thing" in his throat, the top of his head was fuzzy with a little pain, and he had occasional chest and abdominal

pain as well as his back pain. His sleep was disturbed, he was concerned about his bowel movements, and he feared that he might have a carcinoma or some illness that had been missed. His symptoms also included impaired appetite, impaired enjoyment, lost libido, lost interest, moodiness, and a consciousness of bad breath. He felt that he had let people down.

There was past history of back trouble and also of alcoholism. After four convictions for drunken driving, he seemed to have reformed and had had a 7-year period of abstinence or moderation. There had been an episode of heavy drinking and family disturbance in April 1983, and he took beer occasionally but not excessively. He saw himself as "type A" and a tense person. He felt that he could not talk to people, fought rather readily, having done so from his school days onwards, and was irritable. In the past he had had Chordiazepoxide and Thioridazine to control his temper but Diphenyl Hydantoin worked best. He was also a perfectionist.

His father was a skilled person in the same occupation, was a heavy drinker, and got into arguments and damaged property when drunk. He died in 1977 of emphysema at the age of 69. His mother was 69 as well. He sobbed when he talked about her. He was the fourth of six children, all the others being girls. He had been fairly close to the one next after him in age. Altogether he said that he had had quite a reasonable family life, but his father had had the same problem as himself—"too many kids."

He attended school to grade 12, completing only grade 11. He had not been particularly good at mathematics or English. He was proud of having worked from his youth on and having in effect been with his employer for about 27 years. He first married when he was 21, but this only lasted 12 months. Two years later, he started to live with his present wife, and they have been together for 19 years and married for 10 of those. She had two children by her first marriage who lived with them, and there were five more children ranging down to 10 years in age. His wife worked seasonally. They lived on a farm where he had some responsibilities for the upkeep of buildings and pumps, and he found this a burden. He believed that he was the only one who did anything and the children did not help.

On examination his neck movements were good and free, he was in fair general condition, and there was no relevant physical illness. His white beard and hair made him look older than his years. The prominent hypochondriacal complaints and a general air of discontent on his part, coupled with his earlier difficulties of maladjustment and alcoholism, could have supported a diagnosis of personality disorder and hysterical hypochondriasis. Moreover, it looked as if there might have been some dynamic factors involved in the development of his illness and that those would require further assessment. I preferred a diagnosis of endogenous depression, however, because of the evidence of a depressed mood, vegetative symptoms, guilt, and a stable work record. He and his wife were advised, of course, that his pains were real, that they seemed to be related to his mental or emotional state, and that even though medication had previously been tried and had not been very helpful, more should be attempted. He was given a prescription for maprotiline (Ludiomil), a Dexamethasone Suppression Test was arranged, and his past records were sought from other hospitals.

Three things followed from these initial steps. First of all, he showed some improvement with maprotiline, although it was incomplete. Careful attention had to be paid to what he said about this, because on the one hand he said that it made him calmer and on the other that it made him more jumpy. His wife's testimony here was very important, as she emphasized that he was overall much better with this medication.

Second, the diagnosis of depression was supported in two ways. The Irritability Depression and Anxiety Questionnaire of Snaith et al. (1978) indicated a score of 11 for depression (cut-off point for normals is less than 6), as well as mild anxiety and some irritability. The Hysteroid Obsessional Questionnaire of Caine and Hope (1967) interestingly indicated a very reserved, introverted man (score = 12; mean for obsessional/anxious personalities = 17; standard deviation = +6). In addition, a Dexamethasone Suppression Test was positive (serum cortisol = 664 nMol/L at 9 a.m. and 280 nMol/L at 4 p.m. the next day after a preceding dose of 1 mg of dexamethasone; cut-off point = 138 nMol/L at 4 p.m.). This test gave at least some worthwhile support to the idea of a depressive illness being present, although it is not diagnostic and false positives can occur.

The third major set of observations came when other information was obtained from a very capable psychiatrist who had seen him in 1981 and made the following comments:

> He related the stiffness in his neck and the changes in his bowel habits back to November 1980. However, he says that he has felt the pressure on his head over the past 2 years . . . he has entertained ideas that he may have cancer of his bowel. Even as far back as 15 years ago he apparently told his father he would probably die of cancer . . . he feels very tired most mornings and describes his mood as depressed. He feels that nobody cares . . . he has lost interest in everything . . . his personality revealed characteristics of severe obsessionality, of a tendency to be authoritarian, over-controlling, generally cynical and over-critical of others . . . .

This colleague diagnosed him as having a depressive illness presenting predominantly in the form of somatic and hypochondriacal concerns and treated him with amoxapine initially. There appeared to be some improvement but later,

> It became more evident that he was suffering from a total emotional isolation . . . and demonstrated what could best be described as a fairly severe schizoid core in his personality which was making it extremely difficult for him to make social and interpersonal relationships . . . he gave a description of himself as "I am like an island."

This colleague tried to improve things

through a course of individual psychotherapy. In the first two sessions the patient appeared to be showing some movement towards forming a therapeutic relationship, but in the last session he reverted back to most of his physical concerns and complained of some flu-like symptoms. Maprotiline was tried again, and he reverted to the care of his family practitioner. The psychiatrist's final comment was:

> I also found him to be very passively aggressive . . . and at one time he became quite openly aggressive and expressed a great deal of hostility towards myself as his therapist as well as other doctors who have tried to treat him. This seems to be a pattern between him and almost everyone in this world as he feels that he has been treated badly and not given enough attention and consideration by people around him. He, however, has no insight into his own contribution towards these relationships.

My colleague expressed concern that the patient might become suicidal at some time when morbidly concerned with his somatic symptoms.

Evidently maprotiline, which I gave this patient at first, had been tried already. When I reviewed him on the second occasion, I still did not have the latter information, nor did I know that he had had amoxapine, which I gave him next. With both these drugs he improved. While taking amoxapine, ultimately in a dose of 100 mg three times a day, he declared that he was only "20–30% off normal." Then I received the information that neither of these drugs had been sufficiently helpful to him and so decided to try an alternative from another end of the antidepressant aminergic spectrum. The first two drugs had been largely catecholaminergic. This time it seemed more appropriate to try a serotoninergic drug, and chlomipramine was employed in a dose of 150 mg daily. It did not work well, nor did flupenthixol 0.5 mg twice daily. The latter, a very small dose of the drug, which is normally neuroleptic in large doses and considered by some to be antidepressant in small doses, had a rather unusual

effect for it of making him very irritable. He said "It made a monster out of me." After this drug he quit all medications and came back and said, "This way I don't even care to live—to tell you the truth." At this point, a new antidepressant, trazodone, was tried. This gave significant improvement and after 2 months of using trazodone, in a dose of 400 mg daily (100 mg. twice daily, 200 mg. at night), he said it was the best medication he had had. His spirits were much better, he was calmer and not as irritable, and his wife said he was "the best he's been in years." They both agreed that his mood was very close to normal. This man lived some 90 miles from my office and with his improvement in mood he was returned to his family practitioner. At the same time, he said that his pain was no better. A recommendation was made that he should try acetaminophen for it at this point, while continuing to take his antidepressant.

Comment

It may seem unhelpful to colleagues who may read this book but who do not prescribe medication when I describe the drug management of a patient. I have chosen to do so because I think this particular patient illustrates a number of important practical points of which they would wish to be aware. It is probably true that less than 50% of patients in pain clinics will benefit from antidepressants. Many patients in pain clinics do receive antidepressants, most often amitriptyline, which is known to have a good influence both upon depression and, independently, upon pain (Watson et al., 1982). Because of this it is relatively easy to take the attitude that if antidepressants—particularly amitriptyline, which this patient had also had at one time—are not effective and if the patient shows evident maladjustment apart from depression, it is appropriate to proceed to purely psychological techniques.

As indicated here, however, this patient in fact ultimately responded well to medication. Moreover, he was not willing to accept other types of psychological approach. The effort to use traditional exploratory psychotherapy was made by a sensitive and considerate colleague. If he could not form an adequate relationship with this patient for that purpose, it is not very likely that anyone else would have succeeded either. Behavioral or cognitive techniques might have been attempted, but I would not have relished being the individual who tried to persuade this patient of their relevance or usefulness. It had been correctly observed that he was persistently hypochondriacal and had obsessional features besides.

The evidence to support the diagnosis of depression was good, but it tended to be devalued because of the patient's tendency to be hypochondriacal, as well as critical of others, and because of the history that gave some lead towards personality disorder in the past, for example, heavy drinking. Findings that realistically supported the diagnosis of depression in this patient were: (a) his subjective distress; (b) the frequency with which he referred to difficulty in concentration, attention, energy, or enjoyment of life; (c) his suicidal thoughts; (d) his guilt; (e) his psychological test scores; and (f) his dexamethasone test results. Also, the initial response to antidepressants was encouraging although confounded by his persistent dull talk of other physical symptoms, which seemed to cloud for the physician the evident improvement that his wife more easily recognized from his continuing behavior at home.

Another reason for describing this case is to emphasize the importance of supportive psychological measures. The usual notion of supportive psychotherapy involves the idea that the patient's defenses will not be challenged. On the positive side, it requires that things be done to bolster the patient up and to encourage him in constructive views or actions. In this particular case there was clearly no challenge to his views, but there was also very little emphasis on constructive actions by him. This was partly because he was working and remained in work and was encouraged implicitly and explicitly to keep up that role. It was also because, if we were waiting for medication to produce change in his ideas

and attitudes, it seemed pointless to advise the patient to distract himself, concentrate on other matters, stop talking about pain, and so forth. What was done, however, was yet another aspect of supportive psychotherapy. Essentially, this was patient acceptance of him, his complaints, and the seriousness of his condition. At no time in the course of 11 interviews did he demonstrate towards me any of the irritability that he had previously been reported to show. I assume that this was because I was "the good guy" who convinced him that I had accepted the reality of his experiences. In consequence, he became willing to accept psychotropic medication.

Perhaps one of the things that helps to maintain a patient on psychotropic medication is the willingness to discuss with him or her the exact adjustment of the dose. Antidepressants, even the new ones with few anticholinergic side-effects, cannot satisfactorily be given to patients in most cases without careful attention to adjusting the dose prescribed. My personal practice involves explaining to the patient that he or she must help me to find the exact level of medication to be employed. Hence, I usually invite the patient to start the new medication by taking one tablet the first night, two the second, three the third, and so on until he reaches a level at which sleep is adequate or a side-effect appears that he does not like. I warn him about the usual side-effects, such as dry mouth, drowsiness, dizziness on standing up suddenly, etc. The patient is advised further that he must himself decide at what point to reduce the medication from the dose reached to one that is tolerable and that may, after a little while, begin to help him. It is explained to him that he will first find the dose, then come back and review it with me, and then maintain the dose for some while to see if it helps. This is reinforced by arranging an early appointment, usually at a 7-day interval or less to review some of these aspects.

What then transpires is that the patient becomes someone who is taking a physical treatment and whose experience of it has to be reviewed medically. Compliance and acceptance follow relatively readily from this approach. It is also part of the support regimen. Opportunities of this sort are not so readily available to nonphysicians, although some at least are in a position to advise interns and others with less experience of the relevance of psychotropic medication in pain clinics.

Case Study: Physical Illness With Pain And Emotional Disturbance

Mr. C. was born in 1957 and was also first seen in May 1983. He complained of chronic pain in the stump following amputation of his left leg and of psychological symptoms, which he called "repeated nervous breakdowns." What seemed to have happened was that there was pain, followed by insomnia, drink to ease the insomnia, and general depression and restlessness. On one occasion he had been drinking and driving, and a policeman who knew him stopped him and took a lenient view, but told him not to drink and drive again. This made him feel that he was being blocked from any way in which he could relieve his pain on a reasonably reliable basis. Besides that, he had been taking excessive amounts of codeine (11 Tylenol-3 daily). Accordingly, he became desperate and suicidal. He actually swam out into one of the Great Lakes 3 weeks before his first consultation with me, thinking that he would drown. Then he turned around, deciding "God doesn't want me to die."

The following history related to his injuries. Only July 13, 1980, he was driving home down a local street on a motorcycle, when he was hit by a car. It was 1:00 a.m. and he was traveling from Toronto to visit his parents. He suffered a dislocated left hip, subsequent amputation above the knee, a compound fracture of the left forearm, and lost the end of a little finger. He was right-handed. He was knocked out and pinned under the bike and seems to have woken up alone about half an hour after the injuries. The pain was so bad then that he asked to be shot. He said that because of the severe pain he lost consciousness on being lifted off the

ground and that as he lay in the ditch previously, he had thought he was going to die. His next memory was just before his operation, lying in bed while his parents told him what would happen. The next day he was moved to another hospital because of a dislocated hip, which was reduced, the leg later being amputated. He was discharged from the second hospital after about 16 days; at that time he was taking morphine, and he was subsequently given codeine.

He started to walk within 2 months of the injuries, but the pain never subsided and it has never gone away. He said, "It caught up with me a few days or months later. That's when I had my first nervous breakdown." This was marked by exhaustion, with the use of codeine and drink being additional causes. Perhaps some withdrawal of his more effective narcotics contributed. He said that at times in his "breakdowns" he had hallucinated and started thinking about religion, things in general, the way the world is, and so forth. Then he would become morose and cry. This was always marked by a lot of pain and sleeplessness. After those experiences, by about April or May of 1983, he began to drink less, but also to sleep less.

He said that walking on his leg caused pain, that the pain got worse as the day wore on, and that it was not relieved by nerve blocks, cortisone shots, or minor analgesics. Tylenol-3 (acetaminophen, caffeine, and codeine) did help. There was a stump revision in February 1983.

Mr. C. had an unusual background. His father committed suicide when Mr. C. was 9 years old. His mother remarried, but he seems to have fended for himself to a considerable extent since the age of 9 or 10. He had had many changes of school, felt that he knew how to handle himself with different crowds of children, and was proud of the fact that he had worked parttime and fulltime from the age of 15 until the time of his accident. Indeed, he emphasized to me how he made good money in fulltime work in summer vacations and saved towards the purchase of his house. He also had a number of episodes of minor delinquency—riding a minibike on a public road, shoplifting once when he was 15, and drinking beer when he was under age. He did not seem to have been in significant trouble since those juvenile episodes. He tried street drugs to ease his pain, but without effect (except in the case of "speed"). At school he seemed to have been average, he completed grade 12, qualified later as a steam fitter and gas fitter, and since then had taken additional courses in engineering with a view to mechanical engineering. He had had little illness apart from the need for a hernia repair.

When I first saw him, I considered that Mr. C. had no phantom pain, but did have severe stump pain. Walking on the prosthesis would relieve that stump pain temporarily, but then it came back and was worse. He had secondary depression, which is not surprising. I treated him both for pain and for depression with amitriptyline and later added methotrimeprazine (Nozinan), which also seems to have analgesic characteristics. The amitriptyline helped his sleep and seemed to help his pain by day, but only to a limited extent. The Nozinan was not effective enough to justify the side-effects it produced, such as impaired concentration and apathy.

Trazodone, an antidepressant that was not known to have analgesic activities, produced a mild benefit for the pain also. However, it was not enough to justify sustained use. He continued to employ quite large quantities of codeine in the form of Tylenol-3 to control the pain. I wrote to his general practitioner to suggest that he should stop Tylenol-3, but retain the codeine portion of it because the acetaminophen in Tylenol-3 might damage the kidneys if taken long-term and might affect his stomach in any case. Further, I encouraged Mr. C. to utilize cognitive methods of relief of pain, that is, distancing himself from the pain, distracting himself by activity, and even taking exercise when it took his mind off it. Meditation was also encouraged, but did not seem to work particularly well.

In the summer he would work and put himself into terrible pain rather than give up the daily activity on his father's farm, which was economically important to him; he would then sustain increasing discomfort that he controlled with minor narcotics. He would work upwards of 8 hours a day on a tractor with the vibrations steadily exacerbating his stump pain. Previously, in response to the overwhelming misery of his severe pain, he reacted in a fashion that is not uncommon, reaching depths of depression that led him to contemplate and even take steps towards committing suicide. By the time I saw him, he seemed to have all those complaints under control, and my function was to make sure that all relevant treatment methods of a benign type had been employed.

Comment

This is an example of a man with considerable pain and secondary depression following severe physical injuries. Cognitive methods did not help him adequately. He had found many of them already himself—as I think my patients often do. Psychotropic medication was of limited benefit.

This case is described in order to emphasize the limits of psychological and psychiatric treatment. I referred him ultimately to a neurosurgeon who is interested in treatment with implanted electrodes. The neurosurgeon observed that he had not so far had sympathetic blocks and decided to undertake those first and later consider whether implanted electrodes would be appropriate.

Another point to be made about this patient is the use of codeine in order to sustain activity. On compound medication he developed gastrointestinal disturbance from the acetaminophen, which happens frequently in patients who try to push themselves to sustain a day's activity by means of taking compound preparations, perhaps adding them to plain acetaminophen or aspirin as well. Besides the risk of gastric bleeding, such patients are also in potential danger of causing kidney damage to themselves, particularly if the drug employed long-term is aspirin. Nevertheless, there are quite a few who will insist on maintaining their normal level of activity with the help of significant quantities of codeine.

Most pain clinics and most practitioners endeavor to get patients off codeine. I do so myself regularly. However, I have perhaps five patients who take regular doses of codeine, in one instance over 200 mg daily, without raising the dose further. They do this to keep themselves at work and keep pain under control, and that pain is regularly made worse by activity. They make a choice between lying around all day doing nothing or suffering quite a lot of pain that is only partly relieved by the stringently controlled quantities of codeine that they are allowed week by week. When they have a day or two off they usually reduce their dose of codeine significantly by half the total dose or more, suggesting that they are not greatly dependent upon it.

Case Study:
Psychological Management Of A Case
Of Post-Traumatic Headache

In my view, post-traumatic headache has a definite organic basis. The so-called whiplash (cervical sprain) syndrome is associated with a characteristic pattern of pain throughout the head and shoulders, with onset typically a few minutes or hours after an actual injury and gradual remission.

Although it has often been said that patients with compensable complaints do not recover until after their legal claims have been settled, it frequently happens that some patients recover before legal settlement and others persist with symptoms afterwards. Very substantial evidence has now accumulated on these themes (Mendelson, 1981; Merskey, 1984). Besides that, patients with minor head injury or whiplash syndrome tend to have some organic evidence for the persistent dizziness of which they complain, impaired performance on a paced serial addition task (Pasat) (Gronwall & Wrightson, 1974), and other evidence supporting the view that the fundamental syndrome is organic and that legal claims play only a part in the total symptom picture. The present case represents a man who needed a good deal of psychological support until he had a legal settlement. When that settlement freed him from the constraints of a course of action that he found troublesome, he improved significantly, although not completely. To that extent, he contrasts with the argument that I have just offered.

Mr. E., born in 1931, first came to see me in May 1980. He was a TV and electronics technician, had had three jobs in the previous 8 years, and had been with his present company for 2 years. His work, which was skilled, involved matching up to 20 to 30 color-coded wires within one cable. He had not worked for 7 months after an accident that occurred at 3 p.m. one afternoon in November 1980. At the time of the accident he had been in the driving seat of a $\frac{3}{4}$-ton truck, which was hit by a similar vehicle. He had been waiting at a red traffic light, and the second truck pushed his vehicle through the intersection. At the time of the collision he saw stars, flashes, and sparkles. He was not unconscious. After the accident he continued with his work, and he went to work for the next 2 days. Then he developed headaches that were continuous. They were only relieved for a few days at a time with local injection of analgesic. He felt able to put his finger on a point at the right occiput, which was a site of maximum pain. There were also two more tender spots at the occiput and another three on each side of the vertex, distributed from front to back. The pain tended to be worse on the right, he felt that his eyeballs bulged, and he had a feeling of pain deep, in behind the ear. It felt almost as if he could touch the internal pain related to the ear with his tongue. He could live with the pain, although at times it was severe. His sleep was broken, and he would wake after $1\frac{1}{2}$ hours but he was uncertain whether the pain woke him. He described the character of the pain as being like that of "a real bad hangover made worse by attempting to bend over and pick something up—you feel as if you have left your head on the ground." There was no nausea, but his concentration was much impaired and his spirits had been low intermittently.

Eight days after the accident he had been "feeling lousy" with a headache over a weekend and he attended his physician. He took pills for headaches. X-rays were taken and he was put in a cervical collar. He had physiotherapy at one hospital and injections at another for the pain. He emphasized that there was no headache for the first 2 days after the injury but that once it started, it seemed that the cords of his neck got tight and swollen and he could not move his head and neck.

Besides these treatments, he was given diazepam and analgesics by his doctor. His family practitioner referred him to me for additional advice 7 months after the original injury. The doctor wrote,

> The most aggravating aspect is his recurrent severe headaches, which are well localized to specific areas in his scalp. I, therefore, arranged for him to see another doctor for injections of Bupivacaine and steroid. This provided only temporary relief. The episodes are quite upsetting to him and he is feeling quite depressed because of the complete disruption of his life. He previously had no underlying psychological problems. He is now living with a 32-year-old separated woman and their relationship seems quite strong and supportive. Prior to this they both had marital problems but they are both quite satisfied with their present relationship. He has a stable job.

His father was a farmer who died at the age of 51 of a heart attack. The patient was then 27. His mother also died of a heart attack at about the age of 44 when he was 24. It appears to have been quite a happy home, the patient being the middle of three boys, all of whom have done quite well in life. When he was 18 or 19 and had finished grade 13, he wanted to see the world and spent 2 or 3 years in the United States working as a logger. After that he was in the Royal Canadian Navy for 2 years but was given a medical dis-

charge because of a knee injury. His past illnesses have included hiatus hernia, for which he had an operation 10 years ago, and a torn left knee cartilage. He was working as a TV technician at the time of the accident and received compensation, in the form of a permanent disability payment of $83 per month. He had had an operation on his right knee in the 1950s and a cartilage was removed.

He had multiple jobs between 1954 and 1962 but then became a TV technician and electronic technician and worked for three companies for a period of 18 years. He had been with his present company for 2 years. He enjoyed his work. It involved rather fine discrimination between different leads and wires that are color-coded and work with extensive circuit and schematic diagrams.

At the age of 22 he married a woman who was 12 months older than himself and a school teacher. They have two grown children. They divorced 7 years ago, having "just grown away from each other." He had cohabited happily for the past 3 years. In his marriage, however, he drank too much for a short period of about 2 months. Otherwise, he was quite abstemious, did not smoke, and drank very little.

He was a rather young-looking man for his age, with carefully dyed hair, and he had been proud of his physical fitness and his participation in judo. At the time of the interview, there were tears in his eyes and thickened muscular bands were palpable at the tender points.

After 1 month on treatment with amitriptyline he mentioned the occurrence of diplopia. He became extremely depressed. Alternative antidepressants were tried but not well tolerated. Carbamazepine was given to him and was ineffective. He continued miserable and said that his friends had stopped coming to play cards with him, that he was drinking three beers a day, that he was pulling his consort down, and that he did not like himself for it. In the past 3 weeks, the pain, which previously had eased a little, was once more daily and continuous.

At that point he had been ill for 12 months

and off work all that time. He was admitted to a hospital for 3 weeks. He was in the psychiatric ward where he took part in the groups, had individual psychotherapy, and was placed in an exercise program for patients with depression. He left the hospital more cheerful. In January 1981, about 4 weeks after his hospital admission, he reported that the insurance company had paid him nothing for 2 months. His lawyer was supportive and said that there would shortly be an examination for discovery of documents, following which things should be all right again. He went back to his old place of work and asked if they could find some parttime occupation for him. He was told that there was nothing that they could offer him, and he felt they were rather cool. Meanwhile, he was falling out with his consort. He said, "Maybe I should move out . . . I have nothing. No job. No girl. No family." He expressed suicidal thoughts but believed he might get better. His headache and diplopia were unchanged.

By February 1981 he was alone and living in a single room. He wept at interview and said he had split from his consort until he could "get back to work and back to being myself." It was a mutual decision but perhaps with more pressure from her. His savings of a few thousand dollars were gradually declining. He was obviously slow and depressed but denied suicidal ideas. His diplopia continued, and he spent his time sitting, listening to the radio, and thinking. He tried to cook his meals and go shopping. The pain was now greater than previously and bilateral. He took flurazepam to sleep. He bought some whiskey but only took one drink. He tried painting and it turned out horrible. He could not watch TV because it upset his eyes and his stomach. So he listened to music on the radio.

A psychiatric day-care program was provided for him. He expressed anger at some doctors because "They shelved me . . . they couldn't find anything." He was angry with the insurance company, "They are trying to say my headache and double vision are due to the medication and not to the three punks who ran into me." He added, "My depression is being replaced by anger—they aren't the people who lay awake at night with the pain." He was still seeing his consort. Day-care continued for slightly over 2 months. Meanwhile, he cheered up enormously and did not want to see his consort when she tried to make contact with him. He had made friends with another lady. By June 1981 he was cheerful and smiling. He was taking a new antidepressant. His diplopia was unchanged but he was quite content. He had seen a rehabilitation officer provided by the insurance company, but the latter had no suggestion on his behalf. His consort called me, but I could not put her in touch with him against his wishes. In August 1981 he was back seeing her regularly, however. The pain then was worse in his head and also occurred over the left eye.

Insurance investigators were keeping him under surveillance. He said, "I feel paranoid . . . one is watching the motorhome." He felt unable to drive his motorhome any distance for a holiday. He still had not had any money from the insurance company since November 1980 and was hoping for an early hearing of his case. In September 1981 he was talking in a desperate way about how difficult the matter had become. He said, "I need to work. I worked for 30 years. I need it. I am vegetating. I was going to do myself in one day. That scared me; I never thought that I would have thought that way." He stopped because he thought his cat would also die if he was not there to give it attention. He was despondent again about his relationship with his consort, and he wept. His lawyer was not willing to settle the case while he was still as depressed as currently. In fact, he was seen three times in 1 week for supportive interviews and then admitted to London Psychiatric Hospital for 10 days, which he did not enjoy. He came out more cheerful and returned to his consort, and they planned to get married in May. He felt very good about that. Also, the insurance company was talking to him again, and the rehabilitation counselor had been back to see him.

By January 1982 he was living with his

consort again, and ultimately they married in May. In June 1982 he remained cheerful, still had diplopia, and had occasional mild headaches. The adjustment with his wife was very satisfactory. He went back to try to work for $2\frac{1}{2}$ days at his old place of employment but developed muscle spasm from sitting with his head down and forward. After 7 hours work he was worse again, and he gave up that employment. The insurance company had not paid him for 18 months, but currently he was receiving a small government disability pension.

In September 1982 he reported, "An awful lot has happened—most of it good." The insurance company was still not paying him, but he was taking a course at a community college. He felt he could not work in his old occupation because having tried it once more he found that (a) he could not climb a ladder and put his head back to look up to work, (b) he could not work on ceiling wires with his arms above him without developing excessive pain, and (c) he could not work with equipment closer to his eyes than 18 inches and could not handle the colored wires that had to be matched.

In November 1982 he came back severely depressed once more. He was working extremely hard but developing pain in direct proportion to the number of hours he spent in school and because of the way he sat in order to tend to his book and papers. He said he "had a bum neck." The pain was "the normal headache plus all the doubts about myself." In early December, he was still depressed and prophesying bad exam results and failures. At the end of December, he was cheerful again, having obtained three As, a B, and a C in his courses.

His headaches persisted even after the end of December 1982, but in the summer of 1983 a legal settlement was obtained for him. Up to that point he had been pessimistic about returning to work, about being free from his headaches, about living a normal life, and so forth. Suddenly, just before achieving legal settlement he came to a new idea.

He would accept whatever money was obtained. He would not go on with his studies. He had found the effort too much, it would be another 2 years, and he was not sure if he would achieve employment with them. Instead, he would set himself up painting and doing artwork on commission as did his brother, who successfully managed a small business and personal contracts for portraits or scenes. Following this he did not attend again. He was substantially relieved of headache, but his mild diplopia persisted.

Comment

A cynic would say that this patient only thought it worthwhile to have symptoms until he had got money for them and then he relinquished them. The extent of his distress and social disruption at phases after his accident denies that claim. Indeed, the amount of money that he received was less than he would have earned working and he also lost much self-esteem when he did not work.

Psychiatric treatment in some respects was a miserable failure. The drugs used did no good. Hospital admissions tided him over but did nothing fundamental towards his improvement. He declined for a while into poverty and helplessness. The important factors that seemed to produce all this included persistent pain, inability to work, an impaired self-concept, and a striking feeling that he had lost his personal vigor and youthfulness. He was always a man who valued the fact that he looked younger than his years and seemed to be physically fit and able to impress younger women. The interrelationship with his girl friend who became his wife was not greatly helped or hindered by his psychiatric care.

Yet, three people probably made a significant difference to his life and to the remission of most of his symptoms. The first was his fiancee, who married him and who ultimately seems to have made him feel cherished and successful as a spouse. The second was his lawyer, who had known him before his injuries, who supported him with feeling and with energy, and who obtained for him a settlement that enabled him to achieve changes in his life. The third, I claim, was his psychiatrist, who supported him when he was in his worst state, helped find some sort of shelter when he was most depressed, and listened to his outpourings. The nature of the psychological support in psychotherapy was partly reassurance — that he did look young, that he would feel better one day, that he was capable at his studies — and partly the acceptance of his sufferings. Beyond that it extended to interpretations of the importance to him of his wife and his feelings about her. But for the most part, it was essentially a matter of holding the hand of a man who was suffering until such time as he could reconstitute himself with his own plans and purposes.

FINAL COMMENTS

I would emphasize again the importance of not attempting to treat the wrong case. Other doctors sometimes have a bad habit of handing on to psychiatrists or psychologists patients who are not fully understood. A tentative approach is always essential to any proposal that a patient does not have any organic disease at all or that his disease is grossly disproportionate to his complaint of pain. Second, the themes that have been illustrated here have to do with drugs and support. In one of three cases, drugs were very useful; in two cases, they were of no benefit. In other cases not illustrated, they are quite often of some value but insufficient for the patient's needs. For the physician they provide an extra means to a relationship with the patient, as nerve blocks will do for those who provide them. Of course, they should not be used for that alone.

The application of support is very varied. It may involve direct efforts to bolster the patient's self-image (cf. cognitive therapy) or to encourage him to do more physically (cf. behavior therapy). It might comprise help towards obtaining a temporary sickness pension (case 3.) and other financial benefits. It may also comprise encouragement towards action by the patient in the environment or

by others in the environment. Finally, support may not offer the patient insight; but it requires insight from the practitioner.

REFERENCES

Banks, M.H., Beresford, S.H.A., Morrell, D.C., Waller, J.J., & Watkins, C.J. (1975). Factors influencing demand for primary medical care in women age 20–40 years; a preliminary report. *International Journal of Epidemiology*, *4*, 189–255.

Barber, T.X. (1959). Toward a theory of pain: Relief of chronic pain by pre-frontal leucotomy, opiates, placebos and hypnosis. *Psychological Bulletin*, *56*, 430–460.

Beecher, H.K. (1955). The powerful placebo. *Journal of the American Medical Association*, *159*, 1602–1606.

Beecher, H.K. (1956). Relationship of significance of wound to the pain experienced. *Journal of the American Medical Association*, *161*, 1609–1613.

Breuer, J., & Freud, S. (1893–1895). *Studies on hysteria. Complete psychological works of Freud* (Vol. 2). London: Hogarth Press.

Caine, T.M., & Hope, K. (1967). *Manual of the Hysteroid Obsessional Questionnaire (HOQ)*. London: University of London Press Ltd.

Crisp, A.H., Kalucy, R.S., McGuinness, B., Ralph, P.C., & Harris, G. (1977). Some clinical, social and psychological characteristics of migraine subjects in the general population. *Postgraduate Medicine*, *53*, 691–697.

DaCosta, J.M. (1871). On irritable heart; a clinical study of a form of functional cardiac disorder and its consequences. *American Journal of Medical Science*, *61*, 17–50.

Engel, G.L. (1951). Primary atypical facial neuralgia. An hysterical conversion symptom. *Psychosomatic Medicine*, *13*, 375–396.

Engel, G.L. (1959). "Psychogenic" pain and the pain-prone patient. *American Journal of Medicine*, *26*, 899–918.

Goldberg, D.P. (1972). *The detection of psychiatric illness by questionnaire*. Toronto: Oxford University Press.

Graven, P.S. (1924). A series of clinical notes on headache. *Psychoanalytic Review*, *2*, 324–328.

Gronwall, D., & Wrightson, P. (1974). Delayed recovery of intellectual function after minor head injury. *Lancet*, *2*, 605–609.

Hart, H. (1947). Displacement, guilt and pain. *Psychoanalysis Review*, *34*, 259–273.

Jelliffe, S.E. (1933). The death instinct in somatic and psychopathology. *Psychoanalytic Review*, *20*, 121–132.

Lakoff, R. (1983). Interpretative psychotherapy with chronic pain patients. *Canadian Journal of Psychiatry*, *28*, 650–653.

Lewis, Sir. T. (1917). Report upon soldiers returned as cases of disordered action of the heart (D.A.H.) or valvular disease of the heart (V.D.H.) (M.R.C. special report series No. 8). London: Her Majesty's Stationery Office.

Mendelson, G. (1981). Persistent work disability following settlement of compensation claims. *Law Institute Journal*, *55*, 342–345.

Merskey, H. (1975). Psychiatric aspects of migraine. In J. Pearce (Ed.), *Modern topics in migraine*. London: Heinemann.

Merskey, H. (1980a). The role of the psychiatrist in the investigation and treatment of pain. In J.J. Bonica (Ed.), *Pain*. New York: Raven Press.

Merskey, H. (1980b). Some features of the history of the idea of pain. *Pain*, *9*, 3–8.

Merskey, H. (1981). Headache and hysteria. *Cephalalgia*, *1*, 109–119.

Merskey, H. (1984). Psychiatry and the cervical sprain syndrome. *Canadian Medical Association Journal*, *130*, 1119–1121.

Merskey, H., & Boyd, D.B. (1978). Emotional adjustment and chronic pain. *Pain*, *5*, 173–178.

Merskey, H., & Spear, F.G. (1967). *Pain: Psychological and psychiatric aspects*. London: Bailliere, Tindall & Cassell.

Monks, R., & Merskey, H. (1964). Treatment with psychotropic drugs. In P.D. Wall & R. Melzack (Eds.), *Textbook of pain*. London: Churchill Livingstone.

Oppenheimer, O.S., & Rothschild, M.A. (1918). The psychoneurotic factor in the irritable heart of soldiers. *British Medical Journal*, *2*, 29–31.

Parker, G., Tupling, H., & Brown, L. (1979). A parental bonding instrument. *British Journal Medical Psychology*, *52*, 1–10.

Pond, D.A., & Bidwell, B.H. (1959). A survey of epilepsy in 14 general practices. II. Social and psychological aspects. *Epilepsia*, *1*, 285.

Rees, W.L., & Henryk-Gutt, R. (1973). Psychological aspects of migraine. *Journal of Psychosomatic Research*, *17*, 141–154.

Salter, M., Brooke, R.I., Merskey, H., Fichter, G.F., & Kapusianyk, D.H. (1983). Is the temporo-mandibular pain and dysfunction syndrome a disorder of the mind? *Pain*, *17*, 151–166.

Schilder, P. (1931). Notes on the psychopathology of pain in neuroses and psychoses. *Psychoanalytic Review*, *18*, 1–22.

Snaith, R.P., Constantopoulos, A.A., Jardine, M.Y., & McGuffin, P. (1978). A clinical scale for the self-assessment of irritability. *British Journal of Psychiatry*, *132*, 164–171.

Sternbach, R.A., Wolf, S.R., Murphy, R.W., & Akeson, W.H. (1973). Traits of pain patients: The low-back loser. *Psychosomatics*, *14*, 226–229.

Szasz, T.S. (1957). *Pain and pleasure. A study of bodily feelings*. London: Tavistock Publications.

Walters, A. (1961). Psychogenic regional pain alias hysterical pain. *Brain*, *84*, 1–18.

Watson, C.P., Evans, R.J., Reed, K., Merskey, H., Goldsmith, L., & Warsh, J. (1982). Amitriptyline versus placebo in postherpetic neuralgia. *Neurology*, *32*, 671–673.

Watson, G.D., Chandarana, P.C., & Merskey, H. (1981). Relationships between pain and schizophrenia. *British Journal of Psychiatry*, *138*, 33–36.

Wolff, H.G. (1948). *Headache and other head pain*. London: Oxford University Press.

Woodforde, J.M., & Merskey, H. (1972). Personality traits of patients with chronic pain. *Journal of Psychosomatic Research*, *16*, 167–172.

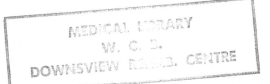
MEDICAL LIBRARY
W. C. D.
DOWNSVIEW REHAB. CENTRE

5 THE INTERDISCIPLINARY PAIN CENTER: AN APPROACH TO THE MANAGEMENT OF CHRONIC PAIN

Richard I. Newman
Joel L. Seres

Chronic benign pain is one of the most serious and baffling health problems confronting contemporary society. Injuries to workmen, and nonindustrial musculoskeletal injuries produce thousands of chronically disabled persons each year in this country. Tons of analgesic medications and tranquilizers are dispensed and consumed daily, and hundreds of hospital operating rooms are scheduled each day for the surgical treatment of chronic pain patients. Millions upon millions of dollars are spent yearly on workers' compensation benefits, time loss, medications, and medical and surgical treatments. Yet, an untold number of patients continue unproductive therapy and fail to be restored to working health (Brena, 1978; Brena & Chapman, 1978; Crue, 1979; Seres, Painter, & Newman, 1981).

There are many reasons for this seemingly insurmountable problem. Our knowledge of the mechanisms, causes, and effective therapies for chronic benign pain remains confused and unclear, in spite of the thousands of published pages on the subject. There are almost as many theories about pain and its causes as there are theoreticians. In order for the individual practitioner to find his way through the massive accumulation of seemingly contradictory and confusing information, he or she must first understand the differences between acute pain and chronic benign pain.

Acute pain is viewed as the transmission of an electrochemical signal through the nervous system to warn the individual of some form of bodily harm or tissue damage (Crue, 1979). In acute pain, generally the person's experience of pain is in some measure proportional to the extent and severity of the tissue damage. Appropriate therapeutic approaches may consist of medications, surgical correction, bracing, splinting, rest, attention, support, and time-out from responsibilities. Unfortunately, most of the evaluative and therapeutic strategies designed to treat chronic benign pain patients follow the general medical model for the treatment of acute pain.

Indeed, a careful review of the medical curricula of most physicians in training shows a paucity of training in the recognition and treatment of pain problems, which may insidiously move from acute to more chronic processes. The continued application of acute pain treatment methods to the chronic benign pain patient not only fails to relieve the patient's suffering, but often aggravates, complicates, and intensifies the patient's disability and severely reduces the chances for successful pain rehabilitation. One does not have to be a pain treatment specialist in order to determine that the continued use of narcotics, tranquilizers and sleeping medications, rest, attention, and support with time-out from responsibilities does little or nothing to solve the suffering of the chronic benign pain patient.

Out of this general medical model framework comes the basic peripheralist's view of pain, which places the etiology of chronic benign pain within the nervous system and the nociceptive stimulation process. The peripheralist believes that if the underlying pain generator or the "organic" mechanism producing the chronic pain can be eliminated, the pain patient's suffering will be relieved (Crue, 1979). To accomplish this process, the peripheralist utilizes such concepts and modalities of treatment as nerve blocks, acupuncture, surgery, injectable steroids, and other potent medications designed to change the neurochemistry of the patient, as well as structural changes with surgical intervention. Such techniques as manipulation of the spine, ultrasound treatments, hot packs, and transcutaneous nerve stimulation follow the general principles of the peripheralists' view in their attempt to reduce the patient's nociceptive stimulations. These approaches are usually carried out in a unimodal treatment program where professionals of one or more specialties share in patient care in a serial or "turn-taking" manner. There is little need for a truly multidisciplinary or interdisciplinary approach in the peripheralist's model, and the serial consultation mode of operation tends to dominate this type of an approach.

By marked contrast, the centralist's view of chronic pain takes into consideration a myriad of factors ranging from the patient's verbalizations of discomfort, socioeconomic variables, family problems, vocational and avocational aspects, emotional and intellectual factors, as well as the cultural context within which these variables occur. For the pain specialist following the centralist's approach, chronic benign pain is more than "the sum of its parts" and a much broader view of the patient's difficulties must be entertained (Crue, 1979; Fordyce, 1979). By necessity the molar nature of the centralist's view leads directly to the need for an interdisciplinary approach. Interdisciplinary pain treatment clinics are an outgrowth of the need for a team-oriented approach. At this writing there are somewhere in the neighborhood of 1,200 operating pain clinics in the United States alone (Crue, 1983).

In 1976 the National Institute on Drug Abuse undertook a survey of pain clinics and pain centers. As a part of this process, 13 programs were described in detail and selected because of their attention to outcome measures and data relative to their effectiveness with this difficult group of patients (Seres et al., 1981). As a result of this blossoming pain industry, the Commission on Accreditation of Rehabilitation Facilities (CARF) has undertaken, with the assistance of the pain community, the establishment of national standards and criteria for pain center certification. This complex process has helped to establish some common framework for comparison of these interdisciplinary pain clinics nationally.

Our present purpose is to describe one such interdisciplinary pain treatment center and to show how the complex process of evaluation and therapy of the chronic benign pain patient occurs in such a setting.

THE INTERDISCIPLINARY PAIN TREATMENT TEAM

The Northwest Pain Center is a day treatment pain clinic designed to evaluate and treat approximately 30 chronic pain patients at any one time. The program has been in existence treating benign pain patients since

1972 (Newman, Painter, & Seres, 1978; Newman, Seres, Yospe, & Garlington, 1978; Painter, Seres, & Newman, 1980; Seres, Newman, Yospe, & Garlington, 1977; Seres et al., 1981). At the outset in 1972 we operated our program as a 3-week inpatient program in a rehabilitation unit of a large urban hospital. At present we operate our program out of a large free-standing clinic with large classroom spaces and treatment areas designed to accommodate an average census of 25 patients with a staff of 33 specially trained and coordinated personnel.

Since the opening of the Northwest Pain Center in 1972, we have had the privilege of evaluating and treating over 8,000 chronic benign pain patients. Our staff of clinicians has an average of approximately 10 years of experience each in the management, evaluation, and treatment of chronic benign pain patients. The medical and psychological leadership consists of co direction by a neurosurgeon and a medical psychologist. A fulltime orthopedist, a fulltime family practice physician, and a parttime neurologist, in addition to the neurosurgeon, complete the physician staff. Three fulltime and two halftime Ph.D. clinical medical psychologists constitute the psychological staff. Two fulltime registered physical therapists, two fulltime registered occupational therapists, two fulltime biofeedback technicians, two fulltime registered nurses, three parttime registered nurses, and an LPN ward clerk round out the clinical treatment team. Nonphysician and nonpsychologist clinical staff are coordinated by a masters'-level trained counseling psychologist with administrative and personnel management skills. The clinical staff is divided into two working interdisciplinary teams, each with equal and appropriate representation of the various pain disciplines. Our teams are interdisciplinary as opposed to multidisciplinary because they operate as democratic sharing units with integration of therapeutic modalities and without deference to some arbitrary hierarchy.

Often a "multidisciplinary" model can be little more than an accumulation of individuals, each performing his or her own area of therapy in a serial consultation or poorly integrated fashion. In our view, the interdisciplinary concept is effective with these difficult patients because it integrates a multiplicity of theories, strategies, and experiences into a single common approach to patient care. There is significant crossover of practice between disciplines. It is not uncommon for the psychologist to be seen engaging in didactic instruction on the anatomical and mechanical aspects of back pain or similarly for the neurosurgeon to be observed helping an angry spouse work through her feelings of frustration in having to cope with a loved one in chronic pain. Although this may seem somewhat strange to the inexperienced observer, the fact is, as a therapeutic team works together daily over the years, there is a tremendous amount of learning and cross-fertilization of ideas and knowledge, which makes each member quite expert in the basic application of the others' disciplines.

Equally compelling is the basic observation that patients' defenses and anxiety often prevent them from dealing with issues directly with the team member who in their minds is "the real authority" on the subject. For example, many of our patients have the covert fear that cancer or some other life-threatening disease may be an underlying and undiscovered cause of their chronic benign pain. They are reluctant to seek an answer directly to these emotionally laden questions from the physician, yet may be more open to discuss these concerns with a physical therapist or a psychologist, thereby "indirectly" informing the team that this issue needs to be addressed.

Our treatment teams meet twice weekly to discuss each patient's progress throughout all aspects of the patient's program. Refinement of the diagnoses, which are often multiple, and of the therapeutic strategies occurs in an orderly and all inclusive fashion. Because the team represents multiple observers in different contexts at different times, a more accurate and complete picture of the patient's limitations and abilities can be obtained than is possible with a unimodal unidisciplinary or serial consultation model. Patients are asked to sign behavioral treatment contracts, and progress toward goal attainment is carefully measured and tracked by each member of the therapeutic team, as well as by fellow patients.

MODALITIES OF THERAPY

As discussed earlier, there are many ways of approaching the chronic pain patient. In our view, active therapies emphasizing patient responsibility, as opposed to palliative or passive treatments, are the key to helping the chronic benign pain patient become rehabilitated and productive again. We will briefly list the primary therapeutic modalities used in our clinic and describe some of the most salient aspects of each.

Physical Therapy

All patients are involved in an active physical therapy program with emphasis on stretching muscles and increasing range of motion, mobility, and endurance. Increasing strength and pain tolerance are integrated in a specialized posture and body mechanics training program that utilizes modeling, video tape feedback, and hours of one-to-one and group instruction from a registered physical therapist with specialization in the treatment of chronic pain. Flexion exercises and instruction in the pelvic tilt, as well as other postural training procedures, are utilized both individually and in group instructional classes. These classes, both individual and group, occur on a daily basis, as well as a modified form of aerobics, walking exercises, and gait training taught in conjunction with video tape or mirror feedback modalities. Specific neuromuscular retraining occurs in conjunction with the use of portable EMG equipment to monitor muscular activity to assist patients in correcting faulty posture and gait. No passive treatments are utilized, such as hot packs, ultrasound, massage, traction, manipulation, or whirlpools. The long-term therapeutic

benefits of these passive treatments have never been proven in the chronic benign pain patient, and they violate the basic concept of a self-help model or philosophy of treatment.

Patients' range of motion is carefully measured and remeasured throughout their physical therapy program and public, as well as chart, records are kept to show each patient's progress in concrete and observable ways. Patients themselves review each other's progress and support one another by reviewing videotape feedback sessions or each other's gait and body mechanics compared to previous weeks' measures. It is remarkable to see the magnitude of the changes that can occur in many of these patients in posture and in pain behavior over their 3-week treatment program. In many ways patients themselves are the most powerful reinforcers for each other's progress, as well as dispensers of appropriate criticism and confrontation for those patients who fail to show reasonable and positive gains (Sternbach, 1978).

Biofeedback Therapy

All of our patients receive training in one or more of the following biological feedback modalities: thermal training, electromyographic training, or galvanic skin resistance (GSR) training. It has been our experience that biofeedback can be a powerful tool in helping patients understand they do have the capacity to control their own bodies in many ways.

Inappropriate muscular bracing and generalized muscular tension are the earmarks of the chronic benign pain patient, and reduction of these maladaptive neuromuscular behaviors can substantially relieve the patient's suffering. Learning autonomic control to the point of controlling one's peripheral skin temperature or the electrical resistance of one's skin has a significant calming effect on the anxious, tense, and depressed chronic pain patient. Additionally, certain specific chronic pain problems, such as migraine, Reynaud's phenomenon, muscle tension headaches, temporomandibular joint syndrome, bruxism, and cervical muscle tension, respond dramatically to biofeedback as a therapeutic strategy.

Portable EMG biofeedback equipment is utilized to do in vivo postural and gait training while patients carry out their normal walking activities, including simulated work samples. More sophisticated multiple-modality monitoring techniques are used to help correct severe neuromuscular problems, such as astasia-abasia or spastic torticollis, as well as to teach the simple "pelvic tilt" for the relief of low back pain. Of course, all patients' progress is quantitatively recorded and used in tracking areas of strength and weakness throughout their program.

Occupational and Vocational Assessment

Most chronic pain patients have serious vocational difficulties, frequently being unable to return to the heavy physical labor that they have performed in the past. A careful and detailed analysis of the patient's interest, aptitudes, intelligence, and work history becomes critical in vocational planning. Many of our patients are resistant to discussing return to work due to their fears of failure and potential loss of workers' compensation, which they frequently see as their only source of financial security. A gentle and interest-oriented approach often "hooks" patients into beginning to explore "what if" issues and reduces their fears of beginning to think in terms of retraining or job restructuring.

Work capacity evaluations and standardized work samples are utilized, as well as a highly sophisticated interactive computer software program (WEST II, IV Systems, and MESA Software System), to psychometrically assess the patient's complete occupational profile from personality and temperament to fine motor dexterity. Integration of these data with objective measures of physical function, as well as dysfunction, from the physical therapy and medicine departments provides a complete database upon which to objectively counsel the patients about their potential for vocational readjustment.

Nursing Services

Team nurses function as the "glue" of the interdisciplinary matrix having a powerful and intensive one-to-one relationship with each patient on their team. Nurses are responsible for the drug reduction and withdrawal program, communications training, nutritional counseling, transcutaneous electrical nerve stimulation (TENS) application and instruction, and many other duties that form the hub of the patients' daily activity program. Relaxation training and stress management skills training are shared with the psychology staff. Nurses are in the unique position of having substantial observational time with patients and provide helpful input to team planning because they have the opportunity to observe whether patients are putting into action what they are learning in other aspects of their treatment program.

Medicine

Team physicians are responsible for monitoring the medical care of the patients by controlling their medications and assessing the need for further diagnostic tests or for outside medical consultation. Because most chronic benign pain patients have been repeatedly examined and treated medically, the physicians in the interdisciplinary pain treatment clinic must adopt a somewhat different role than that of the traditional medical model. The physicians in a pain center must be capable of giving up complete control of every aspect of the patient's care and blending their talents with the talents and experiences of the rest of the interdisciplinary team. They must be capable of accepting the bitterness and frustration that many chronic pain patients have toward physicians in general for their failure to "cure" the patients' pain. Likewise, they must recognize that there is no singular therapeutic approach, whether it be injection, surgery, or pill, that will be completely effective in ameliorating the suffering of the chronic pain patient.

The technique-oriented physician typically does not fare well in the interdisciplinary pain clinic. The physician must help the patients recognize that they themselves are the most powerful agent of change and must restore the physician's role to a more realistic one as a helper and guide with specialized medical knowledge and not a "deus-ex-machina." The demystification of the physician and his role in the treatment of chronic pain helps patients realize, many for the first time in their lives, that their own role in health and sickness is critical to becoming rehabilitated.

The Psychologist

The clinical psychologists in the pain center must have specialized training and experience in medicine, especially in the areas of neurology, neurological surgery, and orthopedic medicine. They must be willing, as well as able, to listen and answer questions and concerns about traditionally defined medical areas. The psychologist who views his or her role as caretaker of the patient's mental and emotional health and refuses to be knowledgeable and aware of the patient's physical problems is certain to fail as an integral part of the pain treatment team.

Chronic benign pain patients in general are almost universally unaccepting of any approach to their problem that suggests a psychological etiology to their pain. They are psychologically unsophisticated and tend toward alexithymic handling of emotions and feelings. They tend to view their pain as physical or mechanical in origin. This generalized antipsychological stance is both a function of the patients' early learning experiences and personality make-up, as well as the covert fear that if their problems are somehow defined as psychological in origin they will be seen as "not real" and, therefore, jeopardize their workers' compensation benefits.

Our population of chronic pain patients has an average educational level of 10th grade and an average of 2.3 marriages, as well as a history of having engaged in heavy physical labor all of their adult lives. As a group, chronic pain patients are reactively depressed, passive–dependent, somatically preoccupied, subassertive, alexithymic, and vocationally without direction. Their family communications, financial stability, and sex lives are a shambles. Their self-esteem is severely damaged because of their physical limitations and the resultant inability to perform their previous occupations. Many of our patients are dependent upon Schedule II narcotics, tranquilizers, sleeping pills, and alcohol as methods of managing their pain, both physiological and psychological.

The interdisciplinary pain clinic approach to chronic benign pain emphasizes a therapeutic approach that addresses the nociceptive, as well as the emotional and psychological, components of the chronic pain experience. As such, one must address the issues of secondary gain, financial compensation, time out from work, and other operant reinforcers, as well as posture, body mechanics, muscle strengthening, and other more physiologic mechanisms of pain. Any singular therapeutic approach to this multidimensional set of variables is likely to leave many patients without the benefit that they deserve. The interdisciplinary team approach places heavy emphasis upon re-education, patient responsibility, and active physical restoration as ways of reducing patients' nociceptive input as well as their psychological symptoms. Patients are actively taught in understandable terms about such topics as the neuroanatomy and neurophysiology of pain, the biomechanics of the spine, drugs and their effects on the body, spinal surgery, family problems in chronic pain, sexual dysfunction, and depression. Therapy sessions range from individual psychotherapy to group psychotherapy and didactic instruction. At all times persuasion, reassurance, support, and confrontation, as well as suggestion and other direct behavioral techniques, are emphasized. Interdisciplinary cooperation and communication are at the hub of our efforts at behavior change, with psychotherapy in its broadest sense being delivered by all staff members from the ward clerk to the neurosurgeon.

Therapeutic strategies are defined and refined in team meetings involving all treatment staff. Antidepressant medications are frequently utilized as an aid to raise patients' subjective thresholds to pain, restore sleep–wakefulness cycles, and make patients more amenable to other therapeutic interventions. Minor tranquilizers, sleeping medications, and muscle relaxants are not used in our treatment program. During the patient's 3-week stay, prescription analgesics are systematically withdrawn without the use of placebos or masked capsules.

Once the chronic pain patient becomes immersed in the therapeutic process, emotional and psychological issues can be addressed as "reactions to" chronic pain. Most of our patients, even the most alexithymic, find this explanation acceptable and thereby make it possible for the therapeutic team to sidestep the issue of causation and help establish a partnership between patients and staff members working together for the betterment of the patient. Similarly, patients themselves are powerful agents of change through the influence of the therapeutic milieu. Because patients are at various stages of their treatment through the 3-week program, there is the immediate installation of hope, as well as a feeling of not being alone, for the new incoming patients. The therapeutic milieu provides a powerful source of imparting information, as well as a mechanism for role modeling in the development of an intense level of camaraderie that frequently goes far beyond the patient's stay in the program.

THE EVALUATION PROCESS

Patient selection and diagnostic assessment begin the therapeutic process of an interdisciplinary pain program. In our hands, patients are seen by both medical, surgical, and psychological specialists. Patients' spouses are interviewed in-depth, and patients complete the Minnesota Multiphasic Personality Inventory (MMPI) and other psychometric tests (Cummings, Evanski, Debenedetti, Anderson, & Waugh, 1979; Wiltse & Roc-

chio, 1974). All of the patients' medical and surgical records are carefully reviewed, as well as most current diagnostic tests and procedures. Occasionally patients are asked to undergo electrodiagnostic studies (EMG) and/or radiographic studies to upgrade and add to the diagnostic database where indicated. Computerized axial tomography, myelography, and other diagnostic tests are employed very selectively when further surgery is being contemplated. Less than 0.5% of our patients are recommended for further surgical procedures relative to their pain.

At the conclusion of each of these evaluations, the combined pain team, as well as the patient and his or her spouse, are seen in an interdisciplinary conference. It is in this conference that the decision to admit the patient to the pain program is made. Patients have the final say in this decision and must show some evidence of willingness to work on their problem from a self-help perspective. Patients and their spouses are clearly told that the examining team feels they can be helped to learn to manage their pain problems more effectively and to enhance the quality of their lives. Specific goals such as learning to manage their pain without the continued use of prescription analgesics and muscle relaxants are discussed. Additionally, vocational alternatives are discussed where appropriate, and spouses are encouraged to participate in the last 2 days of the patient's stay in the program. The spouse's involvement is considered important in helping to alter maladaptive interaction patterns and inappropriate reinforcements of pain behaviors. In addition, communications training and marital counseling are frequently necessary in facilitating new interactional patterns between spouses and family members and in aiding in the transition from pain clinic therapy to the home or work environments.

Approximately 33% of our patients are eliminated and not admitted to the pain program at this evaluation point. Generally patients who are not admitted at this point are unmotivated to help themselves or perhaps view their pain as more of a "solution" to their life problems than a problem in and of itself. A very small percentage of patients may be eliminated because of severe physical limitations to participation in an active physical program. Such patients might have advanced cardiovascular disease, severe COPD, or some other significant physical limitation. Another small segment of patients who are frequently eliminated at this point are "hardcore" drug addicts, individuals who have used pain as an excuse to continue a long maladaptive history of substance abuse. In our experience, attempting to treat a narcotic addict who also presents with pain has been a very unrewarding process. Severe pain behavior or pain disability is not considered grounds for nonadmission to the program. Patients with significant limitations have their programs individually tailored and monitored in order to calibrate and accommodate to the patient's beginning level of function.

All patients participate in the daily lecture series covering such issues as medications, surgery, pain mechanisms, family dynamics, and socioeconomic and vocational implications of pain and disability. Variation in the patients' therapeutic regimen is primarily in the areas of physical therapy, occupational therapy, medical management, and psychotherapy. As individual patients' needs arise, they are addressed as a function of team input and involvement and appropriate modifications of each aspect of the patient treatment program follow accordingly.

Many patients that we see in the pain center have been treated extensively from a surgical perspective and have essentially been devastated, both physically as well as psychologically, by the treatments they have received that were originally designed to relieve their suffering. One such example follows.

Case Study: B.J.C., A 42-year-old Woman With Back Pain

B.J.C., a 42-year-old woman, was contemplating a trip to Europe when she hurt her back at home. She saw her family physician who suggested that, prior to her trip, perhaps it would be wise to at least see an orthopedic

surgeon to be sure that a ruptured disc was not present. Although there were no hard neurological signs, the orthopedist suggested a myelogram to be certain that something wasn't missed that might be helpful and would eliminate the possibility of her having difficulty on her trip. Unfortunately, due to a mixed injection, the patient developed a severe neuritic reaction requiring complete bedrest in the hospital for 3 weeks following the myelogram. Despite the mixed injection and no evidence of neurological dysfunction or positive findings on the myelogram, an exploratory laminectomy was performed 4 months later. With a significant increase in leg symptoms postoperatively, a repeat laminectomy was performed 8 months after the first and an L4-5 fusion 3 months after that. Because of the nature of the persisting pain, it was felt that "central pain" was the source of the patient's distress. In the fall of that same year a dorsal column stimulator was implanted. This resulted in the usual paresthetic sensations in her lower limbs. The patient now noted improvement in some of her foot pain only, but no improvement in the back or leg pain problem. A revision of the dorsal column stimulator was performed 1 month later. Because of persisting difficulty in March of the next year, a revision of the lumbar fusion was performed. The dura was explored and arachnoiditis was found. In June of that year the fusion was taken *down* and a decompressive laminectomy removing the spinous processes was performed. Because of persisting pain, the patient had been considered for a brain implantation procedure. She attended the Northwest Pain Center Program for 3 weeks in the latter part of that year. The following letter was received from her physician at the University of California.

Dear Doctors Seres and Newman:
   Just a note to let you know how much I appreciate your treating B.J.C. She has had an excellent result through your approach to this difficult pain problem. She is much more active now and has considerably less discomfort. She is not on narcotics. I saw her in follow-up 3 weeks ago and she is truly a changed person. . . . (Seres et al., 1981)

The previous example exemplifies the philosophy that "if it hurts, cut it out." This philosophy frequently leads to devastating results for both the patients and their families. In order to help such a person in a pain center, we must first overcome the intense anger that these patients have to deal with, as well as their reactive depressions. Daily psychotherapy and a progressive ambulatory and strengthening program become critical in helping the patients to again gain some feeling of control over their pain-shattered lives.

Another interesting case is:

Case Study: B.L.R., A 24-year-old Woman With Back Pain

B.L.R. is a 24-year-old single female clerk with the legislature of one of the West Coast states. She starting having back difficulties in 1971, sought medical help, and was told that she had a spondylolisthesis. In July of 1972 she had a lumbar fusion, providing her temporary relief of about 6 months' duration. She then began having increased back and leg symptoms and was subsequently told that her first fusion was not solid and that a second fusion was recommended. In April of 1974 she underwent a second lumbar fusion, again with only temporary benefit. At the time of her admission to the pain center program, she was taking 7 to 8 50 mg pentazocine hydrochloride tablets per day and 10 to 20 mg of diazepam per day. She was depressed and spent a substantial amount of her waking day lying down, splinting herself from her chronic pain. She was observed to be a highly intelligent and socially outgoing woman who was quite distraught over her severe physical limitations. Additionally, there was evidence of communication problems in her family and a tendency to inhibit her emotional expression of frustration and anger because of fear of losing control or being rejected by others.

Her stay in the pain clinic was 3 weeks in duration. She was treated with a progressive exercise program, 100 mg of amitriptyline at bedtime, and extensive use of biofeedback, autogenic training and relaxation training, videotaped postural feedback, and psycho-

therapy, which assisted her in bringing her pain under better management. At the time of her discharge, indications were that she had improved quite dramatically and was making heavy use of the autogenic and biofeedback aspects of her program. Following her discharge from the pain clinic she returned home and dealt more appropriately with her family communication difficulties, relocated herself in a large city in the western United States, and in conjunction with some other professionals opened a biofeedback institute for the treatment of other patients with headache and other chronic pain problems.

To this date, this young woman has been quite successful in managing her problems without the use of medications and continues to keep in contact with us. Unfortunately, she has been recently diagnosed as having multiple sclerosis, but continues to maintain a positive attitude and utilizes the tools that she gained while in the pain center program. As of this writing, the patient continues to function at an optimum level. She works fulltime and stated in a recent letter, "I can honestly say that my back has not been a problem for so long now that I rarely consider myself to have a back problem." Unfortunately, not all of our patients are as successful as the previous two examples of highly motivated individuals.

An interesting, but much less successful, example is presented in the following:

Case Study: J.B.R., A 39-year-old Man With Back Pain

J.B.R., a 39-year-old, three-times-divorced male, ex-hod carrier was admitted to the pain treatment program after having first injured his back in 1955 while employed as a hod carrier. In 1956 he underwent a lumbar fusion with poor results, and in 1961 a laminectomy was performed, again with poor results. In 1963 a spinal fusion was performed, followed by "the best period of my life." In 1971 the patient was reinjured falling from a ladder and underwent another spinal fusion in 1972, with reportedly poor results and increasing pain. At the time of his first admission to the pain clinic, he reported pain in his thoracic spine of a stabbing and sharp nature with radiation into both lower extremities, predominantly on the left. He also described disabling headaches of a muscle tension type, which were associated with any kind of physical exertion. At that time the patient was collecting $368 per month from workers' compensation insurance and $308 per month from Social Security benefits, with an additional $48 for each child from Social Security, making a total of $724 per month in disability and Social Security benefits. It is of interest to note that just prior to the patient's injury he was earning approximately $700 per month before taxes, making his injury compensation over 160% more than earned income.

Medications at the time of admission were: flurazepam hydrochloride for sleep; butalbital, 8 to 10 tablets per day; and prednisone, 5 mg three times a day. The patient was depressed, had very little sense of direction vocationally, and was quite bitter about his situation. He had a long history of marital difficulties, having been married three times and having had counseling from a variety of psychologists and psychiatrists over the years prior to his coming to the Northwest Pain Center. His psychological diagnoses were hysteroid personality, social immaturity, drug dependency, poor educational background and minimal job skills, chronic marital and heterosexual adjustment problems, and a low average level of intellectual functioning.

Medically, he was demonstrated to have a solid fusion from L3 to the sacrum and was diagnosed as having chronic lumbar strain and muscle contraction headaches. Following his initial treatment in the pain clinic, J.B.R. did not return to gainful employment. He continued to show poor motivation to exercise and to doing the other things that he was taught in the pain clinic. He eventually returned to the use of the same medications he had been on prior to his admission and in addition began to take secobarbital sodium and acetaminophen with codeine on a daily basis. Four months after his treatment in the pain clinic, he underwent another extensive surgical decompressive laminectomy and revision of his lumbar fusion. The patient's response to this surgical procedure was poor, which resulted in his seeking assistance from a local chiropractor and eventually consulting an acupuncturist for treatment.

The patient was reevaluated in January of 1976 for admission to the pain clinic, at which time he was taking secobarbital, acetaminophen with codeine, amitriptyline, and chlorzoxazone and acetaminophen on a daily basis. His activity level had declined substantially. He spent the largest part of his day reclining and professed being quite desperate for assistance. At that time his financial compensation was roughly the same as it had been in 1974, with some regular increases for cost of living.

The patient was readmitted to the pain program for another 3-week stay. All efforts were made to again reduce this man's intake of medications and to teach him ways of dealing with his problems more effectively. He was stabilized on 100 mg of amitriptyline at bedtime, and he was referred for more intensive vocational assistance and retraining. The patient was enrolled in a local community college and was taking computer programming in hope of again becoming a gainfully employed individual.

Six months after his discharge from his second stay in the pain clinic, the patient "slipped on the ice," aggravating his back condition. He again returned to the use of medications and discontinued his training and schooling program.

J.B.R. was reevaluated once again in 1981, and again an attempt was made to deal with this man through the interdisciplinary pain center program. His hospitalizations, visits to emergency rooms, and other medical costs had become astronomical, which necessitated this third attempt in the pain center setting. At this admission the patient continued to show the same behavioral characteristics and attitudes as before, but his condition appeared to be worsening in terms of the emotional and characterological aspects of his difficulties. Additionally, the patient began to complain of severe vascular headaches and vomiting. He was placed on the following medication: propranolol hydrochloride, 40 mg four times a day; doxepin HCL 150 mg at hours of sleep, and phenothiazine, 2 mg three times a day. He was then withdrawn from all narcotic and other medications that he was taking. He again improved his range of motion, mobility, and endurance during his stay with us.

He left the pain program and within 6 months was consulting a local orthopedic surgeon, requesting another fusion on his back because of what he described as "a bone moving and snapping, causing pain in my back." Dynamic x-rays of his lumbar spine showed movement of a minute nature at the level above his fusion, which resulted in a local surgeon attempting another spinal fusion one level above his previous surgeries. Following removal of his body cast, the patient's abdominal musculature had totally deteriorated. He had bilateral meralgia paresthetica from the pressure of the body cast on his lateral femoral cutaneous nerves. His muscle tension and vascular headaches were described as much worse than prior to his surgery, and he again sought admission to the pain center program.

As an alternative to readmission to the full pain program, the patient was again started on appropriate psychotropic medications and placed in an outpatient psychotherapy group for "hard-core" chronic pain patients. This group meets on a once a week basis and is designed to help patients ventilate their frustrations and discuss in detail their pains and aches. Fellow patients modify one another's pain behavior, and conservative approaches are the rule. It is interesting to see how insightful these "hard-core" patients are about each other's pain behavior and how totally oblivious they are to their own. Since that time the patient has not had continuing rehospitalizations and has essentially stabilized since the awarding of his permanent and total disability. He continues to verbalize the complaint of pain, takes the psychotropic medications prescribed, and occasionally takes some analgesic that he obtains from his wife or some other family member. He has not completed any form of retraining program and shows little or no motivation to improve.

J.B.R. represents a total and complete failure of a system that both financially and medically reinforced him as a disabled person. Pain in his case represented more of a solution than a problem, and he continued to escalate his pain behavior and experience to the point that he became essentially a "professional pain patient." He has effectively defeated the efforts of more than 20 physicians and psychologists who have attempted to treat him over the years and will undoubtedly remain permanently and totally disabled the rest of his life.

Assessing the therapeutic outcome of pain center treatment in more than a few anecdotal cases has been a very important part of our overall research program at the Northwest Pain Center. A number of outcome studies (Aronoff & Evans, 1982, Aronoff, Evans, & Enders, 1983; Newman, Painter, & Seres, 1978; Painter et al., 1980; Seres et al., 1981) have demonstrated that pain center treatment is cost-effective, as well as therapeutically beneficial to many patients who suffer from chronic benign pain.

Long-term follow-up studies have demonstrated that, on average, patients treated in our pain center maintain their gains for an extended period of time or show at least minimal decline. Examination of individual records indicates that one fourth to one third of our patients continue to show progress in pain management skills. However, a similar proportion decline fairly rapidly to preadmission levels of function despite measurable and significant improvement during their treatment programs. It is essential that the reasons for this recidivism or decline be understood (Painter et al., 1980). This group of patients represents a failure of the treatment; and if the regression in treatment is inevitable because of factors peculiar to the individual, then perhaps this treatment should not be offered to this particular group of individuals. If, however, factors extrinsic to the individual are implicated, then overall success for the entire group could be improved by addressing those factors. The very factors causing pain center failure may be those involved in the failure of other therapeutic approaches such as surgery.

In an effort to answer these questions, we conducted a study of 145 previously treated patients from the Northwest Pain Center. On reexamining these patients, 77% felt improved as a result of their pain center experience, with an average reported pain reduction of 35%. Further improvement following discharge was noted by 27% of this sample, with an average further decrease in pain of 21%. Deterioration in function and increase in pain were reported by 27% of the sample. They noted an average increase of pain of 23%. Thus, by subjective report, the pain center experience was helpful for three fourths of our patients. Yet, for almost one fourth, most of the gains were virtually wiped out with the passage of time.

To allow comparisons among nonparametric variables and to highlight differences between the treatment failures and the successful patients, two groups were selected, arbitrarily set at 25 patients each. The group reporting the greatest degree of post-discharge improvement was labeled as the success group, and the group with the greatest deterioration was labeled as the failure group.

On carefully examining these two groups, criterion variables such as pain intensity and limitations imposed by pain demonstrated that the two groups did not differ significantly at the time of admission nor at the time of completing the pain center treatment; thus, the amount of improvement noted during pain center treatment was not prognostic of later regression. The success group continued to show improvement following discharge, whereas the failure group showed deterioration approaching the levels that they had reported at the time of their admission.

Examining the demographic variables of the samples demonstrated that substantially more males appear in the failure group. Marital status is related to group assignment as well; more individuals in the success group report being divorced. This seems paradoxical, because it has been felt that stability in sources of environmental support is important in the alleviation of a chronic pain problem. The difference is a property of the success group, however, in that failure patients were not distinguished from the total group by this factor. Average age was similar for all groups. In fact, although little correlation was noted between age and overall change or regression, it was noted that groupings of age categories did demonstrate some differences. Specifically, the failure group had more individuals aged 20 to 30 and more patients older than 50; the success group and the remainder of the population showed more centralized tendencies, with the bulk of patients falling between 30 and 50 years of age. Another surprising statistic was that patients in the success group had been disabled significantly longer than had the failures or the remainder of the group sample.

Incentive variables demonstrated that approximately 70% of all groups were receiving compensation at the time of admission. By follow-up, only half of the total group and 40% of the success group reported continuing compensation. The total for the failure group was essentially unchanged, with 56% of the failed patients viewing themselves as disabled by pain, a view shared by only 40% of the total group and 25% of the successful patients.

Substantially more of the success group were employed full-time, and the failure group had almost 2 years less education than the success group. Additionally, the success group could be distinguished from failures on the basis of employment history, surprisingly having fewer years of work in a skilled category and more in an unskilled category. The failure group had substantially more skilled work than did the remainder of the sample. Total years of work were similar for all groups.

It was of interest to note that 75% of the

success group appeared to have assumed a self-help approach to their pain problem, no longer seeking medical care. In fact, only 40% of the total group continued in some form of medical care, mostly limited visits to their regular doctors. This is a hopeful sign, in that 100% of these patients had been seeking a cure at the time of admission. The failure group, by contrast, continued to seek medical solutions to their problems.

Subjects rank-ordered aspects of the pain program as most helpful or most negative. The exercise program, biofeedback, relaxation training, education, quitting pain medications, communication, and other such modalities were characterized as "active." "Passive" aspects of the pain treatment program included the treating professionals, other patients, and new medications, getting away from home, and so forth. The groups were similar in endorsing the active aspects of the pain program as being the most helpful. The failure group, however, was more likely to rate active aspects among the negative features of the experience than was the success group. The success group demonstrated a clear tendency to maintain the exercise program more than the failure group—in our experience a critical factor in the long-term success of chronic pain management.

From a psychological perspective, if passivity and dependency are fixed personality traits, then these should be apparent at the time of admission. However, the groups could not be differentiated on the basis of psychological diagnostic impression at the time of admission nor on the basis of MMPI profiles. Depressive symptoms, on the other hand, did appear to be linked to success or failure. Curiously, the success group rated itself as having been significantly more depressed at the time of admission than did the failure group or the total group. Successes showed striking continuing improvement in mood throughout the time period of the study, whereas the mood for the total group stabilized at the time of discharge and failure patients showed considerable regression. Sleep quality and the amount of sleep did not

distinguish reliably among the groups at admission or discharge, but the success group reported substantially better sleep at the time of follow-up and the failure group was doing worse than the remainder of the population. Pain behavior, like other learned behaviors, presumably falls under the control of contingent reinforcers; therefore one would expect that the success group would have a system of reinforcers relating to well behavior and that the failure group would tend to maintain prior contingency relationships. Indeed, this seemed to be borne out by reports of subjects. In fact, the failure group had a tendency to change relatively little in terms of contingent reinforcers following discharge, whereas the success group showed the greatest degree of change in pain behavior.

CONCLUSIONS

The previously illustrated research and our general experience with several thousand chronic pain patients demonstrates that substantial change takes place as a result of interdisciplinary pain center treatment. Significant reduction in pain severity is maintained over time, as long as patients continue to follow through with the active principles of the pain center approach. For approximately 25% of the patients, gains that had been substantial at the time of discharge had all but dissipated after a few months following treatment.

Incentive or financial compensation is a compelling explanatory construct for patient regression. Although groups are compensated equally at the time of admission, the failure group is much more likely to be receiving compensation at the time of follow-up. Inference of causality, of course, is uncertain; one could argue that the presence of the disability itself is the cause of the continued compensation. On the other hand, a variety of findings suggest that regression may be caused by lack of incentive favoring a healthy relatively pain-free way of life. This fact is further illustrated by the observation that multidisciplinary pain centers nationally are heavily attended by industrially injured compensated back patients with proportionately few noncompensated chronic pain patients. One might speculate that chronic benign back pain of a disabling type may have more of a socioeconomic etiology than a medical one.

The high level of employment among the success group may be seen as paradoxical, because the stated reason for not working in many cases is that it increases subjective pain. Instead, it may be argued that working actually decreases suffering and pain. This finding cannot be explained by the assertion that those most severely disabled are those who do not work, because assignment to the success or failure group was not related in the expected way to duration of disability nor to subjective levels of pain or disability at admission or discharge.

Our experience suggests, in fact, that many cannot afford to improve their level of functioning, and this observation is supported by the data. The skilled worker, for example, and particularly the skilled older worker, has less incentive for reentering the job market, because work would often pay him substantially less than he is receiving from compensation. By contrast, the lower skill level among the success group implies that they have greater flexibility in seeking new employment. Furthermore, prospects for employment dim with advancing age. This construct may also explain why men, more often the breadwinner, are less likely to maintain the gains than women.

Although educational level itself does not correlate highly with overall success, it is strongly associated with regression. It would appear that individuals with less education and correspondingly less opportunity for nonphysical work are more prone to regression after initial therapeutic gains.

Patient attitude, which is related to success or failure, is one factor over which pain centers and other treating agents ought to exert some influence. Chronic pain patients typically enter a therapeutic relationship with a passive attitude and implicitly demand cure from external agents. It has been felt that suc-

cess is related to willingness to renounce this helpless victim role. Passivity, which characterizes the failures, may be inferred from their tendency toward greater use of medications, further medical care (including a continued active search for a surgical solution to their problems), and apparent rejection of an active self-help approach to their pain problem.

Psychological diagnoses and psychometric information do not seem to be related to eventual success, a finding that has been reported in earlier research (Seres, 1973). Depression, however, appears to be strongly associated with success or regression. Surprisingly, the success group reported having been significantly more depressed at the time of admission, and their change in mood and improvement was powerfully related to their eventual success with pain center treatment. One might speculate that the failure patients were less depressed at the time of treatment because their pain was more of a "solution" to life's problems than it was a problem itself.

Perhaps the most striking difference among groups is reflected in the changes that they report in lifestyle following treatment. Those who regressed to the point of very little change in patterns of communication or reinforcement after they left the treatment program suggest that patterns that had previously supported their pain behavior continue to do so, contributing to their regression to pretreatment levels of function. The success group, on the other hand, showed considerable change in attitude, communication, and reinforcement contingencies in their general life situation.

In conclusion, it would appear that interdisciplinary pain center approaches to the treatment of chronic benign pain patients have demonstrated effectiveness in implementing changes in a substantial number of patients whose attitude is positive toward a self-help approach. Patients who are unable or unwilling to give up pain as a solution to their lifelong problems are unlikely to benefit from any form of treatment and will continue to escalate in their role as passive recipients of health care services, whether they be surgical, medical, psychological, or pain center. The careful evaluation and screening of patients becomes critical in determining whether patients will benefit from any form of intervention designed to relieve them of their suffering.

REFERENCES

Aronoff, G.M., & Evans, W.O. (1982). The prediction of treatment outcome at a multidisciplinary pain center. *Pain*, *14*, 67–73.

Aronoff, G.M., Evans, W.O., & Enders, P.L. (1983). A review of follow-up studies of multidisciplinary pain units. *Pain*, *16*, 1–11.

Brena, S.F. (1978). *Chronic pain: America's hidden epidemic*. New York: Atheneum/SMI.

Brena, S.F., & Chapman, S.L. (1983). *Management of patients with chronic pain*. New York: Spectrum Publications, Inc.

Bresler, D.E. (1979). *Free yourself from pain*. New York: Simon and Schuster.

Crue, B.L. (1979). *Chronic pain*. New York: Spectrum Publications, Inc.

Crue, B.L. (1983). *The history of pain centers*. Paper presented at the meeting of the American Pain Society, Chicago, IL.

Cummings, C., Evanski, P.M., Debenedetti, M.J., Anderson, E.E., & Waugh, T.R. (1979). Use of the MMPI to predict the outcome of treatment for chronic pain. In J.J. Bonica (Ed.), *Advances in pain research and therapy* (Vol. 3, pp. 667–670). New York: Raven Press.

Fordyce, W.E. (1979). Environmental factors in the genesis of low back pain. In J.J. Bonica (Ed.), *Advances in pain research and therapy*. (Vol. 3, pp. 659–666). New York: Raven Press.

Newman, R.I., Painter, J.R., & Seres, J.L. (1978). A therapeutic milieu for chronic pain patients. *Journal of Human Stress*, *6*, 8–12.

Newman, R.I., Seres, J.L., Yospe, L.P., & Garlington, B.E. (1978). Multidisciplinary treatment of chronic pain: Long term follow-up of low back pain patients. *Pain*, *4*, 283–292.

Painter, J.R., Seres, J.L., & Newman, R.I. (1980). Assessing benefits of the pain center; Why some patients regress. *Pain*, *8*, 101–113.

Seres, J.L., Newman, R.I., Yospe, L.P., & Garlington, B.E. (1977). Evaluation and management of chronic pain by nonsurgical means. In L.J. Fletcher (Ed.), *Pain management: Symposium on the neurosurgical treatment of pain*. Baltimore, MD: Williams & Wilkins.

Seres, J.L., Painter, J.R., & Newman, R.I. (1981). Multidisciplinary treatment of chronic pain at the Northwest Pain Center. In L.K.Y. Ng (Ed.), *New approaches to treatment of chronic pain: A review of multidisciplinary pain clinics and pain centers* (pp. 41–65). NIDA Research Monograph 36. Rockville, MD: National Institute on Drug Abuse.

Seres, N.A. (1973). *Chronic pain and its characteristics*. Unpublished masters thesis, University of Oregon.

Sternbach, R.A. (1978). *The psychology of pain*. New York: Raven Press.

Wiltse, C., & Rocchio, P. (1974). Preoperative psychological tests as predictors of success of chemonucleolysis in the treatment of low back syndrome. *Journal of Bone and Joint Surgery*, *57-A*(4), 478–483.

6 SOCIAL SKILLS TRAINING IN AN OUTPATIENT MEDICAL SETTING

Al S. Fedoravicius
Ben J. Klein

Physicians have realized for many years that a surprising proportion of chronic pain patients report pain in excess of what would seem to be warranted by the tissue damage (Melzack, 1973, Merskey & Spear, 1967). Several studies have reported that perhaps only one half of the chronic pain patients have definite organic findings (Heaton et. al., 1982; Leavitt & Garron, 1979b). Similarly, 30 to 40% of general medical patients are diagnosed as having no organic disruption at all, whereas another 20% have questionable organic findings (Barsky & Klerman, 1983; Ford, 1983). These data strongly suggest that illness complaints, including chronic pain complaints, are frequently disproportionate to the documented organic findings. In other words, complaints of pain or illness are relatively independent of the level of detectable biomedical impairment. Given this weak relationship between biomedical factors and pain or illness complaints, such complaints are very likely to be determined in part by learning experiences and environmental contingencies.

Illness behaviors may be defined as those behaviors or behavioral limitations that patients attribute to their physical conditions or symptoms (Fabrega, 1979; Twaddle, 1974). Chronic illness behavior can be defined as illness behavior that has lasted at least several months, is often characterized by such frequent utilization of medical services that the patient's lifestyle has become centered around illness behaviors, and frequently is accompanied by the following behaviors: helplessness, being demanding, threats, argumentativeness, excessive ingratiation, promises of compliance to treatment, and hostility (Wooley, Blackwell, & Winget, 1978). Pain behaviors, a special category of illness behaviors, can be defined as behaviors or limitations thereof that patients attribute to noxious or unpleasant (painful) symptoms. Chronic pain behavior persists despite standard medical treatment for at least several months (Sanders, 1979).

The term "abnormal illness behavior" has been used to denote illness behavior in excess of the degree of detected biomedical impairment (Pilowsky & Spence, 1975). Abnormal or excessive illness behavior is synonymous with chronic pain or chronic illness behavior to the extent that pain or illness behaviors interfere with one's highest potential level of functioning within the limitations of the biomedical impairment. Regardless of the level of biomedical impairment, higher levels of reinforcement for pain or illness behaviors will strengthen the likelihood that those pain or illness behaviors will excessively limit a person's adaptive functioning.

Evidence exists that chronic pain and chronic illness behaviors are in part learned vicariously through models. For example, diabetics who reported that their parents avoided work and other responsibilities when ill tended to do the same, whereas diabetics with nonavoidant parents did not avoid responsibilities when ill (Turkat, 1982). Turkat and Noskin (1983) found very similar results in healthy individuals for vicarious learning of avoidance of responsibilities when ill.

There is also evidence that the occurrence of certain consequences increases the probability of illness behaviors. For example, persons with irritable bowel syndrome more often reported receiving gifts or food from their parents when they experienced a cold or the flu during childhood than did hypertensives or persons in the general population (Whitehead, Fedoravicius, Blackwell, & Wooley, 1979; Whitehead, Winget, Fedoravicius, Wooley, & Blackwell, 1982). It has also been demonstrated that ill persons will reinforce those around them when the others provide care for them, thereby creating mutually reinforcing relationships centered around illness and caretaking (Wooley & Blackwell, 1975). Perhaps mention should be made at this point that health care providers all too frequently engage in centered relationships, and that moves toward wellness on the part of the patient may be less reinforcing for both the patient and the health care provider than would continued care-eliciting and caretaking behaviors, respectively. Monetary compensation or pending litigation may also be powerful reinforcers of pain and illness behaviors (Beals & Hickman, 1972; Heaton et al., 1982; Wiltse & Rocchio, 1975).

Regardless of whether or not compensation is positively reinforcing, it is possible that avoidance of work or other social responsibilities may be negatively reinforcing for illness behaviors. If avoidance of social or work responsibilities is negatively reinforcing for a person, one might expect that social or achievement situations are uncomfortable for that person. In addition, persons who involve themselves largely in illness-dominated relationships rather than in work or social situations may lack the skills to acquire reinforcement in achievement or social situations, thereby making the illness-centered relationships relatively more rewarding.

It is to this topic of the role of social skills in the development and maintenance of chronic pain and chronic illness behavior to which we turn in the next section of this chapter. With healthy respect for the complexity of defining social skills (e. g., Bellack, 1983), the authors will use the term "social skills" to refer to the range of learned interpersonal responses that, when emitted, typically result in socioculturally adaptive consequences. Social withdrawal, hostile interpersonal interactions, and complaining of illness or pain proportionately more than discussing pleasurable events or everyday life problems would all be examples of social skills performance deficits. We do not believe that social skills performance deficits all stem from anxiety-based inhibition of learned social skills, nor do we believe that all social skills performance deficits result from poor learning of the components of social skills. In any one person, a complex interplay of (a) previous interpersonal behavior learning experiences, (b) current consequences for adaptive interpersonal responses, (c) competing consequences for immediately reinforcing yet maladaptive social responses, and (d) competing consequences for illness-related social responses determine that person's social behavior. "Social skills training," as will be seen, must actually address as many of these determinants of social responses as is possible.

THE ROLE OF SOCIAL SKILLS IN CHRONIC PAIN AND CHRONIC ILLNESS BEHAVIOR

Despite the hypothesis that chronic pain and chronic illness behavior patients may suffer from social skills performance deficits, traditional psychometric instruments such as the Minnesota Multiphasic Personality Inventory (MMPI) and the Rorschach have failed to detect reliable patterns discriminating these patients from other medical patients (Cox, Chapman, & Black, 1978; Leavitt & Garron, 1979a; Louks, Freeman, & Calsyn, 1978; Osborne, 1979; Prokop, Bradley, Margolis, & Gentry, 1980). There are, however, some relationships between psychosocial variables and the frequency and intensity of illness complaints (Pennebaker, 1982). The number of somatic complaints is generally positively correlated with less education, lower socioeconomic class, lower occupational status, ethnocultural group discouragement of emotional expression, self-reported anxiety, and lower self-esteem scores (Barsky & Klerman, 1983; Katon, Kleinman, & Rosen, 1982; Pennebaker, 1982). In general, it appears that persons who complain of more somatic complaints (controlling for organic impairment) are those with fewer opportunities for socially adaptive achievements and less potential for rewarding social relationships.

Some direct evidence exists for the relationship between chronic illness behavior and social skills performance deficits. Chronic illness behavior patients have been found to engage in fewer assertive behaviors and to experience more anxiety in social situations than matched control patients and nonpatients (Wooley, Blackwell, Glaudin, & Lipkin, 1973). Furthermore, chronic illness behavior patients were less likely to request behavior changes from others than was a nonpatient control group (Wooley & Blackwell, 1975).

To summarize, chronic pain and illness behaviors develop and are maintained across all levels of biomedical impairment. Modeling of illness behaviors by parents, reinforcement for illness behaviors, and negative reinforcement in the form of avoidance of social and work responsibilities all appear to contribute to the persistence of chronic pain and chronic illness behaviors. Some evidence suggests that a relationship exists between deficits in adaptive social responses and chronic pain and illness behaviors. Theoretically, the deficits in social skills performance may be accounted for by (a) relatively poor social behavior learning experiences, (b) fewer opportunities or less rewarding consequences for adaptive social responses, (c) competing positive consequences for maladaptive yet immediately reinforcing social responses, and (d) competing positive consequences for illness-centered social responses.

SOCIAL SKILLS TRAINING IN THE TREATMENT OF CHRONIC PAIN AND CHRONIC ILLNESS BEHAVIOR

Many treatment programs for chronic pain patients have reportedly included social skills or assertiveness training as one of the components comprising their treatment programs (Turk, Meichenbaum, & Genest, 1983). These programs, which employ several self-control training and skill acquisition components in addition to the traditional operant contingency management techniques, have generally been equally or more successful than the operant chronic pain treatment programs (Pinkerton, Hughes, & Weinrich, 1982; Turner, 1982; Turner & Chapman, 1982). Several of these multicomponent treatment programs and their outcomes will be briefly discussed below.

Gottlieb et al. (1977) treated chronic low back pain patients with assertiveness training, biofeedback training, physical therapy reconditioning, vocational rehabilitation services, educational lectures, and a socialization milieu. The patients, who were hospitalized for an average of 45 days, improved on all vocational, physical functioning, and clinical assessment measures (one of which was an assertiveness rating). It is, of course, difficult to assess the relative contribution of each of the treatment components to these very impressive results. Elton, Stanley, and Burrows (1978) found that once weekly outpatient treatment sessions for 12 weeks involving biofeedback, hypnosis, and social interaction modification reduced the pain experiences and increased the self-esteem scores of chronic pain patients. Consistent with our hypotheses regarding social skills performance deficits in chronic pain and illness patients, the chronic pain patients scored lower in self-esteem prior to treatment than did a group of pain patients who had responded well to standard medical treatment. Elton, Stanley, and Burrows (1983) reported similarly positive results for an outpatient chronic pain treatment program. Communication skills training was an important part of the program, which also included family participation, stress inoculation training, and imagery and relaxation training.

Several treatment program for chronic illness behavior have also reported positive outcome. In an inpatient setting, Wooley et al. (1978) utilized social skills training, family interaction groups, social reinforcement for well behaviors, and goal setting and self-evaluation to treat patients with chronic illness behavior. Patients made progress on their self-generated symptom, social, family, and life-plan goals; and verbal samples revealed that their verbal behaviors changed from illness versus achievement orientation upon intake to achievement versus illness orientation at time of discharge 1 month later. Fedoravicius, Mariano, Leight, Stehr, and Klein (in press), using similar treatment approaches in an outpatient setting, obtained equally positive outcomes. Morgan, Kremer, and Gaylor (1979) used social skills training, contingency manipulation, cognitive coping skills training, relaxation training, and pharmacotherapy to treat patients whose physical complaints were judged to be either psychophysiological in nature or accompanied by significant contributing psychological components. They reported that patients who increased their use of assertive skills the most as a function of treatment were those who reported the greatest decrease in intensity and frequency of symptoms, whereas no other component of treatment was related differentially to treatment outcome.

In seeming contrast to the findings of the previous studies, Sanders (1983) found that assertiveness training had little effect on treatment outcome in a multi-component behavioral treatment program for chronic low back pain. Relaxation training and social reinforcement for increased activity contributed the most to treatment outcomes. Given the results of this well designed component analysis, one must question the role of assertiveness training per se in the treatment of chronic pain. However, effective social skills training is not to be equated with assertiveness training because a relatively small proportion of interpersonal behaviors are included in assertiveness training. We earlier stated that most treatment programs utilize social skills training to shape a wide array of socially adaptive behaviors and to extinguish illness-centered and other maladaptive social behaviors. In fact, the social skills component of many treatment programs, including our own, subsumes Sanders' effective treatment component—social reinforcement for increased activity.

As will be seen in the next section of this chapter, each patient's performance of social skills must be altered at least somewhat for that patient to be able to adequately utilize each of the other treatment components (relaxation, increased physical activity, vocational placement, etc.). Because improvement is typically inferred from increases in the proportion of socially adaptive behaviors, it would seem that modifications in social responses comprise an important part of any effective treatment approach.

A MULTIDIMENSIONAL CHRONIC ILLNESS BEHAVIOR TREATMENT PROGRAM

Context of the Treatment Program

This section provides a description of the chronic illness behavior treatment approach that has been utilized in the Wooley et al. (1978) and the Fedoravicius et al. (in press) programs. The programs will be called the Cincinnati program and the Albuquerque program, respectively, in accord with their locations. Approximately 800 patients have been treated in the two programs combined, and the senior author served as the clinical director of both programs. The training context and components described in this chapter are based primarily upon the Albuquerque program.

The Albuquerque program is an outpatient day hospital program, whereas the Cincinnati program is an inpatient program. As noted earlier, the two programs have been found to be equally effective (Fedoravicius et al., in press; Wooley et al., 1978). In the Albuquerque program, the patients participate in group and individual therapy sessions in the Behavioral Medicine Program for 3 to 6 hours each weekday for 4 to 6 weeks. (We have found over the past few years that 4 weeks of this treatment often are sufficient, although some patients seem to benefit from an additional 2 weeks of treatment contingent on good progress in the treatment program.)

The Admission Process

Patients are referred to our program from virtually all medical, surgical, and psychiatric specialties in the hospital and its clinics. As Wooley et al. (1978) pointed out, chronic pain and chronic illness behavior patients come with a wide variety of biomedical and psychiatric diagnoses, and many have had numerous and repetitive standard and esoteric biomedical and psychiatric treatments. After receiving the referral, we attempt to determine if the patient indeed fits the criteria for chronic pain and illness behavior described earlier in the chapter and described by Wooley et al. (1978). Because there are no adequate formal assessment methods of chronic pain and illness behavior, our assessment is a clinical one based on chart reviews, discussions with the referring physician, and a thorough clinical interview. We attempt to identify illness behaviors, identify the etiology of such behaviors, and identify the current reinforcers. If the clinical data largely match the criteria for pain and illness behaviors and

their etiology, and we are able to identify the current determinants of such behaviors, then we decide to offer the patient admission into our program.

We explain to the patient that he or she has been referred to us because no adequate biomedical diagnosis and/or treatment has been found for some or all of his or her biomedical problems and that, despite the patient's good intentions and efforts to maintain a normal life style and to be well, he or she has developed an "illness rut." Illness behaviors characterizing the illness rut that were identified by the assessment process are then described to the patient, basically stressing the common behaviors that are found in this patient population (Wooley et al., 1978): helplessness, being demanding, argumentativeness, verbal compliance and ingratiation, and hostility. These behaviors are described to the patient in an empathetic manner that carefully avoids pejorative blaming or labeling. This is an example of such an interaction:

> Your symptoms have had a major impact on you and your life. We frequently find that patients with your symptoms, who have not benefited from medical treatment as much as they were hoping to, get worn out by the symptoms. They get discouraged, feel and become increasingly helpless, and frequently feel that the only way they will be listened to is by being passive or by becoming angry. Frequently, feelings of depression, anxiety, and a real loss of self-esteem develop. As a result, you get stuck in such behaviors. Frequently, others, like family members, become your caretakers; at times they avoid or abandon you. When these events happen you get stuck in an illness rut.

Almost always, the patient begins to agree, especially when we add the following:

> When the illness rut develops, people become even more dependent and disabled by their pain and symptoms than they really need to be. What we hope to offer you is training which will help you get out of the illness rut and, thus, help you control your life. What we are offering you, in the program, is an opportunity to learn how to live with your symptoms.

Approximately 7 out of 10 patients who come in for the assessment interview agree to enter the program. Despite the usual presence of pressure on the patient from the physician and/or family to enter the program, we stress that the decision to enter the program is entirely the patient's. If the patient declines treatment, we encourage the patient to return to us if and when a change of mind occurs. We also inform the physician that we support the patient's decision not to enter the program at this time, and that we are willing to reconsider the patient in the future. In most instances we also make recommendations to the physician on how to manage the patient in order to minimize his/her illness behaviors and maximize coping.

Instructional Set
Provided to Patients

The instructional set we provide to the patients regarding treatment emphasizes that in order for the patients to learn to function despite their pain and other symptoms, they will have to learn several fundamental life skills. Effective social interaction skills (social skills) are identified as the most important skills to be acquired in order to achieve functional independence from their symptoms.

In order to facilitate this instructional set, we share three assumptions with our patients that are fundamental to our treatment approach. First, we assume that clear biomedical answers and definitive treatments are not forthcoming, and that further pursuit by the patient of biomedical cures will most likely be frustrating, fruitless, or even dangerous. Thus, we recommend and offer to the patients an opportunity to deal with their medical problems using alternatives to biomedical treatment. If a patient enters the program, it is with the understanding that no new biomedical interventions will be attempted or sought while in the program. A relatively stable, although not necessarily benign, medical condition is therefore an implicit prerequisite for entry into the treatment program. If the patient is still undergoing active diagnostic evaluations, treatment by us will not begin until all reasonable diagnostic evaluations are completed and the biomedical treatment for the syndrome or disease has apparently stabilized. The active pursuit of biomedical interventions seems to prevent the patient from fully engaging in our treatment process. Whenever we have admitted patients who are undergoing diagnostic evaluations or extensive biomedical interventions, we have encountered enormous difficulties in helping them reduce their maladaptive illness behaviors and develop coping and well behaviors. Frequently, they have left the program more discouraged about psychological treatment approaches and more convinced that biomedical cures are the answers to their problems.

Some elaboration may be helpful at this point regarding the manner in which medical care can be responsibly managed within such a treatment program. Physicians working directly in the program provide whatever care has been deemed necessary, and the limits of this care are established in an agreement between the physician and patient prior to entry into the treatment program. When consultations with care providers outside the program become necessary, consultation discussions take place between the physician and the consultant rather than between the consultant and patient. This procedure, which eliminates needless attention to biomedical symptoms, reduces the reinforcing value of illness or pain complaints. Meetings are scheduled between the patients and their physicians on a regular (once or twice weekly) basis rather than on an as-needed basis, again to avoid the reinforcement for illness complaints that occurs when meetings are contingent on complaints. The patient–physician meetings are kept as brief as possible, and hands-on examinations are held to a minimum. If extensive medical care becomes necessary, the patient is discharged from the treatment program with an invitation to return as soon as the medical interventions are no longer interfering with active work towards the patient's treatment goals.

The second assumption that we share with patients is that many symptoms and illness behaviors are at least in part learned and maintained by psychosocial factors. We carefully emphasize that this learning is most frequently inadvertent, incidental, and without conscious awareness or intent. Because some of the illness behaviors or symptoms are in part learned, we stress that the patient can unlearn them while simultaneously learning more adaptive behaviors for daily functioning and symptom management. (See also Roberts, Chapter 2 of this volume.) The major focus of treatment is thus removed from symptom reduction through biomedical interventions, and is placed on learning to function socially and generally with more meaning and enjoyment despite the presence of symptoms and medical problems. Also, an explanation of the learning and psychosocial factors involved in their illness patterns provides the patients with a "commonsense" explanation of their problems while removing the implication that their symptoms are "in their heads," as if they were imagined, feigned, or created by mysterious forces. Their symptoms are treated as real despite frequently undiagnosable etiology. The phrase "learning to live with the symptoms" is a familiar and often frustrating one that the patients have frequently heard, and the program attempts to help them accomplish this goal.

The last assumption that we share with our patients is that of responsibility. In matters of health, disease, treatment, and rehabilitation, the physician generally makes most of the decisions involving medical care. The patient is usually a passive recipient of such care, and the physician becomes a caretaker of the patient. In the treatment or rehabilitation of people with chronic pain or illness behavior patterns, however, such physician practices appear to strengthen chronic pain and illness behaviors by reinforcing helplessness and the expectancy that the physician will provide solutions to the existing medical problems. The patients with chronic pain or illness behaviors who are referred to us have a long history of such learning and hold such expectancies of themselves and of their physicians.

In order to help reverse the pattern of helplessness and the externalizing expectancies, and in order to better engage the patient in treatment, we communicate to the patient that treatment will be more effective if he or she assumes the major responsibility for identifying treatment goals and for applying the skills learned in treatment to achieving those goals. The responsibility of the program and of the staff is limited to helping the patient identify the treatment goals and to teaching the patient the various skills necessary for reaching such goals.

Translating the last assumption into a workable approach has been consistently and surprisingly difficult. The difficulty, however, has not been for the patients but for the students who rotate through our program and who largely provide the treatment. It has hardly mattered whether the students have been psychology graduate students, medical students, or medical residents or fellows. Despite their agreement with the third assumption and with the intent on avoiding caretaking relationships with their patients, they do in fact easily develop and maintain such relationships. Close supervision of staff–patient interactions and self-monitoring of their interactions have reduced such caretaking–helplessness interactions but have not always eliminated them.

Social Skills Components and Training Techniques

In this section we describe the several components of the multidimensional chronic pain and chronic illness behavior treatment program. The principal focus will be on social skills training. Additional secondary components of the treatment program include stress management and problem-solving training, neither of which will be described in this chapter. They are adopted primarily from stress inoculation methods described in detail elsewhere (Meichenbaum & Turk, 1976; Turk et al., 1983) and from the problem-solving techniques described in D'Zurilla and Goldfried (1971). (See Holzman, Turk, & Kerns, Chapter 3 of this volume.)

Goal Setting

After the patient agrees to participate in the program, we proceed to help him or her establish specific treatment goals to be achieved while in the program. Each patient establishes goals in four general areas: symptoms, social-interpersonal relationships, family relationships, and future life plans.

In the symptoms area, the patient, with the help of a staff person, formulates treatment objectives by identifying symptom-related difficulties that could be reasonably managed behaviorally by the patient without resorting to medical means. Such symptoms or related difficulties may include medication use, sleep patterns, hours in bed during the day, and physical activity. On each goal, the patient establishes a change in symptom-associated behaviors that is clinically reasonable. For instance, if a patient is spending 8 hours lying down during the day, a reasonable goal may be to reduce the number of hours spent in bed during the day to 2 hours by the end of the program.

Analgesic drug use, principally narcotic medications, is frequently targeted for reduction or discontinuation. We use the Wooley et al. (1978) procedure for reducing medications. Because most pain patients return to some analgesic drug use (Wooley et al., 1978), we encourage patients who are overusing medication to reduce their drug use to a reasonable level and not necessarily to discontinue the drugs. A reasonable level is determined in conference with a physician who helps the patient understand the costs and benefits of narcotic use for chronic pain management. Patients who are already using what is considered to be a reasonable amount of medications are encouraged to consider lower levels of drug use or discontinue such medications for pain control. After a specific schedule of medication use is identified, the patient receives a prescription for the medication and then is given the responsibility for its use. Problems with medication use are discussed during one-on-one sessions.

In the social–interpersonal areas, each patient formulates goals related to quality and/or quantity of social–interpersonal functioning. The patients identify specific social relationship problems and the specific behaviors and/or activities they wish to be performing by the end of treatment in order to modify such problems. Goals may include such behaviors as changing emotional reactions (e.g., reducing anger outbursts), spending more time talking to people, and/or being able to disagree with opinions of others.

In family goal areas, the patient again identifies problem interactions and specifies behavioral goals to be attained in order to modify the problem interactions. Such goals may include an increase in the amount of time spent talking with family members, changes in roles at home, changes in emotional interactions during conversations, and/or reductions in the amount of time spent in talking about symptoms. Symptom-contingent interactions are frequently targeted for reduction in family relationships and interactions.

Life-plan goals principally focus on avocational, vocational, and/or educational functioning. Patients are asked to evaluate their activities and achievements in these areas and then to identify specific changes or improvements they intend to make or initiate during the treatment program. Such goals may include establishing an educational program during treatment, or establishing or identifying during treatment hobbies or activities they can pursue during and/or after treatment.

During the program, each patient is asked to evaluate his or her progress on each goal on a daily basis. A standard scale of 1 to 10 is used, with 1 representing the starting point, 5 representing the level that they wish to attain during treatment, and 10 representing the ideal long-term level. The daily ratings of all goals in each of the four categories are then summed each week, and a weekly average is calculated for each of the four categories. A daily goal rating of 5 or a weekly average of 5 in any one of the four categories means that the patient met his or her treatment goal for that day or for that week. Additional goals or new goal levels may then be established in order to keep the patient working in the treatment program.

A Treatment Paradigm

Because the treatment program is based on broad behavioral principles and assumptions, such principles and assumptions are also taught to our patients. In effect, we set out to make "behavioral scientists" out of our patients insofar as their treatment is concerned. We teach them basic principles of reinforcement and the roles of cognitions, emotions, and pain as antecedents and responses.

The S-O-R-C paradigm, adapted from Kanfer and Phillips (1970) and Keefe and Blumenthal (1982), is used as a device with which the patients can analyze their own behavior and its determinants. Of course, the purpose of this behavior analysis is to help the patient learn to generate new and more effective choices. Each letter in S-O-R-C is the first letter of a word that is essential to understanding any particular chain of behavior. The S signifies Situation, including the context in which a behavior occurs and external events that shortly precede or coincide with the performance of a response. The O is short for Organismic factors. These include covert or internal events, and we explicitly state that thoughts are one category of organismic factors; feelings (including affects and physiological responses) are other organismic factors. The R refers to the overt Response that is voluntary in nature and that is partially determined by the thoughts and feelings that one experiences in a given situation. The C signifies Consequences of behavior. The events consequent to overt responses as well as the events that follow thought and feeling patterns are crucial determinants of future covert and overt behavior patterns.

It is often useful to extend the analysis of a chain of behavior by viewing the consequences in one chain of behavior as situational determinants (the S in S-O-R-C) in the immediately following behavior chain. Responses of other people to our overt responses, for example, almost always affect our future responses in similar situations. Those same reactions of others also serve as situational determinants of our very next thought, feeling, and response patterns. It is worthy of note that on follow-up, patients consistently report that this S-O-R-C model is a valuable and frequently used tool to understand and deal with behavior in various situations.

Social Skills Components

The content of our social skills training program is abstracted principally from Alberti and Emmons (1974), Cotles and Guerra (1976), and Lange and Jakubowski (1977). Based on the success of the Wooley et al. (1978) program and the experience that the senior author acquired in that program, we decided to teach the patients the same social skills that were used in the Cincinnati program.

We found that teaching the following named skills required an enormous amount of time. In order for the skills to be learned and used outside of the treatment sessions, it was necessary to repeat frequently the definitions and descriptions of the behaviors and to role-play them frequently. We believe that had we targeted additional social skills for training, we would not have been able to teach them effectively within a 4- to 6-week time period. The social skills that are targeted in our program are assertiveness, expression of feelings, active listening, and behavioral shaping. The shaping skill, which is not a social skill usually targeted in social skill teaching, was included largely to help patients understand and be able to use a graduated approach to skill acquisition or behavior change, whether one's own behavior or that of another.

Criteria for achieving competence in skill use are largely based on each patient's ability to perform the skill several times in group practice and on a report by the patient of successful use of the skill in some social context outside of the program. No other criteria are used to assess competence. We have found that group performance is a highly reliable method of determining adequate skill acquisition, and we make it the responsibility of the patient to apply it outside of the group.

The assertiveness skills that are taught and practiced include saying "no" to requests by others, expressing disagreements, requesting behavior changes, and expressing personal beliefs and opinions. In teaching expression of feelings, we focus primarily on teaching the patient to identify feelings by using situational and cognitive determinants and then teaching them to express the feeling directly and appropriately. The feelings we principally focus on are fear/anxiety, anger, sadness/depression, happiness, and love, or any of their variations. The principal active listening skills that are taught are reflecting back to others what one has heard, asking for clarification, and "listening" to body language. In teaching the behavioral-shaping component, the concept is taught first, followed by teaching the patients to subdivide goal behaviors into smaller steps, and then by teaching the patients to use reinforcement as each step is attained successfully. Finally, each patient is asked to apply the method to one of his or her goals.

The format that we use for social skills training is basically a group didactic and role-playing format. One-on-one sessions are also used to further facilitate skill acquisition. In such sessions, a more personalized treatment focus allows for more specific discussions and rehearsals of the skills. We encourage up to several one-on-one treatment sessions each week. The social skills group, usually composed of two to six patients, is held three times each week for about 2 hours each session. During each treatment session we introduce whatever social skill(s) we are attempting to teach during that session by first describing and then demonstrating the skill(s). We engage the patients in a discussion of the skill or lack of it in their lives, and then help them identify various instances in which the skill could be used.

After the discussion and the demonstration of the skills by the group leader, we start rehearsing the skill by using role-playing procedures in which patients take an active role. Each role-playing attempt is reinforced by the group leader, as well as critiqued by any group member, in order to improve the quality of the patient's skill. In addition to shaping each skill, the role-playing and critique approach appears to have a highly desensitizing effect on the patients' anxiety associated with social performance, and seems to enhance their willingness to participate in the role-playing sessions. To facilitate skill acquisition, we guide the role-playing by first using seemingly less threatening social situations and gradually moving to more relevant and difficult social interactions. For instance, in order to learn to ask someone to change a behavior, we may first have the patient role-play making a request of his child to stop making noise, then role-play asking a relative not to park in the driveway, and finally have the patient role-play a request of his neighbor to keep his barking dogs inside because the barking is annoying to the patient.

The group leader's role is highly important to the treatment process. The group leader explains the various components of treatment to the patients: the S-O-R-C paradigm, the social skills, the self-evaluations. The group leader demonstrates the various social skills and helps to integrate the various components of treatment to facilitate general and personal understanding of the content. Additionally, the group leader must manage the group process, reinforce patients who participate in the group process, and extinguish complaining, nonparticipation, or any other illness behavior. It is frequently tempting to focus on a patient who is behaving in a helpless or even resistant manner and attempt to talk him or her into group participation. Such a focus serves to reinforce illness behavior and needs to be avoided to a great degree.

Whenever the group begins to complain excessively or resist therapeutic activity, it is most probably due to inadvertent attention paid to negative behaviors by the group leader. Systematic training and monitoring of the group leader's behavior are recommended in order to avoid such pitfalls.

At the end of each treatment session, the patients are asked to apply these skills between sessions to their goals and to any other situation they find appropriate. The decision to apply these skills is left to each patient without specific assignments or agreements. Their efforts are reviewed and discussed the next day during the first part of the group session. The group leader's role during this phase is very important. In order to reinforce effort, the major focus of the discussion and review needs to be on those reports that were even minimally successful. Whenever the focus of the discussions and reports shifts to failure or lack of application, we frequently observe an increase in such failure reports and a decrease in skill applications. By focusing on efforts and success, we seem to reinforce application and can avoid formal assignments for overnight activity, making it a natural responsibility of the patient.

Each social skill is presented twice during each patient's participation in the treatment program. Such repetition appears to help the patient apply the skills in progressively more difficult social situations, and occasionally results in a spontaneous emergence of an active "teaching" role by a patient in the group. Group entry in our program is staggered, and newer group members appear to learn from the modeling of the various behaviors by more experienced group members. Whenever a patient begins to actively teach some of the behaviors, it greatly enhances the credibility of our efforts, especially with more skeptical patients during the early phase of their treatment program.

During social skills training, we consistently discuss the application of the social skills to many social and family situations. To facilitate this transfer, role-playing scenarios are frequently chosen from many such situations. We believe that the focus on applications to specific situations facilitates generalizations of learning. In the Wooley et al. (1978) program, such transfer was achieved by inviting the family to participate in aspects of the treatment. In the Albuquerque program such generalization appeared to occur because of the focus on home practice permitted by an outpatient day hospital program. We believe that one of the advantages of an outpatient day hospital program is a more natural generalization of training.

Ending the Program

The program for each patient ends after 4 weeks of treatment. If the patient has progressed adequately during treatment and desires to further improve his or her skills, the program can be extended by 2 additional weeks. Usually, additional goals are identified and the patient proceeds through the program as before. After completing 4 or 6 weeks of treatment, each patient receives a diploma in a "graduation ceremony." During the graduation ceremony, which is attended by all patients and staff members, the patient describes his overall progress, one specific goal he or she achieved during treatment, and the skills or methods that were used to reach the goal. Additionally, the patient identifies one remaining goal yet to be achieved and a plan for attaining that goal. After the patient finishes the presentation, staff members describe their observations of the patient's progress and the specific behavioral changes that were observed. Then, a certificate of achievement is presented to the patient. A follow-up appointment is also scheduled for the purpose of reviewing the patient's progress.

Based on patient request, further one-on-one sessions may be held to facilitate any additional fine-tuning of the patient's skills. If no requests for additional help are made by the patient, no further formal therapy contact with the patient is made by our staff.

CONCLUSIONS AND RECOMMENDATIONS

Chronic pain and chronic illness behavior patterns frequently confront the health care provider. Not only are those behavior patterns costly ones, but they are very difficult to treat using any of several biomedical treatment modalities. Data are beginning to accumulate that suggest that psychosocial determinants increase the likelihood of developing and maintaining pain and illness behaviors, and social skills deficits appear to be among those determinants.

This chapter described a rationale and approach to treating chronic pain and illness patients that principally focuses on social skills training. Although some studies question the value of assertiveness training (e.g., Sanders, 1983), outcome data strongly support the efficacy of programs such as the one which we have described (Fedoravicius et al., in press; Wooley et al., 1978). It is possible that differences in the breadth and amount of social skills training between these programs account for the differences in outcome. Additionally, different subpopulations of chronic pain and chronic illness patients may be participating in such studies due to differing criteria for admission into the programs or due to differing conceptualizations of pain and illness behavior that may underlie selection differences. What is clear is that treatment programs for chronic pain and chronic illness behavior that use social skills training as a part of their treatment strategy, and that are provided on an outpatient basis, report cost-effective treatment outcomes.

We also do not want to miss this opportunity to briefly discuss additional aspects of our treatment approach that seem to have an incredibly powerful effect on the process and outcome of treatment. It seems that the assumptions that we make regarding illness and its effects are communicated sincerely to our patients in such a way that attempts to change themselves are more comfortable to the patients than are their other options (such as pursuing biomedical cures, remaining socially isolated, etc.). The explanation of the illness rut seems to help the patients feel that we understand them and have taken the time to learn about them. The focus on self-understanding within the S-O-R-C model, perhaps the single most important integrating yet pragmatic aspect of our program, allows the patient to become introspective within a relatively short time. Our encouragement to

stop seeking biomedical cures, at least while in treatment with us, helps the patients to become committed to trying as hard as they can to function better regardless of the possible biomedical reality of their symptoms. We also manage to help patients strengthen their beliefs that they can make changes that will increase their enjoyment in life despite the pain, and we do this without minimizing the reality of their symptoms and without demeaning their previous attempts to cope.

In addition to acting in accord with these assumptions and explaining them to the patients, we attempt to listen to each patient and to tailor our discussions and role-plays so as to maximize the meaningfulness of each interaction. The therapist/group leader's skill depends upon his or her own interpersonal skills, belief in the assumptions that we share with our patients, practice in successfully listening to patients' issues, and appreciation of the complex interplay of factors affecting human behavior.

REFERENCES

Alberti, R.E., & Emmons, M.L. (1974). *Your perfect right: A guide to assertive behavior.* San Luis Obispo, CA: Impact.

Barsky, A.J., & Klerman, G.L. (1983). Overview: Hypochondriasis, bodily complaints, and somatic styles. *The American Journal of Psychiatry, 140,* 273–283.

Beals, R.K., & Hickman, N.W. (1972). Industrial injuries of the back and extremeties. Comprehensive evaluation—An aid in prognosis and management. *Journal of Bone and Joint Surgery, 54*-A, 1593–1611.

Bellack, A.S. (1983). Recurrent problems in the behavioral assessment of social skill. *Behavior Research and Therapy, 21,* 29–41.

Cotles, S.B., & Guerra, J.J. (1976). *Assertion training: A humanistic-behavioral guide to self-dignity.* Champaign, IL: Research Press.

Cox, G.B., Chapman, C.R., & Black, R.G. (1978). The MMPI and chronic pain: The diagnosis of psychogenic pain. *Journal of Behavioral Medicine, 1,* 437–443.

D'Zurilla, T.J., & Goldfried, M.R. (1971). Problem-solving and behavior modification. *Journal of Abnormal Psychology, 78,* 107–126.

Elton, D., Stanley, G.V., & Burrows, G.D. (1978). Self-esteem and chronic pain. *Journal of Psychosomatic Research, 22,* 25–30.

Elton, D., Stanley, G.V., & Burrows, G.D. (1983). *Psychological control of pain.* New York: Grune & Stratton.

Fabrega, H., Jr. (1979). The ethnography of illness. *Social Science and Medicine, 13A,* 565–576.

Fedoravicius, A.S., Mariano, M. J., Leight, K., Stehr, D., & Klein, B.J. (in press). Behavioral treatment of chronic illness behavior: An outpatient replication. *Psychosomatic Medicine.*

Ford, C.V. (1983). *The somatizing disorders: Illness as a way of life.* New York: Elsevier Biomedical.

Gottlieb, H., Strite, L.C., Koller, R., Madorsky, A., Hockersmith, V., Kleeman, M., & Wagner, J. (1977). Comprehensive rehabilitation of patients having chronic low back pain. *Archives of Physical Medicine and Rehabilitation, 58,* 101–108.

Heaton, R.K., Getto, C.J., Lehman, R.A.W., Fordyce, W.E., Brauer, E., & Groban, S.E. (1982). A standardized evaluation of psychosocial factors in chronic pain. *Pain, 12,* 165–174.

Kanfer, F.H., & Phillips, J.E. (1970). *Learning foundations of behavior therapy.* New York: John Wiley & Sons.

Katon, W., Kleinman, A., & Rosen, G. (1982). Depression and somatization: A review. *The American Journal of Medicine, 72,* 127–135, 241–247.

Keefe, F.J., & Blumenthal, J.A. (1982). Behavioral medicine: Basic principles and theoretical foundations. In F.J. Keefe and J.A. Blumenthal (Eds.), *Assessment strategies in behavioral medicine* (pp. 3–16). New York: Grune & Stratton.

Lange, A.J., & Jakubowski, P. (1977). Responsible assertive behavior: *Cognitive-behavioral procedures for trainers.* Champaign, IL: Research Press.

Leavitt, F., & Garron, D.C. (1979a). Psychological disturbance and pain report differences in both organic and non-organic low back pain patients. *Pain, 7,* 187–195.

Leavitt, F., & Garron, D.C. (1979b). The detection of psychological disturbance in patients with low back pain. *Journal of Psychosomatic Research, 23,* 149–154.

Louks, J.L., Freeman, C.W., & Caslyn, D.A. (1978). Personality organization as an aspect of back pain in a medical setting. *Journal of Personality Assessment, 42,* 152–158.

Meichenbaum, D., & Turk, D.C. (1976). The cognitive-behavioral management of anxiety, anger, and pain. In P.O. Davidson (Eds.), *The behavioral management of anxiety, depression, and pain.* New York: Brunner/Mazel.

Melzack, R. (1973). *The puzzle of pain.* New York: Basic Books.

Merskey, H., & Spear, F.G. (1967). *Pain: Psychological and psychiatric aspects.* London: Bailliere, Tindall, and Cassell.

Morgan, C.D., Kremer, E., & Gaylor, M. (1979). The behavioral medicine unit: A new facility. *Comprehensive Psychiatry, 20,* 79–89.

Osborne, D. (1979). Use of the MMPI with medical patients. In J.N. Butcher (Ed.), *New developments in the use of the MMPI* (pp. 141–163). Minneapolis, MN: University of Minnesota.

Pennebaker, J.W. (1982). *The psychology of physical symptoms.* New York: Springer-Verlag.

Pilowsky, I., & Spence, N. (1975). Patterns of illness behavior in patients with intractable pain. *Journal of Psychosomatic Research, 19,* 279–287.

Pinkerton, S.S., Hughes, H., & Wenrich, W.W. (1982). Behavioral medicine: *Clinical applications.* New York: John Wiley and Sons.

Prokop, C.K., Bradley, L.A., Margolis, R., & Gentry, W.D. (1980). Multivariate analyses of the MMPI profiles of multiple pain patients. *Journal of Personality Assessment, 44,* 246–252.

Sanders, S.H. (1979). Behavioral assessment and treatment of clinical pain: Appraisal of current status. In M. Hersen, R. Eisler, & P. Miller (Eds.), *Progress in behavior modification* (Vol. 8, pp. 249–291). New York: Academic Press.

Sanders, S.H. (1983). Component analysis of a behavioral treatment program for chronic low-back pain. *Behavior Therapy, 14,* 697–705.

Turk, D.C., Meichenbaum, D., & Genest, M. (1983). *Pain and behavioral medicine: A cognitive-behavioral perspective.* New York: Guilford Press.

Turkat, I.D. (1982). An investigation of parental modelling in the etiology of diabetic illness behavior. *Behaviour Research and Therapy, 20,* 547–552.

Turkat, I.D., & Noskin, D. E. (1983). Vicarious and operant experiences in the etiology of illness behavior: A replication with healthy individuals. *Behaviour Research and Therapy, 21,* 169–172.

Turner, J.A. (1982). Comparison of group progressive-relaxation training and cognitive-behavioral group therapy for chronic low back pain. *Journal of Consulting and Clinical Psychology, 50,* 757–765.

Turner, J.A., & Chapman, C.R. (1982). Psychological interventions for chronic pain: A critical review. II. Operant conditioning, hypnosis, and cognitive-behavioral therapy. *Pain, 12,* 23–46.

Twaddle, A.C. (1974). The concept of health status. *Social Science and Medicine, 8,* 29–38.

Whitehead, W.E., Fedoravicius, A.S., Blackwell, B., & Wooley, S. (1979). A behavioral conceptualization of psychosomatic illness: Psychosomatic symptoms as learned responses. In J.R. McNamara (Ed.), *Behavioral approaches to medicine: Applications and analysis* (pp. 65–99). New York: Plenum Press.

Whitehead, W.E., Winget, C., Fedoravicius,

A.S., Wooley, S., & Blackwell, B. (1982). Learned illness behavior in patients with irritable bowel syndrome and peptic ulcer. *Digestive Diseases and Sciences*, *27*, 202–208.

Wiltse L.L., & Rocchio, D.D. (1975). Preoperative psychological tests as predictors of success of chemonucleolysis in the treatment of low back syndrome. *Journal of Bone and Joint Surgery*, *57-A*, 478–483.

Wooley, S.C., & Blackwell, B. (1975). A behavioral probe into social contingencies on a psychosomatic ward. *Journal of Applied Behavior Analysis*, *8*, 337–339.

Wooley, S.C., Blackwell, B., Glaudin, V., & Lipkin, J. (1973, November). *A new behavioral approach to psychosomatic medicine*. Paper presented to Academy of Psychosomatic Medicine, Williamsburg, VA.

Wooley, S.C., Blackwell, B., & Winget, C. (1978). A learning theory model of Chronic Illness Behavior: Theory, treatment, and research. *Psychosomatic Medicine*, *40*, 379–401.

7 PAIN GROUPS

W. Doyle Gentry
Daniel Owens

Psychological treatment programs specifically designed for chronic pain sufferers have typically been offered on a one-to-one basis tailored to fit the individual needs of the chronic pain patient. Such programs, both inpatient and outpatient alike, have included treatment strategies such as biofeedback, hypnosis, operant conditioning, relaxation training, and cognitive restructuring, all of which have proven effective in helping individual patients manage their chronic pain experience and increase their level of adaptive nonpain behavior.

References to the use of group therapy in treating chronic pain patients, on the other hand, have been scattered and few in number. For the most part, these references have been lacking in detail as regards either (a) a clinical rationale for such groups or (b) the actual mechanics of setting up and running such groups. Neither do these references suggest how pain groups compare with individual treatment approaches as regards their efficacy in altering the psychological aspects of chronic pain experience.

Sternbach (Sternbach, 1974; Greenhoot & Sternbach, 1974; Ignelzi, Sternbach, & Timmermans, 1977; Sternbach & Rusk, 1973) has consistently used group therapy as part

of a comprehensive milieu treatment program for patients hospitalized with chronic benign pain. Sternbach's "transactional approach," which is primarily aimed at challenging "pain games" (Sternbach, 1974; Sternbach, Wolf, Murphy, & Akeson, 1973; Szaz, 1968) played by patients, is well suited to a group format in which staff and other patients alike can expose and disrupt such games. Other references to the use of pain groups in treating chronic pain patients include: Cairns, Thomas, Mooney, and Pace (1976); Newman, Seres, Yospe, and Garlington (1978); and Swanson, Maruta, and Swenson (1979).

In this chapter, we will recount our clinical experience over the past several years with pain groups. Our goal is to share with fellow practitioners (a) our rationale for choosing group therapy as a *primary* therapeutic modality in treating such patients, (b) our thoughts about selection and composition of pain groups, (c) our understanding of the "how to do it" mechanics of conducting pain groups, (d) our view of the changing role(s) of the therapist in pain groups, (e) our summary of what we see as the probable "group dynamics" that account for behavioral changes seen in treated patients, and (f) selected case vignettes to illustrate the type of behavioral changes one can expect of patients exposed to this type of treatment.

Although our experience to date has largely involved treating persons with chronic back pain, we believe it is equally applicable to other types of chronic pain (e.g., tension and migraine headaches), as well as other types of chronic physical illness (e.g., multiple sclerosis; VanderPlate, 1984).

RATIONALE

There are at least seven clinically relevant reasons for considering pain groups as a primary technique in helping patients cope more effectively with the chronic pain experience and associated disability:

1. Although it is certainly true that no two persons cope with chronic pain/disability the same way, they do, as a group, face common problems (e.g., addiction to pain-killing drugs, recurrent depression, excessive dependency). They unwittingly become involved in many of the same "pain games," which as Sternbach (1974) notes are few in number when compared to the large number of individuals involved. Accordingly, they require similar sorts of advice, counseling, education, and therapeutic confrontation. One reason for establishing pain groups, therefore, is to *eliminate therapist redundancy* in dealing with this rather homogeneous patient population.

2. Pain groups also represent a most *economical use of therapeutic resources* by allowing the therapist to treat a greater number of patients than would be feasible using individualized treatment approaches. This, we feel, is an important consideration, given the epidemic nature of chronic pain disorders in our society today. As has been pointed out elsewhere (Turk, Meichenbaum, & Genest, 1983), chronic pain impacts on millions of Americans yearly and may well account for up to 80% of all physician visits.

3. Pain groups provide a means of *ameliorating the abiding sense of social isolation and alienation* common to all chronic pain sufferers. Anyone who has experienced pain continu-

ously for any significant time period (6 months or longer) comes to believe that "I am different from others around me because of my pain!" Over a decade ago, Timmermans and Sternbach (1974) noted that this sense of "interpersonal alienation" included feelings of being helpless and out of control, of being angry and suspicious toward others, and of blaming others for one's difficulties and unhappiness. Such feelings underlie much of the manipulativeness observed in chronic pain patients, that is, "special attempts to influence others" and thereby regain some measure of control over one's life (Timmermans & Sternbach, 1974, p. 807). Pain groups provide a new, much needed source of social support that competes with this sense of alienation. This is, we believe, the reason that patients form pain treatment "alumni associations" (Newman et al., 1978) and frequently carry on with treatment discussions outside of format treatment settings (Greenhoot & Sternbach, 1974).

4. Pain groups offer the chronic pain patient a type of *credible feedback* (confrontation), at least in their eyes, not found in individual treatment. That is, patients are apt to resist feedback from therapists on the premise that the therapist is a *well* person who simply cannot appreciate the extent of their suffering. This is evident in frequently heard statements such as: "You don't understand what it's like to live with pain 24 hours a day!" and "If you had constant pain like I've got, you'd be a bitch too!" Again, as Greenhoot and Sternbach (1974, p. 599) note: "Patients may deceive themselves or the staff, but they do not long deceive other patients with whom they live."

5. Pain groups also provide the therapist with a *different diagnostic perspective*, that is, the therapist has an opportunity to witness the chronic pain patient's behavior in a social context—the group. Our view of pain groups is that they represent a *microcosm* of the real world in which the patient is forced to "play off other persons," thereby displaying adaptive and maladaptive coping strategies *in vivo* rather than (self-) reporting what he or she

would do in such circumstances. Observation of pain patients in the group therapy setting offers new "grist for the mill" in individual therapy and thereby often accelerates progress in the latter.

6. Pain groups allow an opportunity for patients to *define a new reference group* (other pain patients) *and engage in what we call lateral conformity,* i.e., respond to social pressures from other group members to conform to certain shared realities regarding their pain experience and "rules" about living with the limitations established by traumatic injury or disease. This we would contrast with *vertical conformity,* in which the patient is asked to conform to goals and/or behavioral prescriptions set forth by caregivers who are seen as being on a higher plane of health (wellness). The latter, we feel, is more appropriate for persons suffering from an acute pain disorder.

7. Finally, pain groups allow the therapist to *avoid the pitfall of patient dependency,* that is, assuming primary responsibility for "fixing" the patient's problem(s). In the group setting, this responsibility is, at the very least, shared by other members of the group from the outset.

MECHANICS

Several issues pertaining to the "nuts and bolts" of pain groups need to be addressed at this point.

First, how is the patient introduced to the pain group? Basically, all patients are seen initially in individual therapy and then, when appropriate, shifted into the pain group. There are two reasons for holding to this sequence: (a) It allows the therapist time to fully appreciate the patient's suitability and prognosis for participation in the group (e.g., assessing what type of pain games the patient will bring to the group, how much social anxiety is evident, etc.) and (b) it ensures that the patient has adequate ego-strength to face up to group confrontation(s) without feeling intimidated or threatened. With respect to the latter, it is helpful to the new patient entering the pain

group for the first time to perceive a "link" between himself or herself and at least one other person, namely the therapist. On those few occasions where we have failed to build sufficient rapport with the pain patient in individual therapy first, he or she has unfortunately "literally bolted from the group in midsession" or terminated treatment altogether after one or two group sessions.

Second, what are the selection criteria for pain groups? With one single exception (i.e., persons with gross personality disorganization — active or borderline psychosis), we see no basis for excluding any patient from participation in the group therapy program. Nevertheless, our experience thus far does suggest that some patients are more suitable candidates than others.

For example, individuals who score high on the Pd (Psychopathic Deviate) scale of the Minnesota Multiphasic Personality Inventory (MMPI) tend to drop out prematurely, show poor attendance ("Tell the doctor I can't come to group today because my back hurts!"), evidence higher levels of resistance to confrontation, and demonstrate a greater number and variety of "pain games." This observation is consistent with Sternbach's (1974) earlier labeling of patients with an elevated Pd score as "con artists."

Males, we find, are also less likely to engage in self-disclosure in pain groups or to feel at ease in confronting other patients as regards maladaptive coping strategies; their general attitude more often than not seems to be "every man for himself" when it comes to surviving one's chronic pain experience.

Finally, those patients who have been in pain a shorter period of time and/or have not yet had surgery to correct the pain problem seem less motivated to fully participate in group therapy. It is easier, we think, for such patients to deny the reality of their chronic pain condition, that is, wait for it to get better on its own or for some caregiver to "work his magic," than it is for them to accept the harsh verdict that they "will have to learn to live with the pain."

Age, race, educational background, social

class, or marital status do not seem to influence how well patients do in pain groups.

Third, should groups be time limited? We have thus far not seen fit to set time limits (i.e., specific number of sessions) on our pain groups for the simple reason that chronic pain has no time limits, that is, "It is a problem that has a beginning, a middle, but no end; it will be with you until the day you die!" This is not to say that all patients enrolled in the group stay the same amount of time; on the contrary, patients exit at varying points (when they feel they have benefited all they can) and in some cases reenter (on their own initiative) the group for varying periods of time depending on their need.

Fourth, should pain groups be open or closed as regards membership? We have noted that once "group cohesion" is firmly established, it is difficult to introduce new members without disrupting the group process. On the other hand, having new persons introduced into ongoing groups allows (a) those patients who are new and exhibiting maladaptive coping strategies to learn from veteran group members, who have graduated to a higher level of adaptation, while at the same time (b) those veteran patients can feel good about themselves (be self-reinforced) for the progress they have made. Veteran patients can also serve as co-therapists.

Fifth, what is the role of the therapist in pain groups? We see a variety of roles for the group therapist working with chronic pain patients. First, the therapist is an *educator*, for example, explaining to patients (a) what is common to the chronic pain experience—interpersonal alienation and manipulativeness (Timmermans & Sternbach, 1974), (b) what is fact versus fantasy, and (c) what they can anticipate as regards coping in the future (e.g., we stress the point that "depression is always right around the corner," meaning that mood swings accompany all chronic illnesses).

Second, the therapist is a *facilitator* both with respect to social cohesion and confrontation. For example, the therapist may conduct a variety of "cohesion exercises," ranging from simple tasks such as having group members share some personal attribute(s) about themselves (or a designated other group member) to group test-taking (e.g., periodic assessment of levels of depression via the Beck Depression Inventory; Beck, 1967). We believe it is important in this instance that the therapist be an active, full, and sharing participant in such exercises rather than being seen as an "outside agent."

Finally, we see the group therapist as an *observer*, both of group process and of individual change by members within the group. This latter role is perhaps the most important role of all as regards its potential for therapeutic impact in that it allows the therapist (a) to be something other than "a psychologist," (b) to be human, and (c) to be absent from the group while the members set their own session-by-session agenda, engage in confrontation, and take increasing responsibility for managing and/or treating themselves. We see a natural evolution and/or progression of roles from the active, information-giving, didactic role of "educator" to the more passive, commentator role of "observer." To illustrate the *observer* role more fully, we offer the following group vignette:

After a group therapy session in which the therapist had sat quietly for about an hour, the following exchange took place:

Patient: Well, Dr._____, you've been awfully quiet today. We haven't gotten very far in this session, have we?

Therapist: Quite the contrary! I think the group has done a lot today, perhaps more than it realizes.

Patient: (puzzled) What? All we've done is sit around and laugh and tell dirty jokes; we didn't talk much about our problems, pain.

Therapist: I know. That's why I think it's a good session, a milestone of sorts.

Patient: (still puzzled) I don't understand what you mean?

Therapist: It's actually quite simple. What I have been sitting here observing for the past hour are eight people—human beings, laughing and enjoying themselves in a natural, healthy way. What I had to remind myself repeatedly was that you're all here because you're suffering from chronic pain. You haven't, whether you realized it or not, been acting like "pain patients," you know sad, complaining, angry, etc. For once, the group, from the very outset, wasn't focused on pain; it was focused on people, each other. It's nice to see you all laugh, to hear you laugh, in such a natural, unguarded manner. I think the group has given itself permission to enjoy life still, despite the pain. I think that's real progress, don't you?

Group: All affirmative responses. . . .

Sixth, is formal goal-setting or behavioral contracting an integral part of group treatment? The answer is no. We have thus far chosen not to interrupt the ebb and flow of group process with prescribed behavioral assignments, exercises, goal-setting, and so forth. Such activities are normally carried out in conjoint individual therapy and not introduced by the therapist as part of formal group therapy. This is not to say that patients do not occasionally introduce such issues into the group discussion; they do. As we noted earlier, however, our goal is to shift away from the more active role of individual therapist to one of facilitator and observer, which is, in our experience, easier done when structure is at a minimum (e.g., reviewing behavioral assignments from the previous session). We do, of course, find that group members increasingly reestablish and reprioritize (e.g., shifting from "pain reduction" as a primary goal to "coping with pain") their own goals as a function of group therapy, and that group therapy discussions often speed up efforts in individual therapy aimed at goal-setting in the more traditional sense.

Seventh, are spouse, family, and significant others ever included in group therapy for chronic pain patients? To date, we have chosen *not* to include "significant others" in our pain groups. Although we certainly agree that these individuals would benefit from the group process and group discussion(s), we also appreciate the fact that (a) many would be reluctant to participate and (b) their presence, especially early on, would in most cases inhibit group cohesion, self-disclosure, and willingness on the patient's part to acknowledge/relinquish

various "pain games," many of which directly involve these other persons.

We believe, however, that it may be beneficial to meet with "significant others" either in a separate group (i.e., so that they can share their concerns about living with a chronic pain patient, derive support from each other, and acquire helpful information about chronic pain and its effects[s] on people, marriages, and family systems) or as part of our regular group therapy after the group is functioning as a cohesive entity. Just as the group provides a "safety net" for confrontations about "pain games" between patients, we think it can equally serve to facilitate and safeguard similar transactions between patient and significant other(s). As we know already, much of what is seen as chronic invalidism, maladaptive coping, and *painmanship* (Szaz, 1968) can, in fact, result from needs on the part of those who interact with the chronic pain patient, for example, to *deny* the reality of chronic pain in a loved one ("Don't pay attention to what that doctor says, honey; we'll find another doctor who will fix this thing once and for all!"), to *take care of* the pain patient (i.e., fostering dependency), etc.

GROUP DYNAMICS

Our experience clinically tells us that pain groups work to help chronic pain patients learn more effectively to cope or manage their pain on a daily basis and, more importantly, to reintegrate themselves into the mainstream of their social environment. But how is this actually achieved? What is there about the group that enables the pain patients to change their behavior (e.g., to give up their "pain games"), especially in the absence, as we have already noted, of prescribed objective behavioral goals and exercises?

Our best guess at the moment is based solely on clinical observation. As individual treatment strategies for chronic pain give way to group treatment approaches, we hope that systematic research efforts will support or refute our impressions. We see the following only as a starting point for clinical discussion:

To begin with, the group *promotes the concept of universality;* that is, it quickly makes the alienated, isolated, depressed, and withdrawn chronic pain patients aware that they are not alone in their pain experience. As they look around the group, they see "kindred souls" struggling, more or less successfully, with the same problem: chronic pain. Because we have limited exclusion criteria for group membership, they quickly learn that no type of individual or class of people is exempt from this "cursed" disorder; in our groups, they see people of different races, sexes, ages, social strata, etc., all confronted with the same problem: How to survive chronic pain?

Next, the group *provides a forum for shared catharsis.* It represents the one place that they are free to talk about their worst fears (e.g., invalidism, total dependency, addiction), their pent-up hostility towards caregivers (surgeons, psychologists, psychiatrists, and pain clinics) who in the past have failed to make them well, and their resentment of well people (e.g., spouse, family members, friends) with whom they interact on a daily basis. As Sternbach (1974) has noted, it is this shared catharsis that makes for an *esprit de corps* or group cohesion among members of the group, which in turn is a vital enabling condition for meaningful confrontation as regards maladaptive painmanship.

Group therapy also serves as a *place for imparting information and disconfirming myths* about chronic pain. For example, discussions early on include statistics about outcomes of elective back surgery for the initial surgical procedure, as well as subsequent procedures, so that patients can make educated, informed decisions about surgery as an approach to pain relief and/or reduction when and if this opportunity arises. We attempt to educate them as to the fact that surgery does *not* provide pain relief in many cases and in fact may well make them worse off in terms of levels of felt pain, prognosis for return to gainful employment, and general functional capacity (Gentry, 1982).

We also spend a considerable amount of time discussing the appropriate use of pain drugs in managing chronic pain (e.g., time-contingent vs. pain-contingent administration) and the extent of drug misuse in this patient population (Ziesat, Angle, & Gentry 1979). Although we agree with Sternbach (1974) that many "pain games" are motivated by payoffs in the patient's immediate social environment, we also believe that many patients operate out of ignorance and/or on the basis of shared myths (e.g., about the curative effects of elective surgery) about pain and its treatment.

The pain group is a *place for learning and sharing specific skills for managing pain* on a day-to-day basis. Patients share how they have learned to pace themselves in terms of a schedule of daily activities, so as not to inadvertently produce pain by overdoing. Relaxation techniques are shared, for example, playing a guitar, knitting, meditation, and reaching out and touching a loved one during episodes of intense pain. Cognitive restructuring (i.e., what patients tell themselves about coping with chronic pain) is discussed; for example, patients will share perceptions that "You hurt whether you go shopping or not; so the choice isn't between having pain or not, it's a choice between whether you go shopping or stay home!" and "It's not that you can't stand the pain—you can; it's that you don't want to stand the pain. Okay, tell yourself that you don't want to, but you can!" And, patients model changes in the acceptance of and adjustment to chronic pain, for example, increasing their activities outside the home, engaging in pleasurable pursuits (e.g., bingo, bridge, craft work) that conform to their physical limitations, doing volunteer work, and in some cases returning to part-time or full-time gainful employment, for each other. With respect to the latter, we have noticed a "contagion effect," whereby significant positive changes in a nonpain behavior of one group member will shortly be followed by similar changes in several other members.

The pain group *provides a new or renewed sense of hope* as regards both (a) their ability to survive chronic pain and (b) their ability to develop a sense of mastery and pleasure in the course of normal day-to-day interactions. This sense of hope leads to renewed self-esteem, which in turn is accompanied by philosophical and behavioral shifts toward a more *proactive posture* as regards acting on the social environment to meet one's own needs, pain or no pain. As patients become more hopeful, they verbally shift from a negative (I can't . . . because of my pain!) to a positive (I can. . .; I did. . .; I am. . . .) mode of expression. They systematically engage in less and less care-seeking behavior and deal more independently with the world around them. As one group noted in a self-assessment of progress made during therapy, there is an increasing sense that "We are terrific human beings!" even if we do suffer from chronic pain, that "we can and we will survive!"

Next, as we have repeatedly emphasized throughout this chapter, group therapy *provides a new social support system* for the chronic pain patient, who prior to the group therapy experience typically struggled along without meaningful support. As has been aptly pointed out elsewhere (Gentry & Kobasa, 1984; Lazarus & Folkman, 1984), social support — which can consist of some combination of the following: a sense of belonging and emotional support; tangible support (money, assistance); information (advice); appraisal (feedback or social comparison relevant to a person's self-evaluation — is an important mediator of stress–illness relationships.

In this case, we believe social support alters the link between stress/emotional upset and pain complaint/disability. It is the supportive aspect of group therapy that leads most patients to attend on a regular basis, to offer each other assistance in getting to/from group sessions, to inquire about absent members, to engage in regular contact outside of scheduled group meetings, and to accept the confrontational feedback as regards "pain games" offered during therapy sessions. Just how important social support is and how immediate its effect can be felt is illustrated by the following anecdote.

One patient, a woman in her early 40s, was referred to our pain group because of adjustment problems, most notably depression, resulting from chronic pain secondary to back injury and elective surgery, which failed to significantly relieve her pain experience. She rather reluctantly agreed, after several individual therapy sessions, to come to group therapy, stating from the outset that "I don't like to talk about my problems and pain in front of a bunch of other people." In the first session, she was verbal, talking in an angry, emotional tone about her pain, how much she hurt, all the things she couldn't do, and how "unfair" life had been to her. The group was generally supportive, indicating how they also had experienced such feelings, but how they were beginning to feel somewhat more optimistic about their ability to survive their pain and "get on with the rest of their lives" in some fashion. She did not appear at all reassured; rather, she seemed even more upset, having verbalized a lot of suppressed negative feelings in front of these other people.

Three days later, when she came into the office for her next scheduled individual appointment, she started out by stating that she had almost attempted suicide the day after her first group therapy session. She noted that she had in fact been quite depressed and angry for some time, despite claims to the contrary in prior individual sessions, and that this sense of upset and desperation had only been heightened by her experience (behavior) in the group. She felt that she couldn't go on with the pain and all the limitations it imposed, and she decided to kill herself with an overdose of pain-killers.

The morning after group, after she had routinely fixed breakfast and gotten her husband and son off to work and school, she sat down with 75 pills and contemplated suicide. Her first thought was to call her orthopedic surgeon, but she decided "he really wouldn't care or have the time to talk with her." She then thought to call her psychologist "who probably cared, but was most likely too busy to attend to her needs at the moment." Finally, just before taking the pills (an amount and combination sufficient to accomplish her goal of killing herself), she decided to call one of the pain patients "who had appeared to be sympathetic, to understand what she was saying during the group." What she expected from this person, she wasn't sure; but the woman seemed nice, seemed to have the same problem, and seemed to care.

Luckily, she caught the other patient as she was preparing to leave home, they had a very emotional 3-hour telephone conversation, and she was "talked out of killing myself, at least for the moment" and instead agreed to "be more honest" in subsequent individual sessions with her therapist. She never returned to group therapy, choosing rather to work on her psychological problems in individual therapy exclusively, but she credited "the group" with saving her life!

Finally, as we have also already emphasized, group therapy *provides a forum for multiperson confrontation and confrontation by "credible" persons who share the problem* being treated: pain. The sheer "weight of confrontation" experienced by group members when "on the hot seat" as regards some aspect of their *painmanship* is often enough to cause them to terminate or at least reduce their "pain games," that is, "if you can't lick 'em, join 'em."

POINT OF FOCUS

At this point in the chapter, we hope it is clear from the examples, vignettes, and anecdotes we have given that we are primarily concerned with how patients cope with and/or manage their pain experience and how they "learn to live with it," and *not* the pain experience itself. That is, we attend to what patients do behaviorally and cognitively (how they think) on a day-to-day basis, as well as to how they feel emotionally, *as opposed to* whether and how much they hurt.

Accepting chronic pain as we do (something that has a beginning, a middle, but no end. . .), we assume that their pain is always present, that it is a given, that it will ebb and flow in intensity, and that there is little that we can do that will directly influence its character. On the other hand, as psychologists and group therapists, we see our therapeutic

task as directly influencing those things that *psychologically* affect and/or are affected by pain: mood, self-esteem, coping mechanisms, social interactions, and hope. Thus, like some obesity treatment programs, which actively discourage obese patients from continually weighing themselves, we discourage chronic pain patients from constantly assessing their pain (What is my pain level now?) and using this as a basis for all subsequent behavior(s). If anything, this preoccupation with perceived pain, we believe, tends to undermine patients' attempts to "learn to live with it" and inevitably contributes to a sense of despair, hopelessness, and helplessness.

Also, whereas Sternbach (1974) has basically focused on "pain games" (maladaptive coping strategies) and the payoffs they derive in the external social environment, we spend more time and therapeutic energy combating *denial*, that is, the efforts on the part of patients (both cognitively and behaviorally) to avoid partially or totally the harsh unwelcomed reality of chronic endless pain. As we have argued recently (Gentry, 1985), denial, as we see it, is the primary motivating factor behind "pain games," for example, doctor-shopping, addiction, excessive disability, litigation, focusing on the past in day-to-day communications, and externalization of one's pain experience (referring to pain as "it," something outside the otherwise healthy self).

In our pain groups, we — and the patients alike — tend to view all relevant pain and non-pain behavior as reflecting the presence/absence or level of denial operating within the patient and his or her significant others (e.g., a patient's spouse refused to let her purchase a cane to help her in walking long distances, saying "She doesn't need that; that's for old people!"). To successfully cope with chronic benign pain, we feel that patients *must* quit denying the chronicity of their pain experience, stop waiting for someone to "rid them of this awful thing," stop treating it as an acute problem (even after many years and unproductive surgeries), and begin, slowly but surely, to accept and integrate it into their new identity and sense of self. Until they give up their denial, we do not believe therapeutic efforts, no matter what form they take (e.g., individual vs. group therapy, biofeedback, cognitive–behavioral therapy) and/or how skilled the therapist, will prove beneficial.

EXPECTED BEHAVIORAL OUTCOMES

To illustrate the range and degree of altered patient behavior that one frequently sees in pain patients treated with group therapy, we offer the following three cases. These are selected, albeit typical cases; they do not constitute individuals who have done the "best" nor the "worst" in our treatment program.

Case Study 1: A 48-year-old Woman With Chronic Back Pain

This is a 48-year-old, married woman suffering from chronic pain syndrome secondary to an on-the-job injury 7 years prior to seeking treatment. She has had two back operations (lumbar laminectomies) with evidence of pseudoarthrosis at one level of fusion and degenerative disc disease. Her pain was initially described as constant and severe; it was experienced in the following anatomical areas: lower back, right and left hip, right and left legs, and right and left feet. Physical therapy, a variety of pain narcotics, a transcutaneous electrical nerve stimulation (TENS) unit, and antidepressant medication had failed to produce significant pain relief.

She had an 8th grade education, was one of 22 children, came from a rural background, and had been married twice, the first marriage ending after 15 years because of an abusive husband. Early family relationships, because of the large family size, centered on survival; interestingly, the patient received more parental nurturance when she was ill. She had a stable work history for 10 years prior to injury, working at a textile mill; she was in the process of assuming a supervisory role when injured.

At the onset of treatment, approximately 2 years earlier, she gave evidence of clinical depression, anxiety, repressed anger, denial (manifested primarily by her efforts to find a "cure"), social withdrawal (feelings of isolation and alienation), low self-esteem, disturbed body-image, distorted self-concept (saw self as an "invalid"), medication abuse, and excessive pain complaint and posturing at the expense of well, nonpain behavior.

Diagnostically, it was clear that the patient, prior to injury, had basically adopted a hypomanic lifestyle, aimed at providing herself with a sense of mastery and independence through work. This was seen primarily as a compensatory defense (reaction formation) against chronic unresolved dependency needs (Gentry, Shows, & Thomas, 1974), resulting from maternal deprivation during early years of socialization in an unusually large family. She felt good about herself and secure, in essence, only as long as she could work at a high level of performance. Unfortunately, the injury curtailed her ability to work and thus her ability to secure positive reinforcement from her social environment (e.g., from fellow workers). The injury and associated pain/disability also amplified the dependency–independency conflict; gratification of dependency needs became manifest through nonverbal pain behavior (e.g., although she refused to discuss her pain condition with her husband, she stated that "he knows when I feel bad without me telling him"). Her sense of loss, grief, and anger intensified over time, in turn exacerbating her pain experience; a pain–tension–pain cycle had been established.

Initially, she was treated individually with a combination of biofeedback and hypnotherapy, aimed at altering the sensory component of her pain experience. These techniques failed to achieve any change in her reported level of pain or her disability behavior. Six months of weekly individual psychotherapy, both supportive and cognitive–behavioral in approach, achieved some success in stabilizing her emotions and day-to-day functional activity level, but she continued to deny the finality of her chronic pain condition and was at best ambivalent as regards any real attempt to behave in an independent normal manner. At this point, she was enrolled in a pain group.

In general, her style of interacting within the group was to dominate the conversation and draw attention to herself, often competing openly with fellow group participants for the "spotlight." When the focus shifted to other patients, she would characteristically withdraw and appear disinterested. Attempts to confront her "pain game" appeared at first productive, but later became less so in that confrontation still allowed her to seize the group's attention. Group members subsequently shifted from direct confrontation to a shaping program, whereby they attended only to adaptive, nonpain behavior, e.g., positive self-statements, showing interest in others, and involvement in pleasure-giving activities. This latter tactic proved most effective in shifting her investment away from "sick role behavior," in leading to a marked increase in her ability to verbally elicit appropriate support and nurturance (without reliance on body language), and in producing a significant increase in activities involving mastery (e.g., playing the organ, silk flower arranging, and volunteer work) and pleasure (e.g., attending dances, travel).

Table 7.1 shows the concomitant changes in her MMPI profile t-scores over a 16-month period, the first measure obtained at the beginning of treatment and the second following 8 months of group therapy.

Case Study 2: A 38-year-old Woman With Chronic Back, Neck, Hip, And Leg Pain

This is a 38-year-old, married woman complaining initially of chronic pain in her lower back, neck, hips, and legs. She dated the onset of pain to an on-the-job injury 6 years prior to being evaluated; the pain had also worsened as a result of four subsequent back operations involving disc fusions. She reported the pain as constant; the intensity varied from moderate (without activity) to severe (with prolonged activity) on a daily basis. She also complained of marked depression, including feelings of: decreased sexual interest,

difficulty in concentrating, increased irritability, excessive fatigue, sleep disturbance, and frequent urge to cry. She described her life following the onset of pain/disability as "dull, boring, frustrating, and painful!" She reported being virtually housebound 90% of the time, rarely venturing outside because "it hurts when I do." She was no longer working, had terminated all regular social-recreational activities, and was experiencing marital strain with her husband, who also had chronic back pain and was disabled.

To date, over a period of some 17 months, she has participated in a total of 45 therapy sessions, 14 (31%) individual and 31 (69%) group.

Table 7.2 shows MMPI t-score changes at three points in time during the course of treatment. In each case, she showed marked improvement as regards feelings of depression, alienation, excessive dependency, preoccupation with bodily function, anger, suspiciousness, and obsessiveness. Her most recent clinical profile is entirely within normal limits.

Significant behavioral changes during treatment included such things as: significant increase in activities outside the home (social pursuits such as bingo and fishing; volunteer work more than 1 day a week; family trips); marked decrease in use of pain medication;

TABLE 7.1. MMPI t-SCORES FOR CASE 1

MMPI Scales	2/83	6/84
L	63	59
F	53	48
K	57	46
1 Hypochondriasis	68	59
2 Depression	73	67
3 Hysteria	82	70
4 Psychopathic Deviate	55	53
5 Masculinity-Femininity	67	67
6 Paranoia	62	43
7 Psychasthenia	57	49
8 Schizophrenia	60	40
9 Mania	60	52
0 Social Introversion	47	45

increase in assertive behavior; evidence of sustained positive mood and good humor; increased acceptance of fact that "pain will always be with me" and responsibility for "making most days good despite the pain;" and cognitive shift away from an "all-or-nothing" view of life (i.e., categorizing things as either possible or not possible without room for compromise). Most recently she is investigating the possibility of regular part-time (3 days a week) gainful employment. She has widened her social network, including now several members of the pain group, has helped her husband to also venture out more socially despite his bad back, and she feels much better about herself than she had for several years. She reports more energy, less of a sense of guilt over being "handi-capped," is less panic-strickened when the pain gets intense, and avoids conflict (e.g., at home) less, instead choosing to confront and resolve problems as they arise. She has markedly reduced her visits to physicians, no longer requests frequent pain injections, and basically "tries to be my own doctor much of the time." She no longer feels "trapped" by her illness. Interestingly, her level of per-ceived pain has remained the same or, if any-thing, worsened slightly because of markedly increased activity level.

Case Study 3: A 53-year-old Woman With Chronic Back Pain

This is a 53-year-old, married woman also complaining of chronic back pain secondary to an on-the-job injury 3 years earlier, also worsening with two subsequent back surger-ies. At the time of initial evaluation, she was severely depressed: sad affect, pessimism as regards the future, failure to enjoy life, feel-ings of worthlessness, self-dislike, lack of initiative, excessive fatigue, and indecisive-ness. She was totally unable to accept the reality of endless pain and was extremely angry about the fact that doctors were appar-ently making her worse instead of better. Her daily routine was sedentary and she ventured

TABLE 7.2. MMPI t-SCORES FOR CASE 2

MMPI Scales	9/23/83	1/30/84	9/28/84
L	53	50	50
F	60	60	55
K	59	46	53
1 Hypochondriasis	75	67	64
2 Depression	89	69	63
3 Hysteria	91	64	68
4 Psychopathic Deviate	74	57	60
5 Masculinity-Femininity	22	45	42
6 Paranoia	75	44	38
7 Psychasthenia	81	61	56
8 Schizophrenia	96	84	69
9 Mania	55	53	55
0 Social Introversion	53	58	63

only occasionally outside of her home envi-ronment. On a typical day, she stayed in bed late, read the newspaper, did some light housework, and read the Bible. She depended on her husband for transportation every-where and for helping her get out of her ever-present moods.

She had a total of 50 therapy sessions, 20 (40%) individual and 30 (60%) group, over a 21-month period. Table 7.3 shows MMPI t-score changes over this time period.

Her progress in treatment was initially slow, primarily due to her resistance to the idea of chronic pain and the intensity of her

TABLE 7.3. MMPI t-SCORES FOR CASE 3

MMPI Scales	5/3/83	10/28/83
L	60	46
F	55	55
K	57	59
1 Hypochondriasis	78	67
2 Depression	88	59
3 Hysteria	91	70
4 Psychopathic Deviate	64	57
5 Masculinity-Femininity	35	37
6 Paranoia	77	62
7 Psychasthenia	96	58
8 Schizophrenia	83	52
9 Mania	68	50
0 Social Introversion	74	42

depression. At times, she was close to being suicidal; antidepressant medication (imipramine) was tried, but she was unable to tolerate a prolonged course of drugs because of aversive side effects. She reported periods of time when "things were blank," "when I felt as if I were just existing," and when she hoped someone would see that she needed help. She felt that she had been mistreated for her pain problems, that at least "2 years of my life had been robbed from me," and that because of her pain "my life was out of my control."

As her involvement in the pain group increased, she shifted from being a quiet, rather passive participant to someone who openly expressed her feelings and thoughts as regards both her pain experience and mood disturbance. The group was increasingly supportive, and she admitted feeling "protected" by them; their support gave her a renewed sense of "I'm ok, I'm going to be ok!" She noted that she had lost "my sense of being important, of feeling needed," feelings now provided by the group. She increased, slowly but surely, her activities outside the home, became much less dependent on her husband (even to the point of driving herself 200 miles each way to group therapy meetings), and developed increased self-confidence as regards her ability to make sound decisions, carry through with day-to-day tasks, assert herself, and take responsibility for maintaining as best she could (without medication) a positive mood. Pain complaints decreased. She planned for the future and talked increasingly about developing courage to try new things (e.g., cross-stitching, ceramics class) to give her life some meaning and sense of purpose. She reported feeling "like a whole person again" and feeling "proud of what I've done for myself."

Finally, we do not share the rather pessimistic experience of Sternbach (1974) that pain treatment on an outpatient basis, including pain groups, is doomed to failure; in his experience, only 4% of patients showed any improvement after 1 year of therapy. How-ever, as is clear from our case examples, we realize that there is no shortcut to effective treatment and that chronic pain patients may well remain in some combination of individual/group therapy for years. Because chronic pain is an *ongoing*, open-ended experience, we see no reason why treatment should not be also. Some of our patients have, in fact, acknowledged that the treatment principles/techniques learned in inpatient pain treatment programs have limited utility in their home environment; outpatient programs, on the other hand, provide greater *continuity of care* and a local social support system to draw upon.

REFERENCES

Beck, A. (1967). *Depression: Causes and treatment.* Philadelphia, PA: University of Pennsylvania Press.

Cairns, D., Thomas, L., Mooney, V., & Pace, J.B. (1976). A comprehensive treatment approach to chronic low back pain. *Pain, 2,* 301–308.

Gentry, W.D. (1982). Chronic back pain: Does elective surgery benefit patients with evidence of psychologic disturbance? *Southern Medical Journal, 75,* 1169–1170.

Gentry, W.D., & Kobasa, S.C. (1984). Social and psychological resources mediating stress-illness relationships in humans. In W.D. Gentry (Ed.), *Handbook of behavioral medicine* (pp. 87–116). New York: Guilford.

Gentry, W.D., Shows, W.D., & Thomas, M. (1974). Chronic low back pain: A psychological profile. *Psychosomatics, 15,* 174–177.

Greenhoot, J.H., & Sternbach, R.A. (1974). Conjoint treatment of chronic pain. In J.J. Bonica (Ed.), *Advances in neurology* (Vol. 4, pp. 595–603). New York: Raven.

Ignelzi, R.J., Sternbach, R.A., & Timmermans, G. (1977). The pain ward follow-up analyses. *Pain, 3,* 277–280.

Lazarus, R.S., & Folkman, S. (1984). Coping and adaptation. In W.D. Gentry (Ed.), *Handbook of behavioral medicine* (pp. 282–325). New York: Guilford.

Newman, R.I., Seres, J.L., Yospe, L.P., & Garlington, B. (1978). Multidisciplinary treatment of chronic pain: Long-term follow-up of low-back pain patients. *Pain, 4,* 283–292.

Sternbach, R.A. (1974). *Pain patients: Traits and treatment.* New York: Academic Press.

Sternbach, R.A., & Rusk, T.N. (1973). Alternatives to the pain career. *Psychotherapy: Theory, research, and practice, 10*, 321–324.

Sternbach, R.A., Wolf, S.R., Murphy, R.W., & Akeson, W.H. (1973). Aspects of chronic low back pain. *Psychosomatics, 14*, 52–56.

Szaz, T. (1968). The psychology of persistent pain: A portrait of l'homme douloureux. In A. Soulairac, J. Cahn, & J. Charpentier (Eds.), *Pain* (pp. 93–113). New York: Academic Press.

Swanson, D.W., Maruta, T., & Swenson, W.M. (1979). Results of behavior modification in the treatment of chronic pain. *Psychosomatic Medicine, 41*, 55–61.

Timmermans, G., & Sternbach, R.A. (1974). Factors of human chronic pain: An analysis of personality and pain reaction variables. *Science, 184*, 806–807.

Turk, D.C., Meichenbaum, D., & Genest, M. (1983). *Pain and behavioral medicine: A cognitive-behavioral perspective.*, New York: Guilford.

VanderPlate, C. (1984). Psychological aspects of multiple sclerosis and its treatment: Toward a biopsychosocial perspective. *Health Psychology, 3*, 253–272.

Ziesat, H.A., Angle, H., & Gentry, W.D. (1979). Drug use and misuse in operant pain patients. *Addictive Behaviors, 4*, 263–266.

8 A PROBLEM-CENTERED FAMILY SYSTEMS APPROACH IN TREATING CHRONIC PAIN

Ranjan Roy*

Sound clinical reasons for family involvement in the assessment and treatment of psychiatric, medical, and psychophysiological disorders including pain have been offered by many authors (Anthony, 1970; Bishop & Epstein, 1980; Engel, 1980; Haggerty, 1983; Liebman, Honig, & Berger, 1976; Liebman, Minuchin, & Baker, 1974; Livesy, 1972; Meissner, 1980; Minuchin et al., 1975; Minuchin, Rosman, & Baker, 1978; Shanfield, Heinman, Cope, & Jones, 1978). Although family issues germaine to chronic pain have been poorly researched, there has been a mounting interest in the function of family dynamics in the etiology, prolongation, and perpetuation of chronic pain. A common problem shared by chronic pain with other chronic diseases is the impact of the problem on the entire family system. The effects are often of a global nature and can reduce what was formerly a well-functioning family into a chaotic one (Roy, 1984a; Tunks & Roy, 1982). Family factors have long been implicated in the etiology of psychophysiological disorders, and there is evidence, albeit on the

weak side, for the role of family factors in the causation of chronic pain (Roy, 1982a, 1982b). The thrust of this paper will be on intervention rather than on an examination of family etiology of this very complex problem.

A brief rationale for the adoption of family intervention with chronic pain patients and their families is necessary. Apart from the etiological issues, there are two other major reasons for adopting a family therapy approach. The first reason was alluded to and relates to the consequences of having a chronically sick individual within the family system. A well-functioning family can, in a reasonably short time, become almost totally dysfunctional when one of its members gradually assumes the role of a chronic pain patient (Roy, 1984a). Changes seem to occur slowly and imperceptibly to begin with, but over time the pace quickens and dysfunctional elements begin to appear with devastating consequences. As the patient sinks into a chronic sick role and frequently loses his occupational role, the family needs to reorganize with the significant burden of the problem falling on the shoulders of the spouse. There is evidence to suggest that spouses of chronic pain sufferers develop a variety of psychophysiologi-

*I am indebted to Rosalind Husband for her assistance in preparing this chapter.

cal and psychiatric disorders as they are required to cope with changes in their interpersonal relationships, additional financial burdens, and loss of emotional support and sexual gratification (e.g., Mohamed, Weisz, & Waring, 1978; Shanfield et al., 1978).

It will become evident in the course of this chapter that many major dimensions of family function are adversely affected by the presence of a chronic pain patient. The relationship between the spouses and their children undergoes major transformation. One common change is that the disabled or sick individual is "sidelined" from family functions and excluded from decision-making. The affective climate of the family alters for the worst. The chronic pain patient is preoccupied with his or her own problem; the well spouse has to take on more and more responsibility in running the family; and the children develop a great sense of isolation, lack of love, and nurturing.

The second reason for involving the family in the treatment of chronic pain derives from considerable clinical research that has demonstrated the role played by the family members in the perpetuation and prolongation of chronic pain (Block, 1981; Block, Kremer, & Gaylor, 1980; Maruta, Osborne, Swenson, & Holling, 1981; Nichols, 1978; Swenson & Maruta, 1980; Waring, 1977). As this problem has been reviewed elsewhere, only a brief examination is necessary (Roy 1982a; 1982b). The key question is what purpose does the pain serve either for the patient or for the family. Chronic pain in the spouse may relieve the partner of sexual and other marital responsibilities, and the pain may be used to discourage the patient from making demands felt unacceptable to the partner. In addition, the patient's position of dependency may be encouraged by the well spouse, thus reinforcing the pain behavior to his or her own end. It might give rise to undesirable mutuality by removing long-standing conflicts and creating a new homeostasis (Roy, 1984c).

Although the behaviorists have clearly demonstrated the role of the spouse in the perpetuation of pain (Block, 1981), the problem can be viewed from the systemic per-

spective to have a better appreciation of the concept of homeostasis. Jackson (1959) noted that family homeostasis can be understood in terms of communications theory, "that is, depicting family interaction as a closed information system in which variations in output or behavior are fed back in order to correct a system's response" (p. 79). Therefore, it is reasonable that the problem of chronic pain, which frequently persists for months and years, will tend to be associated with repetitive stereotyped patterns of behavior. Steinglass (1980) has observed with great clarity in the context of alcoholic families that "these patterns of behaviour in turn can become integrated in the family's homeostatic mechanisms thereby paradoxically becoming associated with long-term family stability" (p. 214). The notion that a symptom or an illness can provide homeostasis in a family system is well established (Roy, 1984c) and from a clinical perspective is commonly observed. This will become evident in the case example described in the following that involves a newly married couple. The wife's complaint of chronic headache was already giving rise to a pattern of behavior which, unchecked, could have assumed a very stable form.

Family members in many ways reinforce the patient's illness behavior or, more specifically, pain behavior and treat him or her as though he or she was a semi-invalid. Alternatively, family members may take the opposite view that the patient, in the absence of any serious organic finding, in fact does not have a problem. Both these perspectives create considerable difficulties for the family as a whole. In general terms, families do engage in what is described as colluding or pain-reinforcing behavior with chronic pain patients. Swenson and Maruta (1980) reported a very high level of agreement among patients with chronic pain and their families in the areas of duration, location, severity, aggravating and relieving factors, and incidence of pain on other functions. A common phenomenon is that communication emanating from undesirable mutuality and high levels of collusion is a major reinforcer of patient's pain behaviors.

Block et al. (1980) found that patients with solicitous spouses were inclined to report somewhat higher levels of pain than those with nonsolicitous spouses. In a subsequent study, Block (1981) demonstrated that spouses who reported relatively high levels of marital satisfaction also demonstrated greater increases in skin conduction to the painful displays of their mates than did the relatively unsatisfied spouses. Block's conclusion was that in stable marital relationships the well partners tended to reinforce the patient's pain behavior, and the explanation may lie in the fact that the well partners were more sympathetic towards their spouses.

The perpetuation of chronic pain is also attributed to personal factors either as a way of seeking attention or of avoiding responsibilities by the chronic pain sufferer. Conversely, family members frequently treat this person as an invalid and expect less and less from him or her. This then decidedly sets the scene for perpetuation of the problem. Nichols (1978), in a study of marital interaction, noted that in many instances the higher the level of pain complaint, the greater was the degree of marital harmony. The overt maintenance of pain behavior in such a situation was clearly encouraged by the well partner for a whole variety of self-serving reasons, for example, assuming a dominating position in the marriage.

Sick-role homeostasis, individual family member's needs that encourage perpetuation of pain in another member of the family, and secondary gains are some of the common reasons contributing to the perpetuation of chronic pain behaviors. In the final analysis the perpetuation of chronic pain is frequently interactional in nature.

THE PROBLEM-CENTERED FAMILY SYSTEMS THERAPY (PCFST)

First, there will be a brief description of this model. Second, a rationale will be offered for the selection of this approach in treating a couple. Third, its use in treating the couple will be described.

PCFST is the product of over 25 years of research that was started by Epstein and his colleagues at McGill University and continues to date at Brown University. Much of the work, however, was done during Epstein's tenure at McMaster University in Hamilton, Canada. The model has been described in great detail at all stages of its development by its proponents. Several research studies on various aspects of this model have also been reported (Byles, Bishop, & Horn, 1983; Cleghorn & Levin, 1973; Epstein & Bishop, 1981a, 1981b; Epstein, Bishop, & Baldwin, 1982; Epstein, Bishop, & Levin, 1978; Epstein, Levin, & Bishop, 1976; Epstein, Sigel, & Rakoff, 1962; Santa Barbara et al., 1977; Westley & Epstein, 1970; Woodward et al., 1981).

For the purpose of this chapter, only a summary will be offered. This model of family therapy shares one common element with other approaches, such as structural and strategic family therapy, in that they are all predicated on systems theory. Epstein and Bishop (1981a) state that in this approach the family is seen as:

> An open system consisting of systems within systems (individual, marital dyad) and relating to other systems, extended family, schools, industry, religions. The unique aspect of the dynamic family group cannot be simply reduced to the characteristics of the individual or interaction between pairs of members. Rather there are explicit or implicit rules, plus action by members, which govern and monitor each other's behavior. (p. 447)

The PCFST model is based on the following assumptions of systems theory: (a) The parts of the family are interrelated; (b) one part of the family cannot be understood in isolation from the rest of the system; (c) family functioning cannot be fully understood by simply understanding each of its parts; (d) the family structure and organization are important factors determining the behavior of family members; and (e) transactional patterns of the family system shape the behavior of family members.

PCFST has four distinct macro stages. The four stages, assessment, contracting, treatment, and closure, are invariant even though the individual skills of the family therapist may indeed be at different levels. Individual intervention skills are described as micro moves and indeed greatly vary from therapist to therapist. As far as the macro stages are concerned, each stage has an orientation phase, the focus of which is to orient the family to the new stage and what is about to follow.

Understandably, the orientation associated with the assessment phase is critical and is also very comprehensive. Clarification is sought about the expectation of each family member. Each member's expectation and the reason for his presence are explored, and the family is collectively encouraged to assume responsibility for the therapeutic endeavor about to follow. Following orientation, the issue of presenting problem is explored in considerable detail. Plus, it must be remembered, in the context of chronic pain, that the family members frequently need a considerable amount of help in shifting their focus away from the problem of pain itself to related interpersonal and other difficulties discussed earlier.

Through this process, presenting problems are established, following which an overall family functioning is assessed on six dimensions using the McMaster Model of Family Functioning (MMFF): (a) problem-solving, (b) communication, (c) roles, (d) affective responsiveness, (e) affective involvement, and (f) behavioral control. The affective and instrumental types of issues are carefully differentiated, and criteria are established for effective functioning of each parameter of family functioning (Epstein, Bishop, & Baldwin, 1982; Epstein, Bishop, & Levin, 1978).

Seven substages in the problem-solving process are identified. They are described in detail in the following section. On the communications dimension, effectiveness is assessed on two independent parameters, clear versus masked and direct versus indirect.

In the category of role function, a distinction is made between necessary and other types of roles. Again, family roles and functions are subdivided into instrumental and affective areas. Epstein and his colleagues (1982) have defined family roles "as the repetitive patterns of behavior by which family members fulfill family functions" (p. 124). Five essential areas of role function are identified: (a) provision of resources, (b) nurturance and support, (c) adult sexual gratification, (d) personal development, and (e) maintenance and management of the family system. In addition, concepts of role allocations and role accountability are introduced. Role allocation is a function of assigning roles, and role accountability is concerned with ensuring that functions are fulfilled. Role confusion in a family harboring a chronic pain person is considerable. It is also an area that has received rather limited attention. Tunks and Roy (1982) have described in detail the consequences on the family system of a chronic pain patient's losing his or her occupational role.

The next area of family functioning is the affective responsiveness that is designed to explore the "family's potential range of affective responses, both qualitatively and quantitatively" (Epstein et al., 1982, p. 126). The appropriateness of the affect in a given situation underlines this area of family functioning. Two distinct categories of affect are identified, welfare emotions and emergency emotions. Welfare emotions are naturally concerned with more positive feelings, such as joy, happiness, concern, care, and love; emergency emotions represent feelings such as fear, sadness, and depression, generally speaking, negative emotions. The healthy family is viewed as one that has the capacity to express a full range of emotions. In the context of the chronic pain family, emergency emotions tend to supersede the welfare ones (Roy, 1984a).

Affective involvement is defined as "the extent to which the family shows interest in the particular activities of individual family members" (Epstein et al., 1982, p. 126). Six distinct types of affective involvement have been identified: (a) lack of involvement, (b) involvement devoid of feelings, (c) narcissistic involvement, (d) empathic involvement, (e) overinvolvement, and (f) symbiotic involvement. Empathic involvement is a hallmark of a healthy functioning family. Once again, in a family with chronic pain, a common clinical observation is either overinvolvement or lack of involvement on the part of the family members and a somewhat narcissistic involvement on the part of the patient with other members.

Behavior control is defined as "the pattern the family adopts for handling behavior in three different areas: physically dangerous situations; situations that involve the meeting and expressing of psychobiological needs and drives; and situations involving interpersonal socializing behavior both between family members and with people outside the family" (Epstein et al., 1982, p. 128). Behavior control is primarily concerned with rules and standards that the family sets and the degree to which they are able to demonstrate flexibility in handling situations. It is proposed that the family system engages in four styles of behavior control: (a) rigid behavior control, (b) flexible behavior control, (c) laissez-faire behavior control, and (d) chaotic behavior control. In the absence of research data pertaining to chronic pain families, anecdotal and clinical experience suggest that many of these families tend to become chaotic in the area of behavior control.

The last stage of the assessment phase is concerned with clarification and agreement on problems. Clear identification of problems is the first step towards resolution. Roy (1984a), in a recent paper, has described at length the difficulties associated with problem identification in chronic pain families. The patient and the family members alike tend to attribute all their difficulties to the problem of chronic pain.

Following the completion of the assessment phase, the next macro stage is contracting. Conditions have to be carefully stated and delineated; problems must be clearly identified along with the family's expectations and goals as well as the therapist's expectations. Epstein and Bishop (1981a) recommend that an actual contract be drawn up and signed by the family members and the therapist. Not all family therapists find it necessary to actually go through this signing ceremony.

The third macro stage is the actual intervention. A concrete behavioral task is negotiated to clearly delineate the responsibility of individual members and establish a task for achieving the goals. Epstein and Bishop (1981a) have established some guiding principles in negotiating and assigning tasks. Emphasis is on positive and achievable tasks that are meaningful and do not interfere unduly with family schedules and activities. In addition, goals should lend themselves to evaluation. A common method is to encourage the family to appoint one of its members as a monitor who is expected to report on these matters in the following session. The family members are praised when tasks are successfully achieved; but should there be no improvement over a period of two or three successive sessions, then re-evaluation by the therapist becomes a necessity and should either result in an alteration in goals or, not infrequently, termination of therapy. As in all therapy, in the final stage of this model, namely closure, therapy is terminated when all the tasks have been achieved that are stated in the contract. Long-term goals are set and a review session arranged.

RATIONALE FOR ADOPTING PCFST

Given the present state of knowledge about the various modalities of family therapy, it is impossible to claim superiority of one over another. Preference for a model remains a function of one's training.

Nevertheless, a careful evaluation of the family therapy literature will reveal that the PCFST, with the MMFF as its central feature, presents one of the clearest expositions of family functioning that is available to date. The model does not rely heavily on any particular aspect of family functioning. In contrast, strategic family therapy conceptualizes the function of a symptom in a spouse as an expression of hierarchical incongruity. Headache, for example, may be a metaphor for lack of power in a wife (Madanes, 1981).

Strictly behavioral approaches to family problems focus on elimination of reinforcing pain behavior and do not result in an examination of complex interpersonal dimensions of family relationships that may or may not be corrected by rectifying or eliminating the patient's pain behavior. The structural model of family therapy provides a comprehensive conceptual base for examining family interactions (Minuchin, 1974), but this model does not clearly delineate the areas of family functioning. In addition, structural and strategic schools of family therapy subscribe to the axiom that symptoms are a product of family dysfunction, and symptom removal is the primary objective of intervention. Given the complex nature of chronic pain with its biological, social, and psychological dimensions, its etiology cannot be attributed to a single factor or even to as complex a variable as family dynamics. The PCFST does not attempt to establish cause, but the focus clearly is on achieving the most successful ways of dealing with problems that may arise within the family system.

The PCFST model evolved from research with nonclinical families and an understanding of healthy family functioning. It is designed to teach better coping skills to families in difficulty by improving the levels of family functioning. The emphasis on individual dimensions of family functioning provides the family members with tangible direction in their effort to find resolutions to their problems. The usefulness of this model has been demonstrated mostly clinically, not only in the fields of psychiatry but also in rehabilitation, family medicine, and pediatrics (Epstein & Bishop, 1981a). PCFST appears to be a very useful model for practicing clinicans on several accounts, namely, clarity, systemic base, and behavioral orientation.

What follows is the application of PCFST with special emphasis on the MMFF to describe the four macro stages in treating a young couple one of whom had the problem of chronic headache.

Case Study: Mrs. A., A 24-year-old Woman With Chronic Headache

Mrs. A., aged 24, was referred to the pain clinic for chronic head pain. The referring physician stated that she had over the past 2 months not been coping very well with her stress. She complained of frequent frontal headaches, which lasted for 2 or 3 days at a time. She was suffering from some insomnia, waking frequently at nighttime. On clinical examination there were no abnormal findings, and the physician suggested that this intelligent woman seek a means of coping with her stress rather than resorting to psychotropic medication.

Mrs. A. was contacted for an appointment and asked to bring her spouse with her, as this is a standard procedure. She refused to do so, but agreed to come by herself. It needs to be stated that this is not an uncommon response on the part of a patient who views her problem as "medical." The problem of engaging chronic pain patients and their family members in psychotherapy has been described elsewhere (Roy, 1981). It is imperative to impress upon the patient that the involvement of the family in the treatment process is critical, and for most patients a simple explanation to the effect that his or her pain is indeed having an impact on the rest of the family members is sufficient to persuade them to bring their family.

In the case of Mrs. A., however, she arrived alone and categorically stated that her problem was not "psychological." She demanded to see the letter of referral from her physican and was generally angry. She stated that her head pain had nothing to do with whatever difficulties she might have been experiencing in her life. In any event she stated that her problems were quite manageable.

As far as her history of pain was concerned, she presented with a very long history of headache that commenced at age 14. For the most part her headaches did not interfere with her daily living to any significant degree until she reached the first year of university when her headaches worsened and she sought medical help. She refused to take any medication for her head pain and decided that she would try to cope with it in her own way. The pain problem subsided somewhat until just before her inception to the pain clinic.

In the course of the interview she reluctantly acknowledged that she was having terrible difficulties at work. For a young woman of her age she was in a highly paid technical position. She carried an enormous amount of responsibility, and she lived in constant doubt about her ability to function in that job. She also revealed that she had been married for 7 months, but categorically denied that she was having any difficulty with her husband. On the other hand, she revealed that her headaches did interfere with their social life and that her husband must have some feelings about that, although it was never discussed. This last bit of information was used to broach the subject of his coming along with her to the clinic, and she reluctantly agreed to bring him. For her next visit she arrived with her husband. Her husband, a 25-year-old professional engineer, seemed somewhat detached.

The following is a description of how PCFST was used to treat this couple. As was stated earlier there are four macro stages: (a) assessment, (b) contracting, (c) treatment, and (d) closure.

Assessment Stage

The assessment stage has four clear steps: (a) orientation, (b) data gathering, (c) problem description, and (d) clarifying and agreeing on a problem list. Each step will be examined in some detail. The MMFF is at the center of the assessment phase.

Orientation is the critical phase of assessment because at this point the problem that family members and the patient alike view as the patient's problem is reframed in the context of the family. The approach adopted here is somewhat of a departure from that described by Epstein and Bishop (1981a). Instead of asking the family's reasons for being there, an attempt is made to explain why the therapist asked for the presence of family members, in

this particular instance, the husband. As a matter of routine, the rationale used by the therapist is to elaborate on the fact that although indeed the patient has a problem of chronic pain, it is very unlikely that he and their relationship remain unaffected by what is happening to her. It is this simple and common sense explanation that has proven to be extraordinarily successful in engaging chronic pain families in family therapy.

As part of the orientation, once this explanation has been offered, the family members are asked to respond to their view of the problem. To begin with, the therapist commended the patient for being able to persuade her husband to come along. The following is a verbatim report of the conversation that transpired between the two of them:

Husband: All that you have to do is ask. I never say "no." Do I?
Patient: No, you don't. (Turning to the therapist) He is really quite marvelous. But I don't like to bug him about my headache.
Husband: But you know your headaches do bother me. (Turning to the therapist) I don't like to see her in pain.

The headache was no longer the patient's own personal and private problem, and it was very quickly reframed in the context of the relationship. This led to the next stage of assessment, namely *data gathering*. In this stage data are collected in four discrete steps: (a) presenting problems, (b) overall family functioning, (c) additional investigation, and (d) other problems.

The *presenting problem* is probably one of the most difficult of all areas in working with families of chronic pain patients. The problem emanates from a central source, namely, that whatever their difficulties they can all be attributed to the problem of pain. Families experience an inordinate amount of difficulty extricating themselves from their preoccupation with the problem of pain and its impact on the family system. Even in the case of Mr. and Mrs. A., the initial response was that there indeed would be no problem whatsoever if only the medical profession could cure Mrs. A.'s headache.

It has to be acknowledged by the therapist that indeed the problem of pain is a serious one and also that, from the perspective of medical intervention, it has remained refractory. On the other hand, in this instance the couple was reminded about two facts that were known to the therapist: (a) that the patient was having some difficulty at work and (b) that the couple had problems discussing her headaches. In other words, the process of reframing the pain problem in the context of the family remains an ongoing activity. The therapist further reminded the couple that perhaps her headaches were causing other kinds of difficulties that they had not been able to share with each other and that this might be an opportunity to do so.

A shift in focus began to take place in terms of defining the presenting problems. The husband took the initiative by stating that his wife's headaches interfered from time to time with their social activities. Mrs. A. denied this (contradicting an earlier statement) and counteracted by stating that her husband spent most of his evenings watching television. She would be in some other part of the house, and he probably did not even know if and when she had a headache. She challenged him to recall an instance when she refused to engage in any activity because of her headache or used her headache as an excuse. He agreed only in part with her assertion and proceeded to give several examples of how her headache had interfered with their social life.

As Epstein and Bishop (1981a) have pointed out, it is important to explore the presenting problems using the appropriate dimensions of the McMaster model. In the context of Mr. and Mrs. A., it would be imperative to have some understanding about their ability to communicate their difficulties to each other and their efforts at solving these problems.

In feeding back the presenting problems to the family, confirmation was sought by the therapist that he had a reasonable and correct grasp of the problems. In this instance, the therapist identified that: (a) the couple had difficulty talking about Mrs. A's headache problem; (b) Mrs. A. felt that they were lacking in communication and spent too much of their free time doing separate things; and (c) Mr. A. believed that her headaches were interfering to a certain extent with their social life.

The therapist pointed out that although they did not entirely agree about the gravity of each problem, they seemed to be in agreement that these were the major issues. Then, he sought confirmation of his understanding of the problems from the couple. They agreed.

In the next stage of data gathering, using the MMFF the couple was assessed on the six dimensions: problem-solving, communication, roles, affective responsiveness, affective involvement, and behavior control.

The concept of *problem-solving* is a self-explanatory one. It simply refers to the family's ability to resolve its difficulties in a way that allows it to maintain a level of effective family functioning. Epstein et al. (1982) have demonstrated that effective family problem-solving follows seven steps: (a) identifying the problem, (b) communicating with appropriate people about the problem, (c) developing a list of alternative solutions, (d) deciding on one of the alternatives, (e) carrying out the actions required by the alternatives, (f) monitoring to ensure that the action is carried out, and (e) evaluating the effectiveness of the problem-solving process.

In the context of Mr. and Mrs. A., it is imperative to remember the life-stage of this family. They had been married for only 7 months and were therefore still in the process of defining their relationship along all the parameters of family functioning. Needless to say, the ability of the newly married couple to solve their problems in a mutually satisfactory way is a continuous process of trial and error characterized by uncertainty and willingness to acquiesce. The problems in these early stages of marriage are frequently not recognized as problems or, alternatively, are categorically denied. Newly married couples seem to have an enormous propensity for this latter phenomenon.

Hence, when Mr. and Mrs. A. were asked

if they had any problems, their immediate reaction was to reject the suggestion instantaneously and simultaneously. Problems can be subdivided conceptually into instrumental and affective categories. Instrumental problems are the practical ones that people are likely to encounter on a day-to-day basis and may include issues such as social activities, money management, or the decor of the house. Affective problems, on the other hand, are related directly to relationship issues.

Again, experience suggests that a family harboring a chronically sick individual with chronic pain is likely to encounter considerable difficulties in the domain of problem-solving, especially as they relate to the affective areas. Although Mr. and Mrs. A. were capable of solving most of their instrumental problems, they did encounter significant difficulties in reaching agreement on matters of affective import. The picture was further complicated by their response to the question of problem-solving, as they were inclined to externalize the problem and to explain everything on the basis of the patient's headache that, of course, was beyond their solution.

In such a situation the couple has to be steered carefully into the domain of their interpersonal relationships to test their ability to resolve difficulties. An example would be that, whereas both partners acknowledged that they did not like the way they spent their evenings, they also demonstrated a singular inability to resolve the problem. Although the problem may have the appearance of being an instrumental one, the situation was laden with feelings.

To be more accurate, Mrs. A. perceived the situation, that is, spending their evenings in two separate rooms, as a problem; and that is more or less where it stayed until they engaged in family therapy. In Mrs. A.'s judgment, that was an unacceptable way for newly married couples to spend their evenings, whereas Mr. A. regarded the situation as being quite normal. He offered a pragmatic viewpoint, suggesting that they were both tired when they came home after a fairly arduous day's work and needed rest. Watching television was a form of relaxation for him, and he strongly defended his position. He, however, was able to acknowledge, having listened to his wife's side of the story, that he could understand why she felt neglected.

In the course of this segment of the investigation, it became very clear that, although Mrs. A. identified many problems and several areas of disagreement in their relationship, she preferred to remain silent; and Mr. A. was seemingly impervious to most difficulties in their relationship. Affective problems very rarely went past the first step of recognition.

The second dimension, *communication*, is defined as exchange of information in a family. It is further divided into instrumental and affective areas. Types of communication are subdivided along two continuums, clear and masked and direct and indirect. The clear and masked continuum determines the clarity of the message, and the direct and indirect continuum determines the degree of directness with which the message is transmitted to the receiver. Four styles of communication patterns emerge from these two independent attributes. They are: (a) clear and direct, (b) clear and indirect, (c) masked and direct, and (d) masked and indirect.

It has been noted elsewhere that chronic illness and pain can bring about fundamental changes in the communication pattern in a family (Roy, 1984a; Roy, 1984c). The reasons for that are indeed complex and can be in large measure ascribed to the difficulty family members experience in expressing their true feelings about the patient and vice versa. It was clear almost from the very first moment of this interview with Mr. and Mrs. A. that they had considerable difficulty with communication in the affective areas. Until their arrival at the pain clinic, they simply had not spoken about Mrs. A.'s headaches and its impact on their relationship or about Mr. A.'s questions about the headaches.

Although this couple discussed instrumental matters with relative ease, when it came to matters of emotional import they carefully avoided the topic. When Mrs. A. felt neglected and uncared for, especially if she had a severe headache, she tended to withdraw even more but never approached her husband. On his part, on occasion he felt controlled by her because her pain interfered with their plans, but he managed to avoid expressing his feelings. Mr. A. stated that it was hard to get angry with a person in pain in spite of how he felt. Silence and avoidance of emotional issues seemed to characterize their style of communication. In the context of the four patterns of communication, with instrumental issues it was mostly direct and clear, whereas with affective issues the pattern was, for the most part, indirect and masked.

The third area, *roles*, is critical for a number of reasons. In the first place, it can be stated without any fear of contradiction that it is from the performance of a variety of roles that an individual derives his or her sense of identity, and successful role performance also maintains and enhances his or her sense of worth and self-esteem. In the event that a person is either divested of those roles or the roles are compromised through an illness or accident, repercussions vary depending on the duration of time during which the patient either is not able to perform those roles or performs them at a reduced level of efficiency. The question of role complications in a family faced with a chronic pain patient has been addressed elsewhere (Tunks & Roy, 1982). The issue, however, is that the family members are often faced with an enormous dilemma about the patient's level of functioning. There is much inconsistency in role performance on the part of a chronic pain sufferer that can create a great deal of dissension within the family (Roy, 1984a).

Once again, the roles according to this model are divided into instrumental (i.e., provision of resources) and affective (i.e., nurturance and support, sexual gratification and marital fondness, and other affective domains of interpersonal relationships) categories. On the basis of this definition, Mr. and Mrs. A. performed only adequately in the instrumental domain. They were both employed in responsible positions and had a very high joint income. Beyond their professional roles, however, they had a great deal of difficulty in defining who did what, and although they attempted to do things together they had not really defined their respective areas of responsibility. Within a relatively short period of time, this became a serious area of conflict.

The whole issue was further complicated by two other factors. In the first place, Mrs. A.'s headaches with their unpredictable nature and consequences made it difficult for the couple to have well-defined roles because when she was in the throes of severe headache attack, she was virtually incapacitated and unable to do anything. In the second place, given the life-stage of this family, they had not formed any definite rules by which their marriage was governed. Haley (1963) has noted that "the process of working out a satisfactory marital relationship can be seen as working out shared agreements, largely undiscussed between two people" (p. 217). Furthermore, he observed that "the couple must not only set rules, but they must also reach agreement on which of them must be the one to set the rules in each area of the marriage" (p. 217).

It would appear that for a newlywed couple the rules that they bring into their marital situation are frequently the ones that they learned in their family of origin, and role models are also frequently based on their previous learning (Minuchin, 1974). If the expectations of the two individuals are divergent, then the rules established will also be quickly sabotaged. This was experienced time and time again by Mr. and Mrs. A. as they attempted to set rules that in effect determined their roles. Thus, an explicit rule was established that whoever came home first would start the dinner. That only happened when Mrs. A. was the first to arrive. Although Mr. A. agreed to follow that rule, this was contrary to his own learning and he did not follow through. This is an example of a newly married couple's willingness to superficially agree to do almost anything, but in the real situation fail to deliver.

There were similar examples of Mrs. A.'s unwillingness to carry out roles to which she had agreed. This is what Jackson (1965) described as "marital quid pro quo," that is, a marriage based on give and take, but the rules that govern such transactions were inadequate for the As. In essence, two very important aspects of role functioning, role allocation and role accountability, were not being fulfilled. Role allocation is a matter of determining who does what and also who in fact does the assigning. In the context of a contemporary marital relationship, the role allocation is likely to emerge from mutual consensus and determination of individual skills and willingness to carry out the necessary functions within the family. Role accountability ensures that functions are fulfilled. For a newly married couple, this often is a matter of mutual accountability rather than a hierarchical one.

Although Mr. and Mrs. A. were attempting to work out their respective roles and establish rules, the picture was substantially complicated by Mrs. A.'s persistent pain problem. Her pain and her husband's response to it clearly intruded into their nurturing and supportive roles, as well as their sexual relationships, albeit to a lesser extent. In a curious way, both of these people felt neglected by each other. They were abrogating their mutual nurturing role, and Mr. A. clearly experienced a great deal of difficulty in his newly found responsibility that brought about a shift in his identity from being a doting son and "one of the boys" to being a husband. This transition seemed to have been much less onerous for Mrs. A.

Mr. A. also found a rather novel way of implicating the pain issue into the question of satisfactory performance of roles. He observed that although Mrs. A. frequently suffered from headaches that were sufficiently severe to keep her confined to bed for hours on end, she never ever missed work, but unfailingly neglected all her social and personal obligations. When she had a headache, it was not just she who suffered, but he also had to suffer the consequences, for example,

not feel free to go out. The very notion that he could even entertain the idea of going out and enjoying himself when she was suffering was the height of callousness from Mrs. A.'s point of view. Despite this somewhat imperious attitude, she agreed that she did not want him to feel controlled by her headache and that he should feel more free to do as he chose. A careful investigation of the role functioning revealed that: (a) They had rather ill-defined rules of who did what, even when it came to mundane chores; (b) Mrs. A.'s headaches significantly interfered with establishment of rules about role allocation and mutual accountability; and (c) the respective nurturing and caring roles towards each other were in a state of significant jeopardy.

The next dimension, *affective responsiveness*, has, according to the MMFF, two groupings: (a) welfare emotions exemplified by responses such as love, happiness, and joy; and (b) emergency emotions such as anger, fear, and so forth. For successful functioning of the family system, a wide range of emotional responsiveness is desirable. Affective responsiveness is defined as the ability to respond to a given stimulus with appropriate quality and quantity of feelings. Mr. and Mrs. A. displayed more emergency than welfare emotions, and their affective responsiveness was severely constrained. Both of these individuals experienced substantial difficulty when it came to Mr. A.'s feeling of being controlled by her pain and Mrs. A.'s feelings at times that her husband was perhaps not as caring and concerned about her well being as he should be. They dealt with these negative emotions primarily by withdrawal, as has been indicated in a preceding section.

Silence and quiet hostility appear to be a common pattern of interaction among family members harboring a chronic pain patient. It has been described elsewhere how family members' abilities to demonstrate concern for each other, express affection, and be caring are severely challenged in the presence of a sufferer of chronic pain (Roy, 1984a). Generally speaking, welfare emotions are greatly suppressed by the well members of the family, whereas the patient displays a wide array of inappropriate emotions. In the case of Mr. and Mrs. A., it should be emphasized that their problems were due to Mrs. A.'s headaches and the newness of their marriage. Their range of affective responsiveness was restricted and often inappropriate to the situation.

The quality and extent of *affective involvement* that family members have with each other is another area of considerable interest to a family therapist. These are indeed the determinants of the emotional climate of a family. Epstein et al. (1982) have identified six kinds of involvement: (a) lack of involvement, (b) involvement devoid of feelings, (c) narcissistic involvement, (d) empathic involvement, (e) overinvolvement, and (f) symbiotic involvement.

Given this paradigm, the problem then is to determine the specifics of the relationship between Mr. and Mrs. A. The picture that is likely to emerge is complex and multidimensional. Although in broad terms their affective involvement could be described as empathic, and they themselves very definitely viewed their involvement as such, the nature of their involvement was likely to vary somewhat depending on the situation. Given the tremendous investment in their occupational pursuits, and complications brought into this relationship by Mrs. A.'s head pain, the affective involvement at times bordered on lack of involvement. For a young couple, they did very few things together and did not share many common interests. This often led to a great feeling of isolation on the part of Mrs. A., which Mr. A. refused to acknowledge. His position was that he was willing to share her interests only if he knew what they were. They did engage in a few social activities together; but, as was stated earlier, they seemed to spend a good deal of their time at home in individual pursuits. There was some evidence that although their level of sexual gratification was satisfactory, they were lacking in physical contact and proximity. Both of them acknowledged that they had a greater sense of involvement with each other during their courtship. However, their marriage coincided with exacerbation of Mrs. A.'s head pain and more job-related responsibilities that evidently had a distancing effect on their affective involvement.

The final dimension on which data were gathered, *behavior control*, is defined as the standards or rules adopted by a family for handling behavior in the following areas: (a) physically dangerous situations, (b) situations involving meeting and expressing psychobiological needs and drives, and (c) situations involving interpersonal socializing behavior. Four styles of behavior control are identified: (a) rigid behavior control, (b) flexible behavior control, (c) laissez-faire behavior control, and (d) chaotic behavior control.

It should be noted that in the context of marital dyads behavior control has somewhat different implications than in families with young children. For example, the question of physically dangerous situations is not as applicable to a family composed of adults as it is to a family with young children. On the other hand, meeting and expressing psychobiological needs, including sexual drives and interpersonal socializing, are indeed important areas of functioning for a couple. In this respect some interesting problems were observed between Mr. and Mrs. A. As was stated earlier, this couple, quite predictably, was struggling with setting rules. One area of some conflict centered on Mr. A.'s weekly night out with the boys. While he had this night out, his wife never went out alone or had a separate social life away from her husband. She resented his activity in this regard but never expressed it. In this sort of situation it is difficult to define the exact nature of the behavior control that is in effect, other than to observe that rules have not been clearly established. The intent of the couple was very definitely to have flexible behavior control and to establish standards by which they could both live. This couple was in the very early stages of developing such controls.

In addition to the previous information, it may be recalled that Mrs. A. presented with a combination of symptoms that had the appearance of a depressive disorder. She reported a certain amount of anhedonia, sleep disturbance, and general lowering of mood in conjunction with exacerbation of her head pain. This type of presentation is commonly associated with depressive disorders (Roy, Thomas, & Matas, 1984; Roy, 1984b). A detailed mental status examination was conducted to establish the presence of mood disorder, but the overall clinical picture failed to confirm that diagnosis.

Contracting Stage

This stage is a modification of two separate steps defined by Epstein et al. (1981a) as problem description and contracting. For the sake of brevity, these two functions have been combined. The essential task following a comprehensive assessment of family functioning is to identify areas of difficulties and generate a list of problems on which an agreement can be reached by all parties concerned.

Mr. and Mrs. A. engaged in that process actively and with a great deal of enthusiasm. They agreed: (a) that they were to spend part of the evening together and that Mr. A. would be willing to be selective in his television viewing; (b) that Mrs. A. would inform her husband when she had a headache and not simply leave it to his imagination and power of observation to find out; (c) that they should have some planned activities for the weekends; (d) that because Mrs. A.'s headaches never interfered with her work and because she had never taken a day off due to her headache, that she was not to use her headache as an excuse or reason for opting out of social engagements; and (e) that they would both spend an evening away from each other with their friends. These tasks were set to address the problems of combating the feeling of distance, neutralize the negative effects of headaches, and acknowledge their respective needs to maintain a certain amount of autonomy.

Treatment Stage

It was during this stage that Mr. and Mrs. A. began to put into effect the tasks that were identified and agreed upon. Over a period of some 6 weeks during which they were seen by the therapist on three occasions, Mr. and Mrs. A. demonstrated a remarkable ability to achieve the tasks they set for themselves and demonstrated a willingness to go well beyond that. For example, they were not only spending more time in the evenings together, but Mr. A. was paying very close attention to Mrs. A.'s work-related problems and was able to make some valuable suggestions. During this phase of treatment they had not missed a single social engagement due to Mrs. A.'s head pain, and they both seemed to be displaying a greater willingness to undertake responsibility for carrying out household chores. They were beginning to agree on allocation of roles and adherence to the rules. It is also noteworthy that Mrs. A.'s headaches subsided quite significantly during this period.

Mrs. A., who agreed to enter into couple therapy with a healthy amount of scepticism, was indeed surprised that her headache had substantially improved at the point of termination. As was stated earlier, the etiologic factors of her headache are not considered central in this modality of treatment, but some patients do benefit and have the capacity to make a connection between their improved psychosocial situation and the reduction in head pain. It is important to make a distinction between etiologic factors and family factors contributing to the maintenance of symptoms. In PCFST, it is the latter that is the focus of intervention.

Epstein et al. (1981a) have established a number of principles in negotiating and assigning tasks. Some of the key principles include: (a) Tasks should have maximum potential for success; (b) tasks should be oriented primarily to increasing positive behaviors rather than decreasing negative ones; (c) tasks should be behavioral and concrete enough so that they can be clearly understood and easily evaluated; (d) tasks should fit reasonably into the family schedule and activities; (e) task assignments to family members should be balanced so that the major responsibility for completing a task does not reside with just one or two members. Given the nature of the tasks that Mr. and Mrs. A. developed for themselves, it is quite clear that they, by and large, followed the principles.

Closure Stage

A final session was conducted to terminate this treatment, at which time improvements were being strongly maintained, with a provision for a follow-up after 8 weeks. It was stressed that treatment had indeed terminated and that this visit was simply for the purpose of monitoring their progress. Assessment and treatment for Mr. and Mrs. A. consisted of six sessions over a period of 10 weeks.

DISCUSSION

It should be stated at the outset that the case chosen to illustrate this model of family therapy has deliberately been a relatively simple one. Both in terms of the size of the system, that is, a marital dyad, and the chronicity of the headache problem itself, the case has to be viewed at the less complex end of the continuum. Roy (1984a) has discussed, in some detail, a very complex family situation involving a chronic pain sufferer who would meet all the criteria established for a chronic intractable benign pain syndrome patient (Pinsky et al., 1979).

Nevertheless, it should be recognized that, to date, overall experience using this model in treating headache or any other kind of chronic pain remains extremely limited. In the absence of either extensive clinical experience or research, it is premature to make any claims about its success in treating chronic pain syndrome.

In this instance, however, a less complex problem was selected because the situation lent itself to highlighting some key theoretical and clinical issues. In the overall picture of clinical decision-making, the following factors were considered: (a) The life-stage of the family; (b) the function of pain in their marriage; and (c) the question of homeostasis.

Life-Stage of the Family

At the point of inception into the Pain Clinic, Mr. and Mrs. A. had been married for 7 months. From a life-stage perspective, the family was in the very, very early stages of formation. This phase is known to be characterized by a significant amount of instability, and many of the problems encountered by the couple in this early stage are role-related. Both of these individuals had been living with their parents prior to the marriage and brought very different kinds of experiences into the relationship.

Mrs. A. had a tremendously ambitious father who was heavily invested in his daughter's career, and it was clear that she identified with him very greatly. She was a high-calibre scholar and as such was encouraged to pursue her academic activities to the exclusion of any other responsibility within the family. Mr. A., on the other hand, came from a family that was far less invested in his career, and his academic excellence was more or less taken for granted. He had divergent interests outside of his studies and had a close relationship with both his parents. The parents were traditional, and he grew up with a certain view of roles of men and women. In other words, this marriage was between a progressive woman with a high level of commitment to her career and a conventional man who was used to being doted on by his parents and took much of his good fortune for granted.

Haley (1963) has suggested that "marriage therapy seems indicated when a patient has a sudden onset of symptoms which coincide with the marital conflict" (p. 214). Although the symptoms in this case did not exactly coincide with the marriage and predated the marriage by a substantial number of years, there was evidence that the problem of headache had indeed exacerbated in the face of several major changes in Mrs. A.'s life. Marriage was very definitely one of them, the others included leaving home and finding herself in a very responsible job. It was the discovery of these facts in the very early stages of the assessment that led to the decision that Mrs. A.'s problems had to be reframed in the context of the marital situation.

During this phase of marriage, the couple have to work out the rules that will govern their life together in a multitude of areas. It will be largely influenced by their past experiences, and, as has already been observed, these two people brought very different family experiences and role models into the situation. Haley (1963) has identified three kinds of rules, either explicit or implicit, that a newly married couple will follow: (a) those rules the couple has announced, such as the rule that the husband could have a night out with his friends each week; (b) those rules the couple has not mentioned, but would agree to if they were pointed out; and (c) those rules an observer would note, but that the couple would probably deny.

Mr. and Mrs. A. encountered difficulties in establishing any kind of rules. In the first place they did not announce any rules; and, although there was some agreement about what each one might do without the explicit permission of the other, this was an area of considerable dissension. For example, Mrs. A. expressed a great deal of misgiving about her husband's night out with the boys. She stated that she did not so much object to his going out on his own, but that she would at least like to be asked and given the opportunity of saying no. Her husband regarded this as totally absurd, and his solution was that she should reestablish contact with her friends and start having a night out on her own. Similar problems were apparent in the context of household chores. Mrs. A. was quite unaccustomed to what may be described as conventional female roles such as cooking, cleaning, and so forth, whereas Mr. A.'s expectations, mostly unexpressed, were indeed very conventional. Again, this led to a great deal of argument and bickering; but the absence of rules in terms of who did what and the fact that allocation of roles was indeed very poorly defined must be understood in the context of the life-stage of this family.

The Function of Pain in Marriage

It is, of course, very frequently noted that symptoms play a major part in a marital relationship. The spouse with the symptoms has been described as the person with the power or, alternatively, the person lacking in power who therefore uses the symptoms to bring about a balance in "hierarchical incongruity" (Madanes, 1981). The symptom of pain has also been associated with attachment-seeking behavior (Kolb, 1982) and identified as a sign of lack of intimacy in the marital relationship (Waring, 1982).

What specific functions of pain were discernible in the relationship between Mr. and Mrs. A.? A certain amount of lack of intimacy was very evident in this marriage. The behavioral manifestation of that was their separateness at home and indeed absence of common interests. Mrs. A. had a very clear sense of disappointment with this marriage in that she was acutely aware of their lack of intimacy. Whereas her husband was able to maintain a separate life style, she was not. In that situation, the pain did, indeed, serve the function of seeking and receiving a certain amount of succor. Metaphoric use of pain to convey a range of emotion is well established (Roy, 1984c).

Two young people who were enormously invested in their professional careers had very divergent expectations from this union. It is not, therefore, altogether surprising that the more disappointed of the two, namely Mrs. A., experienced an exacerbation of her head pain. The symptom, in addition to being a way of seeking intimacy, was serving as a silent or not so silent protest against her husband's indifference.

The behavioral consequences of pain on a relationship are the only way to establish the functions, and there was enough evidence in this relationship that her headache did add to her sense of isolation and rejection, while at the same time it forced her husband to come into her own orbit. He had to directly deal with the consequences of her headaches and was compelled to pay attention to her. He, in turn, felt controlled by her pain. As they established more acceptable ways of sharing their intimacy and spending more time together, Mrs. A.'s pain complaint subsided quite remarkably.

Another critical function of pain in a marriage is its use as a scapegoat. Minuchin (1974) has described a family in formation where the child was invoked and became the focus of the marital conflict. Similarly, pain can be invoked to justify a whole host of behaviors and, in interactional terms, can provide a powerful rationale for the maintenance of pathological systems. "If only you could take the pain away" or "We never had this problem before his pain started" or, in the case of Mr. and Mrs. A., "Pain gets in the way of having a normal social life" or intimacy, furnish convincing examples of this scapegoating function of the pain complaint.

The Homeostatic Function of Pain

It may be instructive to speculate on the long-term function of head pain in the relationship between Mr. and Mrs. A. There were weak but unmistakable signs of this scapegoating function of Mrs. A.'s head pain. In addition, a pattern of detached behavior, or absence of intimacy in their interpersonal relationship, was finding justification in her pain complaint as well. Pain was beginning to provide homeostasis in this relationship. Many of this couple's difficulties in the various areas of their functioning were being incorrectly attributed to Mrs. A.'s pain problem. The central purpose of intervention was to interdict the emerging homeostasis through a process of renegotiation of their expectations, roles, and rules. In other words, this couple was enabled to move in the direction of healthy adaptation in almost all major areas of family functioning.

Need For Future Research

The application of family therapy in the treatment of chronic pain is a relatively new pur-

suit. Overall quality of research therefore is essentially weak (Roy, 1982b). Liebman et al. (1976) demonstrated the efficacy of structured family therapy in the treatment of abdominal pain in children. The study was uncontrolled, however, and there has been no subsequent effort to replicate the research using more sophisticated design. The findings therefore remain questionable. Russell, Russell, and Waring (1980) reported an outcome study using the cognitive family therapy approach with patients who presented with chronic pain symptoms. The same criticisms addressed to Liebman's work are equally applicable to this study.

In relation to the PCFST, Epstein and Bishop (1981a) have reported one major outcome study. However, they used nonpain subjects; therefore, this study has no direct relevance to the topic under discussion. The conclusion was that, although the project demonstrated the general efficacy of the method for family therapy, it left many questions unresolved. Problems such as therapists' variables, nonrandom selection of families, and lack of control, combined with difficulty in ascertaining outcome measures, made the findings both questionable and debatable.

In general terms, it can be stated without any fear of contradiction that there is a paucity of reliable outcome studies, which prevents drawing any general conclusions about the effectiveness of family therapy in general. In a major review of family therapy research of some years, Wells, Dilkes, and Trinelli (1972) noted the pervasiveness of methodological problems in measuring family therapy outcome; they were able to identify only 18 studies that met minimal standards of validity. Their review revealed the same kinds of methodological issues that Epstein and Bishop (1981a) encountered several years later in their outcome study.

The questionable quality of outcome studies in family therapy in general and the virtual absence of outcome studies in the treatment of chronic pain with family therapy are indeed matters of some concern. Nevertheless, it should be emphasized that the application of family therapy to treat pain is a recent innovation and the absence of research data in support of this particular intervention model should not act as a deterrent. On the contrary, it is hoped, as more and more clinicians begin to adopt family therapy as an adjunct treatment for chronic pain, there will be a corresponding increase in research interest. It is imperative that future outcome studies for family therapy utilize improved methodology that will take into account control groups, therapists' variables, and the critical question of sample selection. It is also imperative that family therapy approaches be compared with other modalities of treatment before any definitive statements can be made about the efficacy of family therapy.

SUMMARY

An attempt has been made in this chapter to describe the problem of headache in a young woman in the context of her marital relationship. A couple's problems were analyzed using the Problem-Centered Family Systems Therapy, the heart of which is the McMaster Model of Family Functioning. Following a comprehensive assessment of the problems, the functions of pain were delineated and behavioral objectives set to alter the emerging homeostasis. Additionally, close attention was paid to the life-stage of this marriage, and many of the problems were explained on the basis of the newly married status of this couple. The couple successfully completed treatment.

REFERENCES

Anthony, J. (1970). The impact of mental and physical illness on family life. *American Journal of Psychiatry, 127*, 138–146.

Bishop, D., & Epstein, N.B. (1980). Family process and disability. In D. Bishop (Ed.), *Behavior problems and the disabled: Assessment and management* (pp. 337–364). Baltimore, MD: Williams & Wilkins.

Block, A.R. (1981). Investigation of the response of the spouse to the chronic pain behavior. *Psychosomatic Medicine, 43*, 415–422.

Block, A.R., Kramer, E.F., & Gaylor, M. (1980). Behavioral treatment of chronic pain: The wife

as a discriminative cue for pain behavior. *Pain, 9*, 243–252.

Byles, J., Bishop, D.S., & Horn, D. (1983). Evaluation of a family therapy training program. *Journal of Marriage and Family Therapy, 9*, 299–304.

Cleghorn, J.M., & Levin, S. (1973). Training family therapists by setting learning objectives. *American Journal of Orthopsychiatry, 43*, 439–446.

Engel, G.L. (1980). The clinical application of the biopsychosocial model. *American Journal of Psychiatry, 137*, 535–544.

Epstein, N.B., & Bishop, D. (1981a) Problem-centered systems therapy of the family. In A. Gurman & D. Kniskern (Eds.), *Handbook of family therapy* (pp. 444–482). New York: Brunner/Mazel.

Epstein, N.B., & Bishop, D. (1981b). Problem-centered systems family therapy. *Journal of Marital and Family Therapy, 7*, 23–31.

Epstein, N.B., Bishop, D., & Baldwin, L. (1982). McMaster Model of Family Functioning: A view of the normal family. In F. Walsh (Ed.), *Normal family process* (pp. 115–141). New York: Guilford Press.

Epstein, N.B., Levin, S., & Bishop, D. (1976). The family as a social unit. *Canadian Family Physician, 22*, 1411–1413.

Epstein, N.B., Bishop, D., & Levin, S. (1978). The McMaster Model of Family Functioning. *Journal of Marriage & Family Counselling, 4*, 19–31.

Epstein, N.B., Sigel, J.J., & Rakoff, V. (1962). *Family categories schema.* Unpublished manuscript, Department of Psychiatry, Jewish General Hospital, McGill University, Montreal, Canada.

Haggerty, J.J. (1983). The psychosomatic family: An overview. *Psychosomatics, 24*, 615–623.

Haley, J. (1963). Marriage therapy. *Archives of General Psychiatry, 8*, 213–234.

Jackson, D. (1959). The question of family homeostatics. *Psychiatric Quarterly, 31*, (Suppl. P. I) 79–90.

Jackson, D. (1965). Family rules: Marital quid pro quo. *Archives of General Psychiatry, 12*, 589–594.

Kolb, L.C. (1982). Attachment behaviors and pain complaints. *Psychosomatics, 23*, 413–417.

Liebman, R., Honig, P., & Berger H. (1976). Integrated treatment program for psychogenic pain. *Family Process, 15*, 397–405.

Liebman, R., Minuchin, S., & Baker, L. (1974). The use of structural family therapy in the treatment of intractable asthma. *American Journal of Psychiatry, 131*, 535–540.

Livsey, C.G. (1972). Physical illness and family dynamics. *Advanced Psychosomatic Medicine, 8*, 237–251.

Madanes, C. (1981). *Strategic family therapy.* San Francisco, CA: Jossey-Bass.

Maruta, T., Osborne, D., Swenson, D.W., & Holling, J.M. (1981). Chronic pain patients and spouses: Marital & sexual adjustment. *Mayo Clinic Procedures, 56,* 307–310.

Meissner, W.W. (1980). The family & psychosomatic medicine. *Psychiatric Annals, 10,* 36–49.

Minuchin, S. (1974). *Families & family therapy,* Cambridge, MA: Harvard University Press.

Minuchin, S., Baker, L., Rosman, B.L., Liebman, R., Milman, L., & Todd, T.C. (1975). A conceptual model of psychosomatic illness in children. *Archives of General Psychiatry, 32,* 1031–1038.

Minuchin, S., Rosman, B.L., & Baker, L. (1978). *Psychosomatic families.* Cambridge, MA: Harvard University Press.

Mohamed, S.N., Weisz, G., & Waring, E.M. (1978). The relationship of chronic pain to depression, marital adjustment & family dynamics. *Pain, 5,* 282–292.

Nichols, E.R. (1978, June). *Chronic pain: A review of the interpersonal and intrapersonal factors and a study of marital interacton.* Unpublished doctoral dissertation, The University of Tennessee, Knoxville.

Pinsky, J.J., Griffin, S.E., Agnew, D.C., Jamdor, M.D., Crue, B.C., & Pinsky, C.H. (1979). Aspects of long-term evaluation of pain unit treatment program for patients with chronic intractable benign pain syndrome treatment outcome. *Bulletin Los Angeles Neurological Society, 44* (1–4 Special Edition), 53–69.

Roy, R. (1981). Social work and chronic pain. *Health & Social Work, 6,* 54–62.

Roy, R. (1982a). Chronic pain and family dynamics. In D. Freeman & B. Trute (Eds.), *Treating families with special needs.* Ottawa: Canadian Association of Social Workers.

Roy, R. (1982b). Marital and family issues in chronic pain. *Psychotherapy & Psychosomatics, 37,* 1–12.

Roy, R. (1984a). Chronic pain: A family perspective. *International Journal of Family Therapy, 6,* 31–43.

Roy, R. (1984b). Migraine and muscle-contraction headache: Psychiatric and personality issues—

A review. *International Journal of Psychiatric Medicine, 14,* 157–170.

Roy, R. (1984c). The phenomenon of "I Have A Headache." Meaning and functions of pain in marriage. *International Journal of Family Therapy, 6,* 165–176.

Roy, R., Thomas, M., & Matas, M. (1984). Chronic pain and depression. *Comprehensive Psychiatry, 25,* 96–105.

Russell, A., Russell, L., & Waring, E.M. (1980). Cognitive family therapy: A preliminary report. *Canadian Journal of Psychiatry, 15,* 64–67.

Santa Barbara, J., Woodward, C.A., Levin, S., Streiner, D., Goodman, J.T., & Epstein, N.B. (1977). Interrelationships among outcome measures in the McMaster Family Therapy Outcome Study. *Goal Attainment Review, 3,* 47–58.

Shanfield, S.B., Heinman, E.M., Cope, D.N., & Jones, J.R. (1978). Pain and marital relationship: Psychiatric distress. *Pain, 7,* 343–351.

Steinglass, P.A. (1980). Life history model of the alcoholic family. *Family Process, 19,* 211–226.

Swenson, D.W., & Maruta, T. (1980). The family's viewpoint of pain. *Pain, 8,* 163–166.

Tunks, E., & Roy, R. (1982). Chronic pain and the occupational role. In R. Roy & E. Tunks (Eds.), *Chronic pain: Psychosocial factors in rehabilitation* (pp. 53–65). Baltimore, MD: Williams & Wilkins.

Waring, E.M. (1977). The role of the family in symptom selection and perpetuation of psychosomatic illness. *Psychotherapy Psychosomatics, 23,* 253–259.

Waring, E.M. (1982). Conjoint marital and family therapy. In R. Roy & E. Tunks (Eds.), *Chronic pain: Psychosocial factors in rehabilitation* (pp. 151–165). Baltimore, MD: Williams & Wilkins.

Wells, R.A., Dilkes, T.C., & Trinelli, N. (1972). The results of family therapy: A critical review of the literature. *Family Process, 11,* 189–207.

Westley, A., & Epstein, N.B. (1970). *The silent majority.* San Francisco, CA: Jossey-Bass.

Woodward, C.A., Santa Barbara, J., Streiner, D.L., Goodman, J.T., Levin, S., & Epstein, N.B. (1981). Client, treatment and therapist variables related to outcome in brief, systems oriented family therapy. *Family Process, 20,* 189–197.

9 BIOFEEDBACK IN THE TREATMENT OF CHRONIC BACK PAIN

Cynthia D. Belar
Stephen A. Kibrick

Over 18 million Americans suffer from chronic painful back disorders (Bonica, 1980). In addition, it is estimated that approximately 10.3 million outpatient visits are made to nonfederally employed physicians each year for back pain, almost one million more visits than for upper respiratory infections (National Center for Health Statistics, 1983). A costly health problem, U.S. expenditures in 1978 for the treatment of back pain have been estimated at 14 billion dollars (Schaepe, 1982). Back pain is the third leading cause of physical limitation (U.S. Department of Health, Education and Welfare, 1974), permanently disabling some 65,000 patients per year (Beals & Hickman, 1972).

Back pain may be a symptom of malignancies, visceral diseases, vascular disease, fracture, infection, ligament rupture, intervertebral disk rupture, paraspinous muscle damage, or congenital defects, to name a few possible causes. Although numerous diagnostic terms are associated with back pain (e.g., lumbosacral strain, myalgia), most are descriptive in nature and have little explanatory value. The term *chronic back pain* (CBP) is commonly used to refer to benign back pain of 6 months or more duration. Its origin is believed to be related to degenerative, muscular, or inflammatory processes, structural abnormalities, or traumatic injuries, although the precise mechanisms are unclear.

Flor and Turk (1984) have recently published an excellent review of research on somatic models and interventions for chronic back pain, concluding that, despite the magnitude of the problem and the abundance of literature, "amazingly little is known about the causes, and hence effective treatment" (p. 106). In their evaluation of research on somatic treatments (including medication, surgery, steroid injections, nerve blocks, physical therapy, transcutaneous electrical nerve stimulation, traction, and prosthetic devices), they note significant methodological problems with respect to: (a) lack of adequate controls, (b) insufficient description of patient characteristics, (c) lack of differentiation between acute and chronic conditions, (d) insufficient measures of treatment outcomes, (e) lack of follow-up, and (f) disregard of psychosocial antecedents and consequences of CBP. Over time, the lack of demonstrated effectiveness of these medical treatments, plus the increasingly accepted view of CBP as involving the interaction of physiological, psychological, and social factors, have led to a multidisciplinary approach to the study and treatment of CBP.

In the past decade, the number of multidisciplinary pain clinics has mushroomed. In these clinics, one of the most frequent problems seen is CBP, ranging from around 30 to 40% (Hallett & Pilowsky, 1982; Pinsky, 1983) to nearly 100% of the clinic populations (Cinciripini & Floreen, 1982; Keefe, Black, Williams, & Surwit, 1981). These clinics usually utilize a variety of the somatic treatments previously mentioned, in addition to group therapies, behavioral management, cognitive behavioral therapies, self-hypnosis, relaxation training, and biofeedback. This chapter will focus on the use of biofeedback in the treatment of chronic back pain, although it is recognized that biofeedback is rarely used in isolation, nor, in the authors' opinion, should it be when attempting to manage a disorder as complex as chronic back pain.

There are two major rationales for the use of biofeedback in managing CBP. One involves the use of biofeedback as an aid in relaxation training. An assumption underlying this usage is that when general arousal is reduced, central processing of peripheral sensory inputs is also reduced. A related rationale for this type of approach is based on the relationship between anxiety and pain. Because anxiety is known to be related to decreased pain tolerance and increased levels of reported pain, relaxation (which is incompatible with anxiety) should result in increases in pain tolerance and decreased distress.

The other major rationale for the use of biofeedback for CBP is based on the pain–spasm–pain cycle described by Bonica (1957). Utilizing this model, treatment is directed at specific peripheral factors believed to be associated with pain (e.g., paraspinal muscle spasm).

Consistent with these models, clinical research in this area has utilized alpha electroencephalogram (EEG) feedback training (Melzack & Perry, 1975), frontalis electromyogram (EMG) (Hendler, Derogatis, Avella, & Long, 1977), and paraspinal EMG feedback (Belar & Cohen, 1979; Kravitz, Moore, Glaros, & Stauffer, 1978; Todd & Belar, 1980) to either assist in achieving a state of general relaxation or to produce control (i.e., ability to relax) of specific muscles whose spasms and/or chronic tension were believed responsible for the pain experienced. However, usually even the latter, more "focal" usage of biofeedback entailed general relaxation instructions as part of the treatment package.

In fact, there are only two controlled outcome studies of biofeedback alone found in the literature. Nouwen and Solinger (1979) demonstrated decreased EMG levels during training of the m. erector spinae near the second lumbar vertebrae, with a subsequent 60% decrease in the pain ratings of the biofeedback group as compared to controls. Flor, Haag, Turk, and Koehler (1983) compared EMG biofeedback to a credible pseudotherapy and a conventional medical treatment for chronic rheumatic back pain. Only the biofeedback group showed significant improvements in the duration, intensity, and quality of pain. Even at 4 months follow-up, the biofeedback group reported a 62% reduction in daily pain ratings.

Although these studies are promising, there are a number of methodological issues that make research in this area difficult to evaluate (see Turk and Flor, 1984). Wolf, Nacht, and Kelly (1982) point out the oversimplification that has permeated clinical treatment and research. They note that not all CBP patients demonstrate elevated paraspinal EMG levels and that EMG activity during movement and different postures has been largely ignored. Given these factors, plus the lack of a documented relationship between reductions in EMG and reductions in pain, absolute decrease in EMG may not be an appropriate treatment goal. Wolf et al. describe a case utilizing EMG feedback to train for symmetry between right and left paraspinal muscle groups and to train for "normal" patterns of activity during static postures and trunk rotation. Indeed, very recent research (Flor, Turk, & Birbaumer, 1984; Sterman, 1984) suggests individualized muscle pattern abnormalities related to position and personal stressors in CBP patients. Identification of these individual patterns is important in the assessment and treatment of CBP, though as yet they are largely ignored in treatment research and clinical practice. A comprehensive review of the relationship between paraspinal EMG and chronic low back pain is provided by Nouwen and Bush (1984).

In clinical practice, however, there is another rationale for utilizing biofeedback on occasion. The utility of this model, although not explored by empirical research, is frequently referred to anecdotally (Freeman, Calsyn, Paige, & Halar, 1980) and is well known to practicing clinicians. This is the model of biofeedback as a facilitator of truly psychosomatic therapy. Lipowski (1984) has described the historical use of this frequently misunderstood term, concluding with a clarification of psychosomatic as relating "to the inseparability and interdependence of psychosocial and biologic (physiologic, somatic) agents of human-kind" (p. 167). Thus, psychosomatic therapy is an intervention involving *inseparable* and *interdependent* psychosocial and biologic aspects. Some patients have an exclusively somatic focus to their presenting problems and have no perception of behavior–emotion–environment interactions that may be perpetuating/exacerbating somatic symptoms. For these patients, initiating treatment with the technology of biofeedback is a potentially less threatening method by which the patient can learn the "physiological insight" through which discovering and dealing with "psychological spasms" can occur.

The following two case descriptions will serve to illustrate how biofeedback training may be utilized as a more "focal" treatment (Case Study 1) or as a means to facilitate general relaxation in the context of psychosomatic therapy (Case Study 2).

The cases will be presented by session, first indicating the clinical procedures employed, then describing the results, followed by an action/plan for the therapist. An analysis of relevant issues follows each session or grouping of sessions. In general, it should be remembered that it is our opinion that one treats not back *pain*, but back pain *patients*, who demonstrate a host of behavioral, cognitive, social, and physiological problems by the time they reach the therapist's office. In our experience, it has been rare that biofeedback as a strategy, even when combined with general relaxation training, has been sufficient psychological management for these patients.

Case Study 1: Mr. B., A 52-year-old Man With Back Pain

Session 1: $1\frac{1}{2}$ hours therapist time.

Procedures. Medical record review; intake interview with patient and spouse if possible; Minnesota Multiphasic Personality Inventory (MMPI); feedback to patient.

Results. Mr. B. is a 52-year-old plumber who injured his back at work approximately 2 years ago. He describes painful muscle spasms with knife-like pain in his lower back, occurring several times a day and increasing with movement and fatigue. He also describes chronic back tension as he "guards" against spasm. He has been treated conservatively (heat, massage, bedrest, corset, William's back exercises, antiinflammatory medications, and muscle relaxants) without significant relief. Married and the father of two grown children, he has worked intermittently since the injury. Currently feeling unable to work (which involves twisting and turning motions), he receives worker's compensation benefits. Repeated myelograms have been normal; neurosurgical evaluations reveal no indications for surgery. Mr. B. carries the diagnosis of "lumbosacral strain, with palpable muscle spasms." Although he denies depression, his wife describes him as having been increasingly more irritable. He reports fitful sleep, with onset insomnia, weight gain, and a decrease in social contacts. Sexual intercourse sometimes precipitates muscle spasms, thus sex has decreased in frequency. His hobbies include fishing, which he has discontinued since he stopped working. He complains about some loss of self-esteem in terms of his role as a breadwinner, but denies other emotional concerns. He appears somewhat angry and defensive about having been referred by his physician to a psychologist for evaluation, although he is overtly cooperative. His wife appears supportive and very protective of her husband.

MMPI reveals significant elevations on scales 1 (Hypochondriasis), 2 (Depression), and 3 (Hysteria), all around T-70 with an F-K of −14. The patient tends to deny strong affect and needs to present himself as very emotionally stable and rational.

Action/Plan.

1. Give general rationale for psychological treatments, providing reassurance that pain is not imaginary.
2. Teach patient how to complete pain diary, with hourly ratings of pain and description of activities. (See Appendix A for a description of the pain diary.)
3. Make appointment for EMG baseline recordings in 2 to 4 weeks.
4. Note potential target areas for interventions: muscle spasms, sleep, social activities, weight, wife's support for pain behavior, management of activity level, sexual behavior, body mechanics, and exercises.

Analysis. In addition to obtaining historical information and completing a general psychological evaluation, the first session is critical in terms of establishing a therapeutic alliance with the patient. Mr. B., as many pain patients, is angry that his physician referred him to a psychologist and quite defensive about the possibility of any emotional concerns. If the patient does not bring up the issue of whether pain may be "all-in-the-head," it is important for the therapist to do so. We always emphasize that all pain is a subjective experience that can be influenced by a variety of factors and that we are interested in finding out about all of those factors

so that we are able to help the patient as intensively and as extensively as would be beneficial. Although we may focus on psychological issues and coping with pain, we are not assuming that the patient is either "crazy" or "imagining" the pain. This theme arises repeatedly in the initial stages of treatment; one cannot assume that a single explanation is sufficient. It must be confronted each time. Until there is at least some resolution, an adversarial relationship with the therapist will result, with the patient having to constantly prove that the pain is "real" and therefore unable to be changed by any psychological intervention. There are several strategies that can be useful:

1. Give information about the relationship between psychological factors and pain (e.g., previous studies; examples from everyday life, such as discomfort experienced from head cold under different conditions: participation in exciting basketball game vs. working on income taxes).
2. Discuss how pain may become "conditioned." (This kind of language appears especially useful for patients who are not psychologically minded.) We frequently use the example of an imaginary lemon that, if described vividly by the therapist, can produce a "real" salivary response on the part of the patient. This in-session experience can be very powerful. We do not go into differences between classical and operant conditioning, etc., but use a "relearning," "deconditioning," and "desensitizing" language throughout treatment, sometimes replacing words such as anxiety with terms such as "nervous system arousal" for the most defensive patients.
3. Communicate empathy for the patient's frustration with previous treatments and understanding of anger if patient had been informed by a (probably frustrated) physician that his or her problem was "psychological."
4. Agree with the "specificity model" of some aspect of the patient's pain (e.g., muscle spasm) while describing a treatment tech-

nique (e.g., EMG biofeedback) that may be useful to the patient in learning to control muscle tension levels.

Another aspect of the first session, which is most important, has to do with how the therapist "postures" with respect to the patient's pain problem. Well-meaning beginners frequently want to "cure" patients and may communicate this intent. The seasoned therapist who accepts his or her limitations communicates to the patient expertise in the treatment of chronic pain problems, but postures as a consultant/teacher, explicitly placing full responsibility for the work of therapy on the patient. The patient's ambivalence about accepting this responsibility will also surface throughout treatment. In our opinion, treatment cannot be successful, nor gains maintained, without the patient working through this aspect; any strategy that highlights the patient's sense of control and active involvement seems to facilitate this acceptance. Strategies to increase active involvement by patients include: (a) keeping pain diaries, (b) graphing own treatment data, (c) making own relaxation tapes, (d) serving as peer counselor for another CBP patient, and (e) reading relevant materials (a patient workbook has been developed to facilitate patients' learning in our programs).

In the case of Mr. B., having him begin to keep a pain diary after the first session was useful for several other reasons as well: (a) It provided an estimate of activity levels and related pain; (b) it provided a data set from which the therapist began to derive hypotheses (we also encourage patients to note good and bad stressors in their diary); (c) it acknowledged the acceptance by the therapist of experienced pain as a problem for the patient; and (d) it provided a concrete data set against which the patient assessed changes over the course of treatment, such as increases in activity without substantial increases in reported pain.

Another appointment was made for EMG baseline. Mr. B.'s description of tension and painful muscle spasms in his lower back had suggested that EMG biofeedback might be a useful aspect of treatment.

The fact that Mr. B. was receiving worker's compensation benefits was not viewed as a contraindication to treatment. Had he been suing someone for liability associated with his back problem, however, the decision to treat would probably have been different. In our experience, disability payments for pain-related problems (although obviously potentially powerful positive reinforcers for sick role behavior) do not necessarily prohibit treatment gains. However, the patient who is in the midst of liability litigations has, in our opinion, more pressures to maintain the status quo until settlement of the suit. Thus, we do not accept such patients for treatment until litigation is completed.

Session 2: $1\frac{1}{4}$ hours.

Procedures. EMG baseline; review pain diary.

Two sets of electrodes were attached to the prepared skin approximately $1\frac{1}{2}$ in. to either side of the spinal cord at L_4–L_5, above the m. sacrospinalis. (Techniques of bioelectric recording are fully described in technical manuals accompanying biofeedback equipment.) Mr. B. was in a prone position and was asked to relax as much as possible for 15 minutes while data were recorded. He was also asked to verbally rate his pain at present. Subsequently, EMG data were collected under the following seven conditions, each 4 minutes in length: (a) cognitive task (serial 7's backwards from 100); (b) imagining a pleasant, relaxing scene; (c) imagining a personally relevant negatively stressful scene; (d) imagining a pleasant, relaxing scene; (e) sitting; (f) standing; and (g) forward flexion (bending 45° forward).

Results. Overall, there did not appear to be asymmetry in muscle tension under the various conditions, that is, right versus left electrode placements recorded approximately the same levels of muscle tension under the different conditions. There was some increase from an average of 4.92 microvolts (Autogen 1700 filter settings of 100–200 Hz, and Autogen 5100 1-minute average) to 5.3 microvolts under the serial 7's condition, and somewhat more (6.52 microvolts) under the negative stressor (which for Mr. B. involved imagining his painful spasms). Sitting, standing, and forward flexion were marked by further increases in average EMG levels (up to 9.41 microvolts). Pleasant imagery conditions averaged around 5 microvolts.

Action/plan.

1. Review baseline data with patient.
2. Explain rationale for EMG feedback training (train for paraspinal muscle relaxation and control).
3. Give support for completing diary.
4. Consult with physical therapy for training in body mechanics and review of back exercises.
5. Review relationship between excess abdominal weight and back strain. Develop weight control program.
6. Enlist support of wife in not rewarding excessive sick role behavior.

Analysis. Had asymmetry in muscle tension been noted, then a biofeedback training for symmetry paradigm (Wolfe et al., 1982) would also be required. In this case, however, simply learning to decrease paraspinal muscle tension was chosen as the initial goal of biofeedback. This reflects a specific usage of biofeedback, targeted at muscles whose increased tension is believed to account for some of the reported pain. However, more general effects such as those obtained from biofeedback-assisted relaxation training would also be likely to result, as would effects due to an increase in perceived control, which in the face of aversive stimulation, has been associated with increased pain tolerance. It was explained to the patient that, although there is preliminary evidence that biofeedback alone may result in some pain reduction, it has been our experience and that of others that best results are obtained from a multifaceted treatment program, because

chronic pain is such a multifaceted and complex problem.

It was noted that Mr. B. could not think of any negative stressor during baseline, thus it was suggested that he focus on his pain for these recordings. We find it helpful to have the patient choose the scene just prior to the recording of that condition, although we do not inquire as to what they had chosen until after the baselines are completed and we have more opportunity to discuss the situation.

Review of the pain diary provides the first opportunity to assess patient compliance. It is noted that in general patient compliance is better predicted by characteristics of the treatment regime than by patient characteristics. If instructions are not followed, rather than make an early interpretation of "resistance," it is important to assess the patient's understanding of instructions and acceptance of the rationale for treatment, continuously supporting his or her active involvement in the treatment process. Appendix B gives a possible script for explanation of treatment. We do not encourage the use of fixed scripts, however, but prefer to tailor our language and examples to the experiential background and cognitive framework of the patient.

Session 3: 1 hour.

Procedures. Progressive muscle relaxation (PMR) exercises, modified to avoid tensing of lower back area; session was tape recorded; diary was reviewed and activities discussed.

Results. Mr. B. reported some cramping of leg muscles, thus exercises were modified to shorten time in tensing these muscles. He also reported some skepticism concerning the relationship between relaxation and his pain problem. Diary appeared to reveal pattern of overdoing it (working on car 3 to 4 hours) and then inactivity (bedrest all day) due to increased pain.

Action/Plan.

1. Explain again the rationale of learning to discriminate levels of muscle tension as

well as the finding that relaxation is associated with increased pain tolerance—even when pain is from a variety of different causes. Explore possibility of "unusual feelings" during relaxation. (Patient denied any.)

2. Continue pain diary; suggest pacing of activities and use of quota system.
3. Elicit and discuss concerns regarding nature of treatment.
4. Instruct to practice relaxation exercises twice per day. Gave Mr. B. tape of session. Enlist wife in supporting home practice and activity pacing. Encourage practice at bedtime given sleep onset problem.

Analysis. PMR training was chosen versus autogenic or imagery techniques because we believed that the rationale related to muscle tension would make more "sense" to this patient at this time. We prefer to tape the relaxation sessions as one of the home practice tapes so we can make modifications particular to the patient and personalize suggestions. Thus, the patient also takes some of the therapy home. Later in treatment we encourage patients to make their own tapes in order to facilitate autosuggestions and to reinforce their active role in treatment. To reinforce the need for home practice, we present a very pessimistic view regarding the long-term effects of treatment without this component. To facilitate compliance, we have the patient record times of practice in the diary, and we enlist the support of significant others within the household.

On occasion, spouses and other family members are invited for conjoint sessions. A day-care program run by the senior author involved weekly family sessions. In other cases, spouses have been a part of the initial evaluation process and have had the treatment regimen fully explained, with only intermittent contacts made subsequently. Spouse involvement is usually, but not always, a prerequisite for treatment. The intensity of contact will depend upon the therapist's assessment of how powerful the home environment is in maintaining sick role behavior.

We have seldom encountered an unwilling spouse. If we do, we may still treat the patient if he or she is informed about potential problems that may arise. We agree to be alert to such issues and to reevaluate treatment goals as needed; sometimes we may "challenge" the patient to behave independently of the spouse.

We do frequently encounter "uncooperative" spouses who either sabotage treatment through well-intentioned ignorance or through competing and counter-therapeutic interpersonal behavior patterns. The former problems are solved early through information-giving; the latter require relationship counseling, which we have already indicated to the patient may become a focus for treatment.

In general, we educate our patients as to our model of pain and the influences on its experience (sensory input, affective states, cognitions, positive reinforcers, negative reinforcers, culture/modeling effects, lack of support for well behavior). We plan treatments to intervene in every area deemed appropriate.

Session 4: 1 hour.

Procedures. Diary review; first EMG biofeedback session.

Mr. B. began training in prone position. The relationship between the two meter readings of microvolt levels and the bilateral levels of paraspinal muscle tension was explained.

Mr. B. was encouraged to experiment with the equipment, increasing and decreasing (as possible) muscle tension via movement, thoughts, "internal manipulations," etc., so that he could fully comprehend the relationship of the meter readings to his internal physiology. For another 10 minutes he was encouraged to reduce his muscle tension utilizing continuous visual feedback from the Autogen 1700 meters.

Results. Mr. B. was surprised that focusing mentally on his back pain could increase his paraspinal tension. He was not successful in substantially reducing his muscle tension, but did note considerable variability. He was uncomfortable in the prone position on our rather hard examining table.

Action/Plan.

1. Plan future sessions in sitting position.
2. Encourage Mr. B. to attend to how often he dwells on pain while at home.
3. Continue home practice and diary.

Analysis. Because there was no paraspinal EMG asymmetry noted on baseline, it would be possible to average the bilateral muscle tension levels and thus utilize various forms of auditory feedback. With back pain patients, however, we find it useful to always separately monitor paraspinal tension, especially given the fact that only one baseline session is obtained. Although one baseline may be an inadequate sample, we have not been able to clinically justify the added cost of multiple baseline sessions.

When we do not rely on dual meter feedback, several different modes of auditory feedback are briefly demonstrated to the patient (clicks, tones, etc.) and the patient is asked his or her preference as to mode and volume. This involves the patient immediately in the treatment.

We usually start training utilizing continuous feedback, under the assumption that continuous reinforcement is more helpful in the early stages of learning. We will switch to a threshold procedure after one or two sessions if no change has occurred within a session. We generally look at several successive 1-minute averages of EMG activity and set the threshold at a level about 10 to 15% below these values. It is best if the patient is able to stay below threshold about 80 to 90% of the time.

One paradigm uses audio signals above threshold with no audio below threshold; the patient learns to "turn off" the audio tone when relaxation below threshold occurs. Another variation is to provide a pleasant audio stimulus (usually recorded music), either of the patient's preference (we have patients bring in cassettes of their favorite "music to relax by") or preselected by the therapist for its soothing properties. In this paradigm, the patient turns on the music by staying below threshold on EMG, and he or she must stay below threshold to continue hearing music. A longer time-constant for signal processing is used to avoid short on–off cycling near threshold. This positive reinforcement technique has the advantage of aiding in later generalization, as patients can take home the music (on cassette) and use it for practice in their home environment. This often helps to "bridge the gap" between clinic practice with the equipment and home practice without it.

We generally do not recommend taking EMG biofeedback equipment home for practice as this tends to foster dependence on the hardware rather than on learning independent control. EMG feedback training gives information about a physiological system in the body that is already under voluntary control and for which the patient already has kinesthetic sensations (proprioceptors, stretch receptors, etc.). If a patient has great difficulty, more frequent clinic sessions can be recommended in the early stages of learning.

We do sometimes utilize home use of temperature monitors when focusing on general relaxation training (or when working with other psychophysiologic disorders). Although many of these devices are not accurate or responsive enough for true feedback training, they do facilitate awareness of different autonomic states. Patients do not have an innate "sense" of these subtle skin temperature changes, and extra information is helpful. Patients may be asked to record temperature data in their pain diary and can thus readily see under what conditions (persons, places, thoughts) their bodies are responding.

Session 5: 1 hour.

Procedures. Diary review; EMG feedback training (sitting position): 5 minutes presession baseline (no feedback); 20 minutes continuous feedback; 5 minutes post-session (no feedback).

Results. Mr. B. demonstrated a good deal of variability in his EMG levels. For a few minutes it seemed as if he was able to decrease muscle tension, but these trends were quickly reversed. He reported trying very hard.

Mr. B. was able to fall asleep better at night utilizing his relaxation tape.

Action/Plan.

1. Discuss with patient need to not "try too hard"; discuss relationship between pressure to perform and increased muscle tension; inquire about pressure to perform in home/work situations and patient identifies similar situations; discuss sense of failure due to patient's not working and his feeling that it is not appropriate to engage in recreational activities if "disabled"; discuss negative effects of decreased social/ recreational activities and encourage more involvement.

2. Support patient in learning to relax muscles as a skill that may take time to learn; suggest that patient might experiment with pleasant imagery, encourage patient to bring in cassette of his favorite relaxing music to play as background during imagery; patient can then play this music during home practice as well.

Analysis. All potential relationships among behavioral strategies ("trying too hard"), feeling states ("pressure"), and muscle tension are explored. How the patient approaches the biofeedback task is a sample of how he or she may approach other performance tasks. Patients frequently inhibit relaxation by "working at it"; the therapist can encourage them to "let it happen" or to utilize distracting imagery (e.g., pleasant scenes, limp muscles) with only occasional attention to the feedback signal.

Many patients who are not working feel that they should also then not engage in social or recreational activities; this results in increased isolation and inactivity that perpetuates the chronic pain syndrome. The therapist can utilize the leverage of professional expertise to give permission or "prescribe" more activities, even if other agencies/ family members have not been supportive of this. Explaining the rationale to family members is important.

Sessions 6-13: 1 hour each, twice a week.

Procedures. Diary review and discussion; EMG feedback training.

Results. Mr. B., by the end of the 7th session could decrease his muscle tension to around 3 microvolts, but could not sustain this without feedback at the end of the session. Beginning in Session 8, feedback was withheld at intermittent intervals during the training trials.

Mr. B. reported that when his back muscles were the most relaxed they felt "loose." This language was utilized in future discussions of his relaxed state, and he was encouraged to use this term as a cue to facilitate relaxation outside of therapy. He began to report fewer episodes of spasm, stating that he could now sometimes identify earlier "twinges" and institute his relaxation before onset of the spasm.

As therapy progressed, a more trusting relationship developed with the therapist. Diary review and informal chit-chat while attaching and unhooking electrodes led to the discovery of several problem areas:

1. Mr. B. and his wife have a limited repertoire of sexual behavior, yet his common pattern of male superior intercourse aggravates his back pain, which resulted in less frequent sex and decreased self-esteem.

2. Mr. B. is resentful that his grown children, who visit weekly, never offer to help his wife with any of the heavy chores, now left to her for management.

Discussions of alternate sexual positions and strategies for assertion were incorporated into the session.

When Mr. B. seemed able to lower his muscle tension without feedback and to maintain these low levels for 5 minutes or more, we began practice under stress conditions (e.g., imagining a muscle spasm) as well as standing and forward flexion positions (45°), first with feedback and then without.

Analysis. The criteria utilized for deciding when to move to the next step in training are arbitrary. We do find it helpful, however, to assure that the initial relaxation response is overlearned before proceeding to other tasks in training. It is also noted that almost without exception, intrasession variability of the physiological response decreases as control is learned.

As in any other therapy, there may be plateaus of seemingly little progress. These are normal, but sometimes progress can be facilitated by a simple change in strategies (e.g., continuous feedback to threshold training, visual feedback to auditory feedback). Patients are urged repeatedly to view their training as analogous to learning a sport or mastering a new musical instrument. In addition to fostering independent practice at home and placing responsibility for success on *their* efforts, this approach also makes it easier to deal with setbacks when they inevitably occur. Reference is made to a "learning curve," which may show "ups and downs" in any given period, but can still indicate generally upward progress. Comparisons to the "off" day of a well-trained athlete, or other similar examples, prove helpful in maintaining motivation. We do consider 10 to 12 sessions as an adequate trial of biofeedback training and would recommend cessation of this aspect of treatment if no gain were noted.

In chronic back pain patients such as Mr. B., some asymmetry might be noted during more complex tasks, such as forward flexion, which was not picked up on baseline. This should be watched for, and "balance" training instituted should it be noted. "Balance" training involves maintaining equality of left and right paraspinal EMG during standing and forward trunk flexion movements versus simple relaxation of bilateral muscle tension. The patient makes use of independent feedback meters to internally coordinate muscle activity.

Training for generalization and maintenance are paramount. Strategies to facilitate generalization include:

1. Moving from continuous to intermittent to no feedback conditions within sessions;
2. Varying the conditions under which relaxation can be produced (standing, sitting, under stress) in sessions;
3. Developing "cues" for relaxation that can be utilized in the environment (e.g., self-statements such as "stay loose"; reminders on watch, refrigerator, auto dashboard, etc.);
4. Practicing relaxation training at home with tapes made in sessions, then with tapes made by patient, and finally without any taped instructions.
5. Practicing relaxation, and scanning for tenseness, in a variety of increasingly difficult extra-session situations.

There are no studies comparing the variety of methods and schedules of EMG feedback training for the treatment of CBP. Thus, although biofeedback may seem to be a more "scientific" psychological treatment, much of the application remains a clinical art, requiring judgment and sensitivity to the individual patient's needs.

Sessions 14-18: Follow-up and booster sessions; 1 hour; biweekly and then quarterly until 18 months; diary discontinued at 16th session.

Results. Mr. B. continued to do well, with a greater than 50% decrease in daily ratings of pain while concomitantly increasing his activity level substantially. He began working in a plumbing supply store parttime, though he could not return to full employment as a plumber due to the numerous twisting and bending positions required. He was arranging with worker's compensation to support him in a vocational training program in small appliance repair. He still had difficulty relaxing his paraspinal muscles after a spasm had started, but felt he was much more able to prevent spasm onset. His wife described him as less irritable and more loving.

Analysis. Follow-up sessions are designed to provide practice with the equipment and discussion of problem areas based on individual patient needs. They also provide the opportunity to reinforce strategies for maintenance, especially home practice. Phone-in checkups and "alumni" groups can also be used to facilitate maintenance.

Case Study 2: Mrs. L., A 34-year-old Woman With Neck, Shoulder, And Back Pain

Session 1: $1\frac{1}{2}$ hours therapist time.

Procedures. Medical record review; intake interview with patient; MMPI; feedback to patient.

Results. Mrs. L. is a 34-year-old nurse who strained her back and neck while reaching to catch her child who was falling off a piece of playground apparatus. This precipitating incident occurred 9 months ago and coincided with her transfer to a new unit in the hospital that placed increased work demands on her. She describes continuing episodes of painful spasms in her neck, shoulders, and back, which have caused her to miss work. She has received supportive treatment (heat, massage) from the physical therapy department at work and has relied on increasing doses of muscle relaxants and pain medication prescribed by "helpful" colleagues. Divorced and the mother of two school-age children, she has continued to work despite episodes of increasing pain.

Physical exam findings were negative; neurological consultation also was unremarkable. This patient was self-referred, as she found herself no longer able to work without relying on medication, a situation that she found increasingly intolerable, as the dosages she was now taking interfered with her alertness at work. She noted that her symptoms were much worse on "high stress" days at work. She denied depression or other "psychiatric" symptoms, but did report some sleep disturbances.

She denied significant symptom-related problems in her social life away from work, although she admitted that she was less able to engage in physical activity with her children and that she had stopped playing tennis and hiking with friends on the weekends. She was "annoyed" that her medical colleagues had found no "organic" basis for her complaints, but stated she was "willing to try anything." She specifically requested biofeedback treatment, as she was interested in "handling this on my own" and eliminating what she feared was an increasing dependency on drugs. MMPI was within normal limits, with moderate elevation on scale 2, Depression (T = 68). Results indicated high ego strength and only moderate defensiveness. Patient describes herself as very rational and perfectionistic.

Action/Plan.

1. Assure patient that pain is not imaginary and that her goals in treatment are realistic.
2. Instruct patient in keeping pain diary with hourly ratings of pain and activities.
3. Schedule appointment for baseline session in 1 week.
4. Note potential target areas for intervention: muscle spasms, sleep, increased social activities, body mechanics, reduced drug use, more assertive behavior with supervision at work.

Analysis. This patient is educated, knowledgeable about human physiology and clinical pharmacology, and moderately sophisticated about psychological matters. She is not seeking compensation for a work-related injury and appears highly motivated to learn self-control pain management techniques. Her elevated score on the Depression scale of the MMPI is largely due to endorsing many somatic items on this scale. High ego strength and the facts that symptoms have a clear onset and that this pain pattern has not been of long duration (less than 1 year) are all positive prognostic signs for successful biofeedback treatment.

Session 2: 1 hour.

Procedure. EMG baseline; review pain symptom and diary.

A spaced (differential) EMG electrode array was applied to forehead (frontal) area of patient's head. A Biotrode strip was applied horizontally, centered 1 in. above nasion. Autogen SCL electrodes were attached to the three middle fingers of the dominant hand. EMG was monitored with Autogen 1700 and data were integrated on Autogen 5100. SCL was monitored on Autogen 3400. (See equipment manuals for detailed procedures used.)

Patient reclined in a reclining chair with her eyes closed in a sound-attenuated temperature-controlled room. After 10 minutes of adaptation, averaged EMG and SCL readings were taken at 1-minute intervals for 20 minutes, during which patient was instructed to "just relax" and no further verbal instructions were given. Data were then collected as patient was taken through the following conditions: (a) mildly stressful cognition task (subtracting 7 serially from 100); (b) imagining a very pleasant relaxing scene; (c) imagining a personally relevant negatively stressful scene; (d) imagining a pleasant scene; (e) sudden loud sound startle stimulus (hand clap); (f) quiet, relaxed, easy breathing; and (g) 15 seconds of hyperventilation. Conditions a, b, c, d, and f were all 2 minutes in length.

Results. Patient appeared to be able to relax under conditions (b, d, f) of mildly pleasant arousal (average EMG = 1.27 microvolts, bandpass of 100–200 Hz). She showed significant elevation in frontal EMG (average EMG = 3.51 microvolts) for a mildly stressful cognition task (serial 7's), however; and patient remarked that she wanted to be sure to "get them all right."

Skin conductance level (SCL) data indicated high levels of autonomic arousal (average = 15.7 microohms) during condition of mild cognitive stress (serial 7's). Levels dropped to 8.1 during pleasant imagining, but increased to 26.9 during hyperventilation, and hit a high of near 30 microohms in response to startle stimulus (hand clap).

Action Plan.

1. Review baseline data with patient.
2. Explain rationale for EMG training (general relaxation of skeletal musculature; frontal area sometimes useful as index of overall body tension; describe possible future monitoring sites: bilateral upper trapezius, bilateral lumbar paraspinal muscles).
3. Explain rationale for SCL training (autonomic hyperarousal to mild stress induces generalized state of tension, leading to muscle spasms, and associated pain; vicious cycle).
4. Give support for completing accurate pain diary, log of concurrent activities, thoughts, and feelings, and medications log (very important in this case).
5. Enlist cooperation of patient's physician (with permission from patient) to prescribe medications only for a fixed interval schedule, i.e., three or four times a day — not on an "as needed" basis. Plan to fade pain medications as patient progresses in treatment.
6. Enlist support of patient's medical colleagues in the hospital (with patient's permission and support) to not engage in "handing out" extra medications or in reinforcing pain behavior.

Analysis. Both EMG and SCL were monitored for this patient, as it appeared that both central nervous system (CNS) parameters as well as autonomic nervous system (ANS) responses were involved in the etiology of her CBP syndrome. A frontal site (forehead) for EMG monitoring was chosen because she was complaining of head and neck tension and pain, which often exacerbated her upper and lower back pain. We have found this to be a good site to begin training upper-body relaxation, and once patients have begun to learn to lower EMG levels monitored from the frontal area, they are usually able to transfer this learning to other muscle groups in the body. Once a patient is able to relax one set of muscles at will, even in the presence' of pain symptoms from nearby areas, they find it much easier to transfer this learned skill to other muscle groups. Low EMG values (less than 1.0 microvolts) during mildly pleasant arousal conditions indicate that this patient can already relax when not particularly stressed—a very positive sign for treatment. Chronically tense patients are often unable to lower EMG levels even under low arousal baseline conditions and often require many more sessions of training to be able to lower EMG to values approaching 1 microvolt (integral-averaged, 100–200 H_2 bandpass).

SCL values are often used (as here) to give an indicator of overall autonomic arousal and can be read as an index of overall level of emotional arousal. The values from this patient are typical of those seen in "anxious" patients, and the lability of these readings (8.1 microohms to 30 microohms) is generally a good prognostic sign. Patients who demonstrate high (20 microohms) stable ratings generally require longer periods of training to lower their autonomic arousal levels at will; patients whose values are low (less than 5 microohms) and stable generally do not benefit significantly from SCL training. Behaviorally, this patient also demonstrates the perfectionistic tendencies seen in many of this type of CBP patient.

Session 3: 1 hour.

Procedures. Introduce relaxation training exercise; provide patient with tape of session; review pain diary, activities, thoughts, and feelings log, and medication log.

Results. The patient reported increased pain and "tension" at work. She misses "as needed" medications and has some skepticism

that this approach will work. Her pain diary and logs revealed a perfectionistic attitude towards her work and much negative thinking about her supervisor.

Action/plan.

1. Explain rationale for learning to increase ability to discriminate *small* changes in muscle tension (much easier to relax if one can "catch" neck, shoulders, and back before they are painfully tense). Explain again concept of relaxation—pain incompatibility, that one cannot experience pain when deeply relaxed.
2. Discuss feelings about reducing reliance on drugs, possible withdrawal symptoms.
3. Continue pain diary and activities log.
4. Instruct patient to practice relaxation exercise at least once per day, preferably twice a day. Make time for herself at home, tell children this is her time for herself.

Analysis. It is very important to engage this type of patient in a technique that he or she can practice on a daily basis at home. We have found that a 15 to 20 minute relaxation exercise is best for regular home practice. The audio cassette tape is introduced as a guide, to help pace the practice and to help in the transfer of learning behavioral self-control skills from the clinic to the home environment. Exercises longer than 20 minutes often seem to provoke more resistance in patients who "can't find the time" to practice. The ·importance of regular daily practice is stressed, with an explanation of the superiority of "distributed" (i.e., 20 minutes daily for 1 week) over "massed" (i.e., $2\frac{1}{2}$ hours of practice on Saturday) practice for effective learning of a new skill.

Discussing openly the patient's skepticism and/or resistance to this behavioral treatment is essential. Patients are urged to experience "whatever they can" in each practice session and not to strive for a "perfect" session each time. Encouraging busy "Type A" patients to schedule this time for themselves is often helpful.

Giving lots of encouragement and praise for the patient's decreasing use of pain medications is helpful, but the therapist should not push for rapid withdrawal, as this is likely to provoke more resistance. Consultation with the primary physician may be necessary. Likewise, the patient should be reassured that "distracting thoughts" are common and that she need not try to stop them but just allow them to flow and they will decrease with time.

Session 4: 1 hour.

Procedure. First biofeedback session — feedback given for EMG only, monitor SCL; review diary and logs; EMG feedback was both audio (pulsed analog tone) and visual (analog meter).

Results. The patient could readily control EMG level for brief periods. She experienced some difficulty with intrusive thoughts, fear of failure, perfectionistic striving, and a need to "look good" for the therapist. EMG levels ranged from initial 3.44 microvolts to a low of 1.13 microvolts. SCL ranged from initial level of 10.4 microohms to low of 7.8 microohms; one brief SCL response showed elevation to 14.5 microohms. The SCL data were discussed after feedback session, and it was found that the high response coincided with intrusive thoughts about her supervisor. The patient was pleased that she could demonstrate some "control" over EMG, but was somewhat puzzled by SCL responses.

Action/plan.

1. Continue diary and logs.
2. Continue feedback for EMG only for 2 to 3 more sessions, then move to SCL feedback.
3. Continue daily relaxation progress.

Analysis. We usually begin multi-modal biofeedback training with EMG feedback alone, even if other modalities (Thermal TEMP, SCL) are to be emphasized later. This is because EMG levels are already under voluntary (CNS) control, and the patient can readily experience the correspondence between his or her "efforts" at raising or lowering EMG levels and the changes in the biofeedback signal. When monitoring another modality, in this case SCL, no feedback is given and the therapist merely observes and records the values during the session. Some discussion after the EMG feedback training may be indicated, but no detailed discussions are needed until the new modality is introduced with feedback.

EMG feedback is usually begun with both visual and auditory feedback (eyes open). As patients progress in training, patients generally move to an eyes closed condition, which necessitates auditory feedback alone. We recommend using an EMG feedback unit that provides a choice of several auditory signals, as varying the type of auditory feedback employed is often necessary to avoid patient fatigue and adaptation (i.e., they stop listening to the signal). Auditory feedback in later sessions can be a musical selection from a battery-operated tape recorder switched on when patient is able to stay below the selected EMG threshold.

SCL levels in this patient reflect her emotional lability. In later sessions, SCL training will be directed towards her having more voluntary control over producing a low arousal state in the ANS, with accompanying emotional feelings of calm and quiet.

Progress in Later Sessions:

In Session 5, the patient showed good ability to decrease frontal EMG to levels below 1.0 microvolts threshold and maintain these levels for more than 5 minutes. Audio feedback was made contingent on threshold level. In Sessions 6 and 7, electrodes were moved to bilateral trapezius sites, and EMG feedback was continued. Patient showed rapid learning of relaxation response and ability to maintain trapezius EMG below 1.5 microvolts for periods exceeding 5 minutes. Threshold training was introduced, and the patient was instructed to bring in a cassette of her favorite classical flute music. This cassette was played on a battery-operated tape recorder interfaced with the Autogen 1700 (Ext. Audio In, rear-panel jack). The EMG unit was set to provide audio (music) *only* when EMG levels were below threshold. Using this paradigm, the patient was able to stay below 1.5 microvolts for long periods (greater than 10 minutes). She was then instructed to play this same music cassette at home, while practicing relaxation without the recorded instructions.

In Session 8, SCL feedback was introduced. The patient was also introduced to autogenic training (cf. Schultz & Luthe, 1969). This exercise was recorded in the session and given to the patient for home practice. SCL feedback was visual only (from Autogen 3400 panel meter) in this session. Diary review indicated decreased pain frequency, but occasional episodes of pain almost equal in severity to original symptoms. These periods coincided with confrontations between the patient and her supervisor or physicians at work. Medication use was decreased, and the patient was adhering to a twice daily schedule.

In Sessions 9 through 12, SCL feedback was continued, and the patient was introduced to some simple assertive strategies. She reported that her sleep was improved, and that she generally felt more positive in outlook. Medication usage was down to once a day in the morning before work. Her social activities had also increased, and she reported deriving more pleasure from activities with friends.

In Sessions 13 through 16, the patient reported markedly reduced frequency and severity of pain episodes, down to less than three times per work week. Medication was discontinued after Session 15. She reported that she is more able to deal directly with her supervisor at work and that her relationships with physicians have improved. She reported that she no longer feels defensive about her "problem". She reported more satisfying interactions with children.

The patient continued in bi-weekly 1-hour follow-up sessions. Feedback was given only intermittently, and the patient was instructed to visualize stressful situations at work. She generally demonstrated good control over both EMG and SCL even with imaginal stressors.

OVERVIEW

The preceding two case summaries have been chosen to illustrate not only the technical procedures involved in biofeedback treatment of CBP patients but also the different rationales for the use of biofeedback training. Case 1 is an example of a nonpsychologically-minded individual for whom the initial goal was self-control of the paraspinal muscle tension thought to be related to his pain experience. General relaxation usually accompanies such training, and patients often report increasing awareness of how their behavior affects their pain (i.e., sleep habits, posture, emotional states). Environmental influences on chronic pain behavior are also considered and treated as necessary.

Case 2 illustrates the kind of patient in whom psychological factors (frequently characterized by ANS hyperarousal but little psychological insight) are hypothesized to play a larger role in the maintenance of the CBP symptoms. These patients often present with no clear-cut pathophysiology but have difficulty with direct expression of negative emotions. They may express frustration and anger via somatic symptoms and then attempt to treat themselves for what they perceive as a somatic problem. In this case, medication was utilized to relieve pain, but it also resulted in more emotional distress (and thus increased pain) as the patient became aware of her increasing dependence on the medication. (Medication, especially the more potent analgesics, can also directly reinforce pain behavior via the "high" that some patients experience.)

Successful treatment of such cases involves psychosomatic therapy; that is, integrating biofeedback, relaxation training, supportive counseling, medication management, restructuring the social environment to remove social reinforcers for pain, and providing the patient with new coping skills (assertion training). In this case, biofeedback served as an aid in general relaxation training as well as a nonthreatening avenue for the patient to be able to establish a therapeutic relationship in which emotional and behavioral factors involved in the pain problem were first identified and then dealt with. Biofeedback treatment is often more consistent with the patient's initial perception of the problem; too early attempts at other verbal and behavioral therapies often result in resistance.

In our experience, a feature common to all users of biofeedback treatments, whatever the initial rationale, is that learning more physiological self-control ultimately leads to a sense of psychological mastery and understanding. It is then much easier to introduce new concepts such as autogenic training, assertion training, cognitive restructuring, stress inoculation, etc. This sense of control is also hypothesized to affect the pain experience itself via the cognitive and affective components of pain. For example, positive expectations concerning one's ability to monitor pain facilitate placebo effects. In addition, a sense of control in an aversive situation such as pain is associated with decreased anxiety and depression. It is especially noteworthy that the biofeedback training process can be arranged so that the patient will only experience success.

It is also noted that, rather than being merely a technical procedure administered to a passive patient, biofeedback actively involves the patient. Technically oriented individuals (who are often defensive about getting psychological help) are fascinated by the hardware and enjoy manipulating the machines and the feelings of control and mastery that ensue. Less sophisticated patients often must be disabused, via demonstration sessions, of magical beliefs regarding the equipment and how it will cause his or her pain to vanish with no effort on his or her part.

Sometimes, "Type A" individuals fear transformation into relaxed (i.e., lazy), calm (i.e., dull) individuals, but therapists can emphasize that patients will actually be learning more control, and will thus have a wider range of choices once they master physiological self-control techniques.

Thus, active participation and assumption of responsibility for change and for development of coping skills are explicit features of the patient's role in biofeedback treatment. Indeed, it may be that these aspects of biofeedback treatment not only enhance, but may actually account for, the treatment effects noted clinically. Work with headache patients has suggested that "it is less crucial that headache sufferers learn to directly modify EMG activity than it is that they learn to monitor the insidious onset of headache symptoms and engage in some sort of coping response incompatible with the further exacerbation of symptoms (Holroyd, Andrasik, & Noble, 1980, p. 38).

In a well controlled study, Andrasik and Holroyd (1980) concluded that it was increased coping ability rather than reduction of frontalis muscle tension that accounted for the relief from pain in headache sufferers. The importance of these factors in outcome might be underscored by the inconsistent findings associated with the relationship between paraspinal EMG and back pain. Nevertheless, we caution against premature conclusions with respect to the importance of either cognitive or physiological variables in treatment outcome.

Perhaps even formulating our questions in this manner is unfortunate, as it reflects a continuation of dualistic thinking that may impede the development of better biopsychosocial models. In our opinion, chronic back pain patients are a heterogeneous population, and the report of pain is multiply determined. The relative importance of various determinants will vary from patient to patient, necessitating individualized assessment and treatment protocols. We do believe that biofeedback can be a highly effective component of treatment. It is noninvasive and has few known risks if utilized for appropriate patients and with clinical sensitivity.

Relaxation-induced anxiety is currently receiving more attention in the literature (e.g., Heide & Borkovec, 1984). It is noted that some conditions involving hypotension, diabetes, or a significant psychopathology would require close monitoring and interventions as necessary.

SUMMARY

The treatment of chronic back pain patients requires assessment of sensory, affective, and cognitive components of pain, as well as positive and negative reinforcers for pain and well behavior. The specific rationales for utilizing biofeedback as a treatment technique include: (a) to facilitate control of a physiological variable (sensory component) thought to be related to the pain experience (e.g., reduction of paraspinal muscle spasm, correction of "abnormal" paraspinal EMG patterns); (b) to facilitate reduction of general muscular or autonomic activity that would reduce central processing of peripheral sensory inputs (sensory component) and be incompatible with anxiety (affective component); and (c) to facilitate truly psychosomatic therapy, integrating all relevant psychosocial and biologic interventions in the management of CBP patients.

It has been our experience that, whatever the initial rationale for incorporating biofeedback in treatment, there are powerful cognitive effects of utilizing these procedures that can decrease pain and enhance (or even account for) treatment outcome. These include facilitating a sense of mastery and self-control, learning to discriminate when to institute coping skills, and having a conceptual model that integrates and promotes the understanding of biopsychosocial phenomena such as pain.

It is our belief that effective clinical use of biofeedback with CBP patients requires not only a knowledge of physiology and elec-

tronics but also a solid background in psychological therapies and behavior change. One cannot employ a fixed script or rigid set of procedures for all CBP patients. One must meet the patient at his or her own level to engage them effectively in this approach to self-management of chronic pain. For maximum results, however, it must be combined with other approaches.

APPENDIX A: PAIN DIARY

Our pain diary is a simple recording of pain level by hour for each waking hour, where "0" = no pain and "5" = excruciating incapacitating pain. Activities are recorded for each hour, along with medication usage and relaxation practice as appropriate. Thus the patient creates a graph of pain levels throughout the day, as follows:

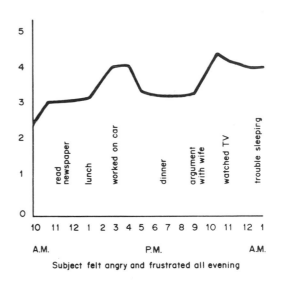

Subject felt angry and frustrated all evening

Although we recognize that a focus on hourly recording is not always reliable, we encourage it, especially in the early stages of treatment in order to highlight the variability of the response and to focus on the analysis of behavior–pain relationships. Follick, Ahern, and Laser-Wolston (1980) present promising reliability and validity data on the daily activity diary method.

APPENDIX B: PATIENT INSTRUCTIONS

As we have discussed, biofeedback is one treatment approach for your back pain that has been helpful for many patients. Whether it proves beneficial for you depends largely on how much time you put into practicing with the exercises we will be working with. Biofeedback is not a treatment where something is done *to* you (such as injections, pills, or surgery) or where things are done *for* you (such as massage, or physical therapy). Biofeedback is a learning process, and we will work with you, somewhat like a coach or music teacher, to help you learn how to have more control over your back pain and associated symptoms (poor sleep, fatigue, etc.).

The process is a lot like learning any new physical skill, like learning to play tennis, ride a bicycle, or play the piano. You will need to put in regular periods of home practice, every day, to really learn this new skill. Just as you will not learn how to play the piano well if you only play at your weekly lesson with the teacher, you cannot expect to master these new self-control skills merely by coming in for a weekly biofeedback training session.

As we mentioned, the biofeedback equipment merely provides information about how different systems in your body are responding. It doesn't make anything happen. Think of the equipment as a learning tool. You will be learning how to control the muscle spasms that are producing your pain. When you are learning to ride a bicycle for the first time, it is often helpful to attach "training wheels" to the bike to help keep you from falling over while you learn to balance while riding. Once you learn to do it, you don't need the training wheels anymore. In the same way, once you learn to sense the first beginning signs of a muscle spasm and how to "let go" of that un-

necessary tension, by using the information from the very sensitive equipment to help you, you don't need to rely on the equipment anymore. The real goal of biofeedback training is for *you* to learn the skill, that is, to make the equipment unnecessary.

EMG Electrodes

I'm going to place these sensors [we try to avoid the term "electrodes," as it has negative connotations for many patients and arouses fear of shocks, etc.] onto your skin over the muscles that are tightening up and causing you pain. They merely stick onto the skin like this. [Demonstrate on self.] They will pick up the tiny electrical signals produced in the muscles as impulses from your nerves cause individual fibers in the muscles to contract. These are very tiny signals, on the order of one-millionth of a volt. Think of a flashlight battery, which produces about $1\frac{1}{2}$ volts. The signals produced in your body are a million times weaker than that, so we need to make a very good contact with your skin. I'm going to clean your skin with some alcohol, just to remove the oils that tend to interfere with a good signal. Remember, there are no needles here and nothing that will be uncomfortable. The gel I'm placing in these sensors also helps make good contact with your skin. [Apply electrodes.]

Now the cables from the equipment attach to these snaps in front. [Attach cables to sensors.] Now the equipment amplifies these weak signals from your body about a million times, so we can see and hear these subtle changes in your muscles, as they happen. Most people find that with this additional information, they can more easily learn to control these signals and thereby control (relax) their muscles more quickly and easily.

SCL Electrodes

Now I'm going to attach these sensors to the fingertips of your dominant (preferred) hand. [See equipment manual for detailed procedure.] This machine picks up tiny changes in the activity of your sweat glands. These changes reflect overall changes in the arousal level of your autonomic nervous system. You can think of the feedback signals from this machine as reflecting a general index of your level of emotional arousal. It cannot tell us anything about what kind of emotional change you may be experiencing, but high readings generally indicate that you are experiencing some kind of emotional arousal (anger, frustration, fear, sexual arousal, joy, etc.). Lower readings are generally associated with the emotional experience of quiet, calm, peaceful, and relaxed feelings.

This equipment, like the EMG unit, is extremely sensitive and can help make you more aware of very small internal changes in your autonomic arousal level. This is a very different part of the nervous system from that which controls your skeletal muscles. Training with the EMG unit helps you control (relax) your muscles. Training with this equipment (SCL) helps you learn to have more control over your emotional feelings. You can learn exactly which people, situations, or thoughts produce the largest autonomic responses in your body and then find out which self-control exercises help you lower the feedback signal and produce calmer, more peaceful feelings. As with EMG feedback, once you learn this control you don't need to rely on the equipment anymore.

REFERENCES

Andrasik, F., & Holroyd, K.A. (1980). A test of specific and nonspecific effects in biofeedback treatment of tension headache. *Journal of Consulting and Clinical Psychology*, *48*, 575–586.

Beals, R.K., & Hickman, N.W. (1972). Industrial injuries of back and extremities: comprehensive evaluation — An aid in prognosis and management. *Journal of Bone and Joint Surgery*, *54*, 1593–1611.

Belar, C.D., & Cohen, J.L. (1979). The use of EMG feedback and progressive relaxation in the treatment of a woman with chronic back pain. *Biofeedback and Self-Regulation*, *4*, 345–353.

Bonica, J.J. (1957). Management of myofascial pain syndromes in general practice. *Journal of the American Medical Association*, *164*, 732–738.

Bonica, J.J. (1980). Pain research and therapy: Past and current status and future needs. In L. Ng & J.J. Bonica (Eds.), *Pain, discomfort and humanitarian care* (pp. 1–46). New York: Elsevier.

Cinciripini, P.M., & Floreen, A. (1982). An evaluation of a behavioral program for chronic pain. *Journal of Behavior Medicine*, *5*, 375–389.

Flor, H., Haag, G., Turk, D.C., & Koehler, H. (1983). Efficacy of EMG biofeedback, pseudotherapy and conventional medical treatment for chronic rheumatic back pain. *Pain*, *17*, 21–31.

Flor, H., & Turk, D.C. (1984). Etiological theories and treatments for chronic back pain. I. Somatic models and interventions. *Pain*, *19*, 105–121.

Flor, H., Turk, D.C., & Birbaumer, N. (1984, September). *Paravertebral muscular reactivity during stress exposure in chronic back pain patients.* Paper presented to the International Association for the Study of Pain, Seattle, WA.

Follick, M.H., Ahern, D.K., & Laser-Wolston, N. (1980). Evaluation of a daily activity diary for chronic pain patients. *Pain*, *19*, 373–382.

Freeman, C.W., Calsyn, D.A., Paige, A.B., & Halar, E.M. (1980). Biofeedback with low back pain patients. *American Journal of Clinical Biofeedback*, *3*, 118–122.

Hallett, E.C., & Pilowsky, I. (1982). The response to treatment in a multidisciplinary pain clinic. *Pain*, *12*, 365–374.

Heide, J., & Borkovec, T.D. (1984). Relaxation induced anxiety; mechanisms and theoretical implications. *Behavior Research & Therapy*, *22*, 1–12.

Hendler, N., Derogatis, L., Avella, J., & Long, D. (1977). EMG biofeedback in patients with chronic pain. *Diseases of the Nervous System*, *38*, 505–514.

Holroyd, K.A., Andrasik, F., & Noble, J. (1980). A comparison of EMG biofeedback and a credible pseudotherapy in treating tension headache. *Journal of Behavioral Medicine*, *3*, 29–39.

Keefe, F.J., Black, A.R., Williams, R.B., & Surwit, R. (1981). Behavioral treatment of chronic low back pain: Clinical outcome and individual differences in pain relief. *Pain*, *11*, 221–231.

Kravitz, E., Moore, M., Glaros, A., & Stauffer, T. (1978, March). *EMG feedback and differential relaxation training to promote pain relief in chronic low back pain patients.* Paper presented at the Ninth Annual Meeting of the Biofeedback Society of America, Albuquerque, NM.

Lipowski, Z.J. (1984). What does the word "psychosomatic" really mean? A historical and semantic inquiry. *Psychosomatic Medicine*, *46*, 153–171.

Melzack, R., & Perry, C. (1975). Self-regulation of pain: The use of alpha-feedback and hypnotic training for the control of chronic pain. *Experimental Neurology*, *46*, 452–469.

National Center for Health Statistics. (1983, March). 1981 summary: National ambulatory medical care survey. *Advance Data*, No. 88.

Nouwen, A., & Bush, C. (1984). The relationship between paraspinal EMG and chronic low back pain. *Pain*, *20*, 109–123.

Nouwen, A., & Solinger, J. (1979). The effectiveness of EMG biofeedback training in low back pain. *Biofeedback and Self-Regulation*, *42*, 103–111.

Pinsky, J.A. (1983). Psychodynamic understanding and treatment of the chronic intractable benign pain syndrome—treatment outcome. *Seminars in Neurology*, *3*, 346–354.

Schaepe, J.L. (1982). Low back pain: An occupational perspective. In: M. Stanton-Hicks and R. Boas (Eds.), *Chronic low back pain* (pp. 15–24). New York: Raven Press.

Schultz, J.H., & Luthe, W. (1969). *Autogenic therapy: Vol. 1. Autogenic methods.* New York: Grune & Stratton, Inc.

Sterman, R.A. (1984, September). *Relationships between strength of low back muscles; contractions and reported intensity of chronic low back pain.* Paper presented to the International Association for the Study of Pain, Seattle, WA.

Todd, J., & Belar, C.D. (1980). EMG biofeedback and chronic low back pain: Implications of treatment failure. *American Journal of Clinical Biofeedback*, *3*, 217–224.

Turk, D.C., & Flor, H. (1984). Etiological theories and treatments for chronic back pain. II. Psychological models and interventions. *Pain*, *19*, 209–234.

U.S. Department of Health, Education and Welfare. (1974). *Vital and health statistics. Limitation of activity due to chronic conditions, United States, 1974.* (Series 10-No. 111). Washington, DC: Government Printing Office.

Wolf, S.L., Nacht, M., & Kelly, J.L. (1982). EMG feedback during dynamic movement for low back pain patients. *Behavior Therapy*, *13*, 395–406.

MEDICAL LIBRARY
W. C. B.
DOWNSVIEW REHAB. CENTRE

10 HYPNOTIC ANALGESIA

Joseph Barber*

There are many pain conditions that are not amenable to cure by either medical or conventional psychological treatment. Certain ongoing pain syndromes, such as migraine headache, trigeminal neuralgia, or osteoarthritis, involve recurrent nociception; and when the best medical care cannot significantly reduce pain, psychological intervention is today often undertaken to help the patient live with an ongoing pain problem. Although cognitive and behavioral treatments may be critical to the rehabilitation of such a patient, these approaches do not have as the focus or goal the elimination of pain itself. Although the majority of patients who undergo comprehensive pain clinic cognitive and behavioral programs learn to be more active, to take less medication, and to function better in other ways despite their pain, the problem of the pain itself generally persists (Fordyce et al., 1973). Giving such patients mood-altering analgesics (e.g., narcotics), even if such medication could continue to ameliorate the pain, which it cannot, is clearly undesirable because of the damaging side effects of such medications (e.g., psychological dependence, physical dependence, tolerance, dysphoria, constipation, pruritis). For such patients, what is needed is

psychological intervention that can: (a) eliminate or at least significantly reduce pain; (b) do so without untoward psychological side-effects, such as operantly increasing the level of perceived pain or reducing activity levels; (c) enhance the other treatments the patient is receiving; and (d) enable patients to learn to use it themselves so that they are more self-reliant and less dependent on the medical—psychological system for their continuing health care.

Hypnosis is just such a clinical tool. No other psychological technique is as efficacious in creating comfort out of discomfort, with none of the adverse side-effects associated with medical treatments of comparable efficacy. Using hypnosis effectively in the management of a chronic pain condition, however, requires more than a simple "application" of a hypnotic induction followed by suggestions for pain control. Many people turn to hypnosis with the expectation that it is a magic treatment for chronic pain, just as many regard it as a sole treatment to cure compulsive problems, sexual problems, or anxiety. It cannot. To be effective for such complex problems, hypnosis must be wisely incorporated into a broader psychotherapeutic intervention (Barber, 1982; Edelstien, 1981). When it is so incorporated, however, hypnosis can be a uniquely powerful part of treatment.

Although hypnotic phenomena have probably been used in clinical treatment for as

*I thank Cheri Adrian for her generous attention to this manuscript.

long as there has been clinical treatment, the modern history of medical hypnosis begins with the work of the Austrian physician, Franz Anton Mesmer. Despite the fact that Mesmer's explanation for the effect of hypnosis, animal magnetism, was incorrect, he did attempt to use modern science to account for powerful and previously inexplicable phenomena. The use of hypnosis in medicine continued through the 19th century, most dramatically in the operating room. As early as 1850, James Esdaile, an English surgeon working in India, reported successfully using hypnoanesthesia for a variety of major surgeries (Esdaile, 1857). Since then, there have been numerous accounts of surgery performed with hypnosis or self-hypnosis (Rausch, 1980) as the sole anesthetic. In recent years, hypnosis has been increasingly employed in the treatment of a multitude of pain problems and psychophysiologic disorders, including the acute pain of burns, surgery, and malignancy, as well as chronic pain syndromes such as trigeminal neuralgia, peripheral neuropathies, and thalamic pain syndrome (Barber & Adrian, 1982; Crasilneck & Hall, 1975; Hilgard & Hilgard, 1983).

Hypnosis is an altered state of consciousness characterized by a markedly increased receptivity to suggestion, the capacity for alteration of perception and memory, and the capacity for direct control of a variety of usually involuntary physiological functions (such as glandular activity, vasomotor activity, etc.). All of these features of altered cognitive functioning can be useful in the control of pain, but clearly the most important are alterations of perception and physical functioning.

With respect to alterations in perception, individuals who are hypnotized can experience both positive and negative hallucination. Positive hallucination refers to the capacity to perceive something that one would not otherwise perceive. Negative hallucination refers to the capacity to not perceive something that one would otherwise perceive. Such hallucination can occur in any sensory modality. As will be illustrated in the following text, it is the capacity for such perceptual alteration that allows the development of hypnotic analgesia or anesthesia.

Some people believe that hypnosis is only effective in treating pain because it is associated with relaxation; in fact, some believe that hypnosis is merely an exercise for creating relaxation. Muscular relaxation, however, is not a useful treatment for chronic pain unless of course the pain is specifically caused by muscle spasm (McCauley, Thelan, Frank, Willard, & Callan, 1983). And, in fact, hypnosis is not relaxation, nor need it even induce relaxation. The two phenomena can occur quite independently; their association is largely the result of the artifact of using relaxation suggestions in traditional hypnotic inductions. Far from being merely relaxation, hypnosis involves a dramatic shift in consciousness; it is this shift, presumably, that permits the change in pain perception (Shor, 1965; Orne, 1976).

It is the utilization of the capacities made available by the shift in consciousness that distinguishes hypnosis from cognitive strategies for pain control. Hypnosis is not cognitive therapy, in the sense that a clinician teaches a patient how to think differently about a problem. A patient who experiences hypnotic analgesia or anesthesia feels both the change in perception of pain (either sensory or affective) and the automaticity of that change.

Frequently, patients who experience hypnotic anesthesia or analgesia do not believe they have been hypnotized (for reasons usually having to do with false expectations about the experience) and may have no awareness of any change in their cognitions or in any other aspect of their experience except for the reduction or absence of pain. For instance, one patient, who endured an ordinarily painful dental procedure (root canal treatment of a vital tooth) with hypnosis as the sole anesthetic, believed he was not hypnotized ("because I can't be hypnotized") and explained to his bewildered dentist that he was not hurting because "you didn't do anything to me that would hurt." Another patient, being treated for chronic back pain, came to the first appointment insisting that he needed to be hypnotized and that he could not be. At the termination of treatment (after six appointments, during which he had shown ample evidence of his talent as a hypnotic subject), he was relieved of his pain. He left, declaring that his only disappointment was that he never had been hypnotized. Though conscious cognitive changes may be part of hypnotic treatment for pain, they are not essential to it and may be entirely unnecessary to pain relief.

Some attempts have been made to understand the neurophysiological mechanism by which hypnosis operates to produce analgesia. Although such a mechanism has yet to be identified, certain hypotheses have not been confirmed. Goldstein and Hilgard (1975), Barber and Mayer (1977), Finer and Terenius (1981), and Spiegel and Albert (1983) each independently found that hypnotic analgesia is apparently not subserved by the endorphin system. Sternbach (1982) was unable to confirm another promising hypothesis, that acetylcholine underlies hypnotic analgesia. Presumably the mechanism is more complex than can be understood by reference to the action of a single neurotransmitter.

Whatever its underlying mechanism, it is clear that the rate and the degree to which hypnosis enables the modification of pain perception and concomitant suffering are quite dramatic. The hypnotic elimination of both experimental and clinical pain, whatever its nature, history, or intensity, has been fully documented (Crasilneck & Hall, 1975; Hilgard & Hilgard, 1983). Further, such elimination can occur immediately in response to hypnotic suggestion. Research over the past 30 years has demonstrated that hypnotic subjects (including college students, children, and older adults) are able to reduce or eliminate a variety of experimentally-induced pain, including ischemic, cold-pressor, electric, and thermal (Hilgard & Hilgard, 1983). Careful investigation has established that such hypnotic pain control is uniquely su-

perior to that achieved by other psychological means (Hilgard & Hilgard; Orne, 1980; Turner & Chapman, 1982). For a full account of this research, see Hilgard and Hilgard, 1983.

The critical clinical question is under what conditions hypnosis can be used to achieve such effects. Recent research has explored the conditions under which hypnosis is clinically useful. Neither gender nor intelligence is relevant to the development of the hypnotic state (Hilgard & Hilgard, 1983). Nor is age a factor; much work has been done with the hypnotic treatment of children in pain (Gardner & Olness, 1981; Hilgard & LeBaron, 1982, 1984; Kellerman, Zeltzer, Ellenberg, & Dash, 1983; Schafer, 1975; Wakeman & Kaplan, 1978; Zeltzer, Dash, & Holland, 1979).

It is well known that individuals differ in the degree to which they respond to hypnotic treatment (Hilgard & Hilgard, 1983). An issue that remains as yet unresolved is the relevance of measured hypnotic responsiveness to clinical hypnotic responsiveness. This issue is partly clouded by the difficulty in discriminating treatment responsiveness from hypnotic responsiveness in a clinical setting (Hilgard & Hilgard, 1983); and experimental investigations of this issue have yielded differing results. Because "Who can benefit from hypnosis?" is an important clinical issue, it is worth considering what is known to date.

The belief that only some individuals are responsive to hypnosis is based partly on the old and clearly unsupportable belief that only persons of inferior intellect or of "weak personality" could be hypnotized (and on the assumption that hypnosis requires giving up control of one's mind to the hypnotist). More important, however, are experimental and clinical investigations that seem to suggest that only a minority of individuals are able to achieve clinically significant hypnotic states (Hilgard & Hilgard, 1983). (A clinically significant state is one in which clinical treatment might be effected, as opposed to a measurable but insignificant state.)

In the typical study, hypnotic responsiveness is measured by reference to an individual's performance on a standardized test, such as the Stanford Hypnotic Susceptibility Scale (Weitzenhoffer & Hilgard, 1959) or the Harvard Group Scale of Hypnotic Susceptibility (Shor & Orne, 1962). Such tests create a setting in which an individual has the opportunity of responding to a hypnotic induction and to several suggestions for hypnotic behavior. The number of behaviors the individual exhibits becomes the numeric measure of hypnotic responsiveness. It has been shown, for instance, in a study by Hilgard and Morgan (1975), that the correlation between such measures and an individual's ability to hypnotically reduce pain is significant ($r = .50$). However, Hilgard and Morgan also reported that 44% of low susceptible individuals were able to reduce their pain by 10% or more and concluded:

> This means that the relation between pain reduction and hypnotic responsiveness is probabilistic, with a greater reduction of successful pain reduction for those highly responsive to hypnosis. The data do not mean that those unresponsive to hypnosis, as measured by the scales, have no possibility of help through suggestion. (Hilgard & Hilgard, 1975)

Although it is clear that there is a wide range of hypnotic responsiveness among individuals, there is evidence that another significant variable in determining clinical effectiveness of hypnosis is the particular approach to the patient by the clinician (Alman & Carney, 1981; Barber, 1977, 1980, 1982; Fricton, 1981; Gillett & Coe, in press; Price & Barber, unpublished). These reports indicate that an approach to the patient based on suggestions individualized to the needs of the patient, rather than on standard suggestions, is more likely to be successful with individuals performing poorly on tests of responsivity. (Although such an approach has been characterized in the past as "indirect," as distinct from "direct" [Alman & Carney, 1981; Barber, 1982; Fricton, 1981], I believe such a characterization is too simple and misses the fundamental difference between sugges-

tions communicated in a standard way, e.g., through a test of responsivity, and those communicated in a nonstandard but more individualized way [Price & Barber, unpublished].)

Individuals differ in the degree to which they can understand and respond to any idea; more individuals understand and respond when the idea is communicated in a way carefully addressed to them. An individual who responds minimally to a test of hypnotic responsivity may require special communication of the principles of hypnotic induction and suggestions for treatment. The case of Ben, described later in this chapter, is an example of the treatment of such an individual.

One explanation for this disparity in research findings with respect to the analgesic capacities of low susceptibles might be that high susceptibles are better able to reduce the sensory-discriminative component of pain and low susceptibles are able to reduce the motivational-affective dimension (Melzack & Wall, 1973). The disparate findings might be accounted for by the fact that these two components are rarely measured independently.

Price and Barber (unpublished) sought to assess this possibility. In the Price and Barber experiment, thermally induced pain was measured independently on both the sensory-discriminative and the affective-motivational dimensions, using a visual analogue scale (Price, 1983). Low-susceptible subjects were as able to reduce both the sensory-discriminative and the affective components as high-susceptible subjects. This finding confirms earlier reports that the use of a nontraditional, individualized hypnotic technique elicits clinically significant analgesia from low-susceptible subjects.

Another unresolved issue is that of the experimentally verifiable effects of hypnosis compared with clinical reports of hypnotic effectiveness. Most of the clinical literature shows hypnosis to be more effective as an analgesic (and more frequently so) than experimental reports suggest (Crasilneck & Hall, 1975; Haley, 1967; Hilgard & Hilgard, 1983).

Part of the explanation for this difference lies in the obvious differences in motivation of the subjects and patients. Experimental subjects are significantly less motivated to experience a hypnotic effect than are clinical patients who are seeking relief from suffering.

There are also significant differences in the behavior of experimenters as compared with clinicians. Experimental protocols usually require rigid adherence to a well-operationalized, standardized induction and set of suggestions. Rarely is the purpose of an experiment the search for optimum hypnotic effect. However, that is precisely what is involved in the clinical situation. Effective clinical use of hypnosis requires an individualized approach. Rarely is a standardized set of procedures followed, and the clinician is normally focused only on doing what works and may vary or repeat procedures until success if obtained. While this may lead to successful clinical outcomes, it is usually difficult to assess the precise nature of the causal link between what was done and what resulted. In this regard, Orne (1980) suggests that effects of the context of the situation, both direct and indirect, must account for at least a part of what would otherwise be taken to be the hypnotic effect. For instance, the meaning of the clinician's attention is very different from that of the experimenter's. As Diamond (1984) suggests, the relationship between the hypnotist and subject is a powerful determiner of the hypnotic effect. The relationship between an experimenter and a subject is significantly less personal — sometimes "hypnosis" is even administered by a tape recorder — than the sometimes dramatically personal (and, thereby, more potent) relationship of a clinician and a suffering patient. Whatever the explanation, it is clear that clinical success with hypnosis requires innovative experimental procedures that can investigate reports of dramatic hypnotic effect.

Though the issue of what best predicts hypnotic responsiveness is still far from resolved, there are very good reasons not to use susceptibility tests to "screen" patients for potential hypnotic treatment. Because the evidence suggests that such screening would not reflect actual capacity for response, and because of the potentially discouraging effects of such tests, I would argue that such screening be done only under very carefully considered circumstances.

Effectively using hypnosis in the treatment of a chronic pain condition requires individualizing the hypnotic treatment and integrating that treatment into the larger psychotherapeutic intervention. This means that the first step is to assess the patient's personal style, expectations, and attitudes toward hypnosis, and to choose hypnotic induction procedures and suggestions for pain relief accordingly. In general, a patient's chronic pain can be reduced by hypnotic means. (Hypnosis is generally ineffective in the treatment of psychogenic pain, but such a condition is quite rare.) How hypnosis is used for such reduction, however, is a very complicated issue and requires assessment, in general, of the consequences of pain reduction for the patient. For instance, I would use hypnosis to initiate pain reduction if the following criteria were met:

1. Will the patient be harmed by using hypnosis? That is, will the patient be motivated to see the use of hypnosis as an excuse for being harmed in some way? Some relatively disturbed patients, for instance, might use the opportunity to ignore pain that signals harm and might thereby injure themselves further. Such patients might also neglect to take necessary medication. In extreme cases, such patients might behave in a "trance-like" fashion in inappropriate circumstances (e.g., while driving). In general, if a patient tends to have more than the usual side effects from medication, or has a history of developing complications from medical procedures, I think it wise to defer the use of hypnosis.

2. Will the patient's life be improved by pain reduction, without significant loss (of esteem, of secondary gains, of stability of the family system, etc.)? If such pain reduction would be disruptive, the use of hypnosis ought be deferred until other therapies can take care of the patient's other needs.

3. Is the patient willing to take the respon-

sibility to initiate his or her own treatment? (Use of hypnosis for pain reduction requires significant effort on the part of the patient; an inability to initiate such effort renders the effective use of hypnosis unlikely.)

It is beyond the purpose of this chapter to describe hypnotic induction techniques or to discuss the complexity of choosing appropriate suggestions, although the broad issue of hypnotic phenomena that can be used for pain control will be discussed below. The reader interested in hypnotic training should inquire at universities and medical schools, and about the training programs offered by Division 30 (Psychological Hypnosis) of the American Psychological Association, by the American Society for Clinical Hypnosis, and by the Society for Clinical and Experimental Hypnosis. There are a number of books that teach hypnotic techniques (e.g., Crasilneck & Hall, 1975; Gardner & Olness, 1981; Hartland, 1971). Bowers' *Hypnosis for the Seriously Curious* (1983) is a wonderfully lucid general introduction to the subject.

What follows, then, is a description of the kinds of hypnotic phenomena that may be successfully used for obtaining pain relief once a patient has been effectively hypnotized.

HYPNOTIC TECHNIQUES FOR ANALGESIA

Patients who require treatment of chronic pain nearly always have an organic basis for the pain, though it may not be physically treatable. Since hypnosis is capable of altering either the sensory or the affective dimensions of pain, then any of the following techniques may be helpful, depending upon the circumstances. How one chooses the particular technique in any given situation is a clinical judgment that should be based on what will best meet the needs of the patient. (The experienced clinician has a large repertoire of approaches, of course. Erickson [Haley, 1967] reported a variety of unorthodox but often remarkably successful hypnotic treatments for pain.)

There are five techniques used to create hypnotic analgesia: (a) anesthesia; (b) direct diminution of pain; (c) sensory substitution; (d) displacement of the pain to another, less vulnerable body area; and (e) dissociation.

Anesthesia

Hypnotic suggestions can evoke a hallucination of anesthesia that renders a body area insensitive to pain. In such a case, the patient is unable to feel the pain, but instead feels numbness—just as if a local anesthetic had been injected.

Anesthesia can be suggested, as for example, "it can begin to feel as if [the painful area] is becoming numb, with no sensation at all." The accomplishment of this requires a positive hallucination of numbness and, in my experience, is a relatively difficult phenomenon to achieve, compared with other techniques.

Direct Diminution

Direct diminution is a simple technique for reducing sensory pain. A suggestion might be made, for example, that "you can continue to enjoy feeling increasingly well, with each breath you take. . . almost as if the discomfort is somehow gradually going away." Suggestions focus on the diminution of the intensity of pain; one might suggest that the "volume" of the pain can be turned down. Metaphors for turning down volume, dimming brightness, cooling heat, and so on are most effective when matched to the patient's own phenomenology of pain intensity or quality. Asking the patient to scale pain intensity and to discover the apparent change in that intensity level is another diminution technique.

Sensory Substitution

Hypnotic suggestions can be used to create sensory substitution, or a reinterpretation of sensations. A sensation of intolerable burning, for instance, can be unconsciously substituted by another sensation, not necessarily pleasant, such as itching, or coldness, or tingling. Such a substitute feeling has several virtues: (a) It allows the patient to know the pain is still there (so the cancer patient, for instance, does not have to be concerned that he or she will forget that cancer still persists and thereby discontinue proper medical attention); and (b) it is not particularly pleasant, so it is more plausible than, say, a sensation of pleasure. A third virtue is that if one is still feeling uncomfortable — but not in agony — many secondary gains associated with pain can still be obtained without suffering. (Such a clinical strategy would probably be used temporarily, as a means of eventually diminishing debilitating secondary gains.)

Sensory substitution might be accomplished with the following kind of suggestion (successfully used with a 42-year-old paraplegic patient suffering burning dysesthesia in the legs):

> The feelings that you describe as hot needles stabbing you can begin, oddly enough, to seem as if the needles are becoming more and more blunt and broad, almost as if they have become tiny, massaging fingers — what an interesting sensation you can begin to have: thousands of warm fingers buzzing, massaging your legs. Not entirely pleasant, but perhaps a welcome relief.

Again, suggestions are most effective if they incorporate the qualities of the patient's personal experience of pain, and suggest a plausible modification of quality.

Displacement

Displacement of the pain from one area of the body to another can be accomplished in well-localized pain that is primarily disabling because of its location (e.g., abdominal pain is more disabling than limb pain). This is also a valuable temporary technique that can serve to increase the confidence of a patient who is skeptical about his or her hypnotic abilities. A suggestion for creating displacement, for example, is:

> You may have already noticed that the pain moves, ever so slightly, and you can begin to notice that the movement seems to be in an outwardly spiralling circular direction. As you continue to attend to that movement, you may not notice until later that the pain has somehow moved out of your abdomen and seems to be staying in your left hand.

The effectiveness of such suggestions may be increased for some patients if they are left free to choose the direction or location of movement, or if the phenomenon is made more plausible by some discussion of the interconnections of the nervous system. The primary goal is to change the locus of pain experience so that the pain is less disabling or threatening or frightening (and, thus, more tolerable). An important implication of such modification, however, is that if pain can change in location, it may also be changeable in other dimensions (and, ultimately, may be eliminated entirely).

Dissociation

Aside from creating the kinds of sensory alterations just described, hypnotic suggestions can also create a dissociation from the pain. In such a case, the patient is able to accurately describe the still-persisting pain — but with no affective involvement. That is, the pain is still perceived, but the patient no longer suffers from it. Dissociation is often useful in a situation in which the patient is relatively immobile (e.g., during surgery or some other painful procedure, or for a bedridden patient). A suggestion to create dissociation might be as follows:

> It is unnecessary for you to have to stay here, in bed, conscious of all the routine that occurs. I wonder if you might prefer to enjoy a kind of vacation from this room. You might like to imagine yourself, for instance, stepping out of the room, moving down the hall, and settling nicely into the solarium. Or, later today, you might prefer to feel as if you are enjoying a lovely sunny afternoon resting on the beach at Maui. Your body can remain here, in bed, in order that all the routine things can be done for you; but your

mind can take you far away, and you can enjoy whatever you'd like, with nothing to bother you.

EXTENDING RELIEF

The fact that a patient can be comfortable during a hypnotic treatment obviously has limited usefulness. For the patient whom we would like to activate and rehabilitate, we use posthypnotic suggestions as a means of extending the duration of the hypnotic effect. A posthypnotic suggestion is one that is intended to have effect after the hypnotic state has ended and the patient has regained normal waking consciousness. In general, posthypnotic suggestions include a cue that initiates the suggested experience (or behavior). For instance, one could suggest that, "Whenever I lift your arm, you will discover, at that moment, how really comfortable you feel." If successful, this suggestion would create analgesia whenever I lift the patient's arm. This strategy has instructive value for the patient because this effect can be generalized to other experiences. (e.g., if the patient's arm can become analgesic, then potentially any area of the patient's body can become analgesic, including the area affected by chronic pain.)

The cue can also be made a function of context. For example, one might say, "Whenever you need to feel relief from this pain, you'll suddenly notice that in fact you are beginning to feel relief. And that relief will last throughout the day." In this way, the patient's own recognition of the need for comfort is the cue, and no behavior on the clinician's part is necessary.

Different patients may need different kinds of cues, some more elaborate than others. For instance, an independently functioning individual can discover that he or she can create his or her own cues, and can create hypnotic analgesia in a variety of ways the clinician may not have described. A less independent patient may need more careful, circumscribed suggestions, such as, "When you are in your bedroom, lying in your bed, you can know that just closing your eyes and taking a deep breath will allow you to suddenly notice how really comfortable you have become."

SELF-HYPNOTIC MANAGEMENT

The most effective means for creating both independence for the patient and long-lasting pain relief is through self-hypnosis. Most patients can learn self-hypnosis quite readily, and can learn to apply their skills to the development of analgesia over increasingly greater lengths of time (Barber, 1982; Sachs, Feuerstein, & Vitale, 1977). (A patient's interest in learning and willingness to use self-hypnosis is a valuable index of the patient's motivation for recovery, as well as a means of assessing broader psychological issues.)

As a patient becomes more and more independent of the clinician, and increases his or her mastery of self-hypnotic skills, follow-up becomes increasingly important. Patients need to know that help is available in the future, however infrequently they may need it. Sometimes, many months go by during which a patient successfully uses self-hypnotic management of pain. Then, for a variety of reasons (including sudden onset of environmental stressors), he or she finds increasing difficulty in managing the pain. At such a time, a "booster" treatment may be all that is necessary to return the patient to independent functioning.

Because hypnotic effects are not as reliable or predictable as one would like, it is necessary to be persistent when treating chronic pain. If what seemed like one's most brilliant clinical strategy is not succeeding, then it is time to try another. The creativity of the clinician is as important in hypnotic treatment as it is in any other treatment. If the pain is not eliminated (and if that was the goal), this need not be assumed to be a failure. Rather, this result can be used as evidence for the patient of the modifiability of the pain—and perhaps of the need for reexamining the patient's needs. (The example of Susan, below, illustrates this.) Although it may seem appropriate to focus on sensory-perceptual alteration, it is also valuable and necessary to focus on alteration of the affective dimension. A strategy that succeeds only temporarily may need to be subsequently replaced by yet another strategy. (And, sometimes, yet another. . .and another.) The following clinical examples are included to illustrate the principles described earlier.

Case Study: Isadora, A 77-year-old Woman With Thalamic Pain Syndrome

Isadora was a 77-year-old woman who presented with a 2-year history of excruciating hemicorporeal pain secondary to cerebrovascular accident (CVA). Her diagnosis was thalamic pain syndrome, for which the only remedy is thalamotomy—the likely consequences of which she was unwilling to choose. She had traveled to several pain centers on the east coast and in the midwest and had received a variety of treatments, including hypnosis, physical therapy, analgesic medications (including some experimental ones), acupuncture, and transcutaneous electrical nerve stimulation (TENS), all to no avail. In addition to the pain, the CVA had left her with hemiparesis, so walking was very difficult for her. She was, however, an extraordinary individual; vivacious and lively, she hoped that she would eventually find curative treatment. A retired college professor, she had filled her life prior to the CVA with travel and friends. Now, with movement difficult, and every waking moment filled with the perception that the left side of her body was "being squeezed in a red-hot vise," she was virtually house-bound.

She was taking no analgesic medication, since none affected the pain. She simple endured the pain and suffered mightily. She was unable to enjoy any activity, because the intensity of the pain was so great as to take up most of her awareness.

The first appointment was taken primarily with assessment of Isadora's psychological status, with a particular interest in her pain, how she coped with it, and what relation it bore to her life, and a review of her medical history pertinent to the rehabilitation treatment she had received.

It was clear from Isadora's demeanor that she was quite depressed. She was fatigued, sad, sometimes crying during the interview, and expressed an unusual degree of hopefulness about my treatment of her pain. She had read an article in a magazine that led her to conclude that I would be able to successfully return her to a pain-free life. My own reaction to Isadora, primarily in response to reading her chart, but also in response to her depression, was one of hopelessness. She was clearly distressed by the high level of intense pain and seemed highly motivated for relief. Her life had become increasingly constricted by her disability, so that her once-active life had now been reduced to watching television for most of each day in her home. My immediate impulse was to return her to her own town and find someone there who could care for her. She had said that she planned to be here for 2 weeks; I told her that would not be enough time to properly treat her and began suggesting alternatives for care back home. She quickly discounted that possibility and said she would make arrangements to stay as long as necessary. Feeling no choice but to try to help Isadora, I suggested that we would make an appointment for the following day, at which time I would begin showing her "how to retrain your nervous system and begin feeling more human again." I explained that I would use hypnosis to alter her sensory processing and that it might not be immediately effective.

At the second appointment—the first treatment appointment—she was hypnotized, given an explanation of her pain, based on the understanding of the consequences of an infarct to the thalamus, and told that over time her nervous system could "reroute" nervous impulses through other pathways, just as her motor system had done. (In the 2 years following her CVA her paresis had improved markedly, though it was now stable.) This suggestion for diminution was intended to counter her belief—and fear—that her pain was merely imagined. Furthermore, especially with such a highly educated individual as Isadora, such explanations were expected to increase the plausibility of treatment success. Suggestions were given that she could not reasonably expect full relief from pain to last throughout the day and certainly not to last until the next appointment (2 days hence). However, she was also given suggestions that *some* relief could be expected during that period of time. Suggestions were also given her to increase her confidence in her ability to endure, no matter what the outcome of treatment, and posthypnotic suggestions were given to facilitate the redevelopment of hypnosis at the next appointment.

At the termination of the hypnotic treatment, she expressed some surprise that her arm and chest didn't seem to hurt as much as usual. I asked in what way they felt different. She indicated that both the temperature and pressure of the vise had somehow decreased. Arrangements were made for her to return in 2 days for the next appointment.

At the second treatment appointment, Isadora arrived looking significantly more cheerful and reporting that she had been hurting less. Specifically, she reported that her arm and chest had felt unencumbered and comfortable following the previous treatment, and that this relief had lasted throughout the day. She slept comfortably and without sedatives for the first time since her CVA. The next day, however, she awoke feeling nearly as much pain as was usual for her. The pain had remained unchanged throughout that day, she had taken medication to sleep that night, and was now feeling her usual amount of pain.

I induced hypnosis using a relaxing image of sitting at a lakeside (an image she had suggested when describing enjoyable vacations at a particular lake) and deepened the hypnotic state by inducing catalepsy in her unaffected (right) arm. I then discussed the importance of the analgesia she had created 2 days previously and emphasized the implication of that: She had the power to alter her pain experience. If she can do it for a day, then a day

and an hour wouldn't be too much to expect. And a day and an hour isn't so much less than a day and an hour and a half, of course. . . . So that, within a few minutes, suggestions were given for increasing the amount of time she could expect comfort. I then reinforced the previously given suggestion that she could retrain her nervous system to reroute sensory processing through other pathways, isolating the damaged pathways, and thereby avoiding the need for processing "painful impulses." In order to begin the process of independence for Isadora, I also gave her posthypnotic suggestions such as the following:

> This experience, right now, of comfort and peace, is your experience, not mine. And the ability to create this experience is your ability, not mine. And you can enjoy learning how to use your ability to create this experience whenever you need to. For instance, whenever you're feeling very fatigued, or uncomfortable, and would really like to reexperience this pleasant comfort, all you need to do is lie down in a bed, close your eyes, and recall to your mind this lovely lakeside setting that you know so well. I'm going to stop talking right now, and I want you to just enjoy as fully as you like the comfort and peace you can bring yourself from just sitting here, looking out at the water, or enjoying the scent of flowers from that garden over there. [This is, of course, a suggestion for dissociation.]

At the end of this second treatment session, Isadora was excited and surprised that she had no awareness of any discomfort at all. As she left, I suggested that it would make for a more pleasant stay in the city if she were to remain relatively comfortable over the next 4 days until our next appointment.

At the third treatment appointment, Isadora reported that she had had no pain since she left my office, 4 days before. She was quite dramatic in her expression of delight and gratitude at this turn of events. She had slept well without need for sedation, as well. Hypnosis was used at this appointment to reinforce the gains that had been made and to reemphasize the importance of her own independent use of this skill — so that she could remain comfortable back home, far from my office.

The fourth, fifth, and sixth treatment appointments were used to consolidate these gains and to increase Isadora's confidence in her own hypnotic abilities, independent of my clinical intervention. She had had six treatment appointments in $2\frac{1}{2}$ weeks and was now ready to return home. Although I tried to refer her to someone near her home for follow-up care, she declined this and we agreed that we would keep in touch by telephone and through the mail.

Follow-up contact revealed that she maintained her pain-free condition for over 7 months, at which time she suffered a serious fall, spraining an ankle and causing a return of her pain to nearly pretreatment levels. We arranged that she would return for treatment, which she did — 1 year after the first series.

Continued treatment of Isadora's pain was complicated by other factors. Although the first treatment alleviated her pain, it was clear that Isadora was quite depressed. She remained for 2 more weeks, and treatment for her depression was initiated, as well as hypnotic reinforcement of her analgesia. I attempted to engage her in treatment for her depression with a psychiatrist near her home, but she resisted this. Follow-up contact was again maintained by telephone and through the mail, and Isadora continued to do well, although her depression remained without much relief; and despite my urging her into treatment, she remained untreated. I maintained contact with Isadora; she returned for treatment once more, 2 years later. Her phone conversations and letters had reflected some dementia — poor memory, frequently misunderstanding communications, some slight paranoid ideation — and her visit clearly indicated a mixture of her depression and sometimes cloudy thinking. Her pain was no longer a serious problem, and she continued to resist anyone's help with depression and with the increasing difficulties of living as an elderly, now somewhat infirm, person. Isadora died a year later following another CVA.

This case illustrates the complexity of treating chronic pain and the unique value of hypnosis in such treatment. Isadora's hypnotic treatment included: (a) suggestions for directly reducing the sensory dimensions of her pain (e.g., by imagining a rerouting of the sensory signals); (b) suggestions for reducing the affective dimension (e.g., not being bothered by whatever sensations she did notice); and (c) training in self-hypnosis so her relief could be maintained independently.

Case Study: Ben, A 56-year-old Man With Osteoarthritis

The application of hypnotic treatment principles differs considerably depending on the patient and the nature of the pain problem, as the case of Ben demonstrates.

A 56-year-old man referred by his rheumatologist, Ben suffered mightily from pain in his left hip that radiated down his leg into his ankle. A civil surveyor by trade, Ben was highly intelligent and well-read. He had been off work for 6 months due to his pain and took aspirin with codeine, about three tablets a day, when the pain became unbearable. He spent most of his time in his garage-shop, fashioning a cello, which he intended to learn to play. (He taught himself to play the piano, which he enjoyed playing quite well.)

His rheumatologist wanted Ben to have hip replacement surgery, and believed that was the only satisfactory treatment for the very severe degeneration of the head of the femur. Ben refused to take anti-inflammatory medication, because when he had taken it previously, it caused very severe side effects (intestinal blockage that required emergency surgery). Ben also actively resisted the idea of surgery; he reasoned that because of his relatively young age the prosthesis would need to be replaced two, possibly three, times over his lifetime — and he did not want to risk that much surgery. Ben's rheumatologist wanted me to convince Ben to go back on the medication or to have the surgery. Ben wanted me to hypnotize him so he would no longer have pain. His preference was to be able to go back to work, not take medication, and not have surgery.

At Ben's first appointment, I knew upon first seeing him that we would have trouble. As I opened my office door to show him in from the waiting room, he was standing there, glaring at me, his pipe in hand. He said to me with unconcealed ire, "What am I supposed to do with this?" He was referring to his pipe (and to the fact that my secretary had told him smoking wasn't allowed in the office).

Ben was a severe man, suspicious of the medical community (primarily because of his ordeal with the anti-inflammatory medication). During the history-taking, I noticed his increasing agitation: frequent sighing and other expressions of irritation in response to my persistent questioning. I explained that I needed to know a lot about him in order to know how best to help him. Nonetheless, with questions about his father's health, his wife's employment, his children, where he went to school, he became more convinced than ever that clinicians were not going to help him. It was only the fact that he had been told, for over 2 years, by several different people, that he should come to see me and that it was certain I could help him, that he endured my seemingly irrelevant questions.

Ben believed that hypnosis could reduce a person's pain, but he also believed that he could not be hypnotized. He had taken a course in hypnosis at a local community college; during the course he and his colleagues were given a hypnotizability test and he was found to be clearly unhypnotizable. He had later gone to a psychologist for the purpose of being hypnotized to relieve his pain and, he said, he found it to be a total waste of time; he did not respond to the suggestions. He was quite articulate and emphatic, though, in his belief that hypnosis might be able to help him under the right circumstances. He had been

told independently, by three individuals, over the past 2 years, that he should be treated by me. So, he had finally concluded, he would "give [me] a try."

It seemed clear that Ben was a healthy, highly functioning man, motivated to be rid of his pain. Ben also had a strong streak of skepticism in him and was unwilling to be hoodwinked by some mysterious, mystical force. I thought it best to be clear and straightforward with him and to educate him about the nature of hypnosis—in order to defuse his skepticism and provide him with needed information. The goal of treatment was the reduction of his pain (though I thought it likely that such reduction would provide inspiration for Ben to follow his rheumatologist's recommendations for surgery). I recommended a book for Ben to read about hypnosis (Bowers, 1983), and made an appointment for the first treatment.

The following week, Ben arrived with difficulty in walking due to a particularly severe pain. I asked him why he didn't use a cane to relieve some of the pressure from his beleaguered hip joint; he replied that he wasn't a cripple. He was particularly sour on this day, responding to any comment or request by me with a scowl and an unpleasant remark. I looked at him without speaking long enough to get his attention. Then, "You're a grumpy old bastard, aren't you?" His shock and amusement at my confrontation felt to me like the first real contact we'd had.

Ben: "Well, you'd be grumpy too, if you felt like I did."
Me: "I'm sure you're right; and I'd want someone to get through my grumpiness and help me to feel better. I actually like your grumpiness, but I suspect it gets in the way of your getting help."
Ben: "Do you think you can hypnotize me?"
Me: "I have no doubt at all about your ability to be hypnotized. But I don't know if you're going to bestow upon me the honor of being present while you're hypnotized, but we'll see."

Because Ben had previously had disap-

pointing experiences with hypnosis, I began
an induction that would be too complicated
for him to monitor—and thus would provide
the opportunity for new responses:

Ben, I want you to close your eyes as you
settle back in the chair now, so that I can
talk to you without interruption. I don't
really expect much to happen today, given
the kind of experiences you've had previously. It might take many, many appointments for you to get any benefit. I know that
will be expensive, but you are very persistent. [This paradoxical suggestion was
intended to stimulate Ben's already existing
concern about the cost of treatment and thus
increase motivation for a more rapid success.] Today you can expect to be appropriately disappointed that you haven't been
hypnotized, but that can afford you the
opportunity of experiencing some other kind
of relief without knowing how or why. It is
very important that you pay as much attention as you possibly can to the experience of
breathing. I know you can attend to whatever you want, and I want you to pay attention right now to your breathing. Really
notice what it feels like, each time you
breathe in, each time you breathe out.
Notice the rising and falling of your chest,
notice the change in tension of the material
of your shirt as your chest fills with air with
each inhalation, notice that the air is cool as
it enters your nose, and warm as it leaves. It
has been warmed by the very process of your
life.

And in a moment I want you to begin
counting your breaths, each one, either as
you inhale or as you exhale, it doesn't really
matter. I'm going to keep talking to you for
a while, but I want you to pay direct and
complete attention to counting your breaths.
Begin now. Count each breath. If you
become distracted and forget, just bring
your attention back, and resume counting.
If you don't remember at which number you
forgot, that's okay . . . just start over again
at the beginning. Just keep count-
ing . . . don't pay attention to me, I'm not
saying anything important at the moment
anyway, and it will be difficult to determine
when I do, so just keep counting. And while
you're counting, I'm going to talk to you

about some experiences you might have, if
you knew how, and you do; and I'm going to
suggest various experiences to you . . . and
you can respond to those suggestions in a
variety of ways. You might respond fully,
or partially. You might respond quickly, or
with some delay. You might respond predictably, or you might surprise yourself. I
don't know how you'll respond, and I hope
you'll allow yourself the opportunity of responding in more than one way. And keep
counting. . . .

I continued to suggest that Ben could
ignore my suggestions or could respond. In
general, I emphasized the autonomous nature
of his relationship to me. This was done
because I believed he would have an easier
time responding to suggestions if he were
more secure in his independence.

Next, I also suggested that he couldn't reasonably expect much to happen that day.
This was because, in the past, he had
expected results and had gotten none. With
no expectation, he could not be disappointed.
Further, no expectations would allow room
for new responses. I believed that his characteristic monitoring was largely responsible for
his previous lack of hypnotic success. Then
suggestions were given to allow for a possible
pleasant surprise (e.g., pain reduction). Ben
knew intellectually that hypnosis could reduce
pain. He also knew that he had not been able
to be hypnotized, and that his hypnotizability
score was low. However, he must have had
some idea that he could get results, or he
would not be in my office. I needed to capital-
ize on that hope, while disarming his skepticism. The following suggestions were given:

You know how to explain a lot of things.
Some things you don't know how to explain,
but you can enjoy them just the same. For
instance, you don't need to understand principles of optics in order to be absorbed by
the beauty of a sunset. You don't have to
know anything at all about reflection or
refraction or spectra in order to really enjoy
the vivid golds and reds and pinks and pur-
ples and blues of a sunset. And you certainly
don't have to be able to explain why it hap-

pened in order to enjoy the comfort you can feel later today. Because later today, and I don't know precisely what time it will be— How can I know precisely what time it will be?—later today, you will have the opportunity to suddenly discover how really well you are feeling—without any need to explain how it happened. It might be 2 o'clock this afternoon, or 5 minutes after 3, or 15 minutes after 4, or perhaps exactly 5 o'clock. I don't know what time it will be—in fact, it may not have to do with the actual time on the clock, it may seem more related to what you are doing. You might be untying a shoe, or lifting a glass to your lips, or turning the page of a magazine—I don't know what you will be doing when you'll have the sudden awareness that you are feeling better than you expected. And you will not have any way to explain it, nor will you need to. For some reason, you'll just realize you're feeling better, with nothing to bother you, and nothing to disturb you. And you won't even have to memorize the fact that I've told you this. And you won't even have to believe that you've been hypnotized. After all, who's to say that you were? In fact, if you are asked, later today, if you were hypnotized, you can take comfort in the fact that you can say you really don't think so. You really don't think you were hypnotized. And who is to say that you were? The fact that you are feeling better might be accounted for in a number of other ways. And you don't even have to think about it. But when I see you next time, I'll be really interested in any surprises you have had . . . particularly pleasant surprises.

Now, in a few minutes, I'm going to suggest that you take a very refreshing breath, or even two, and open your eyes and enjoy how very wide awake you feel. And, when you leave my office, although you will certainly feel alert and awake, it is possible that you might also feel very dry and thirsty, just as if you have been working out in the hot sun all morning. Because you have been working hard. And you can enjoy how easily you can get a drink of cool water. And when you are lifting the glass to your lips, you can really enjoy how nice it is that you can quench your own thirst, that you can satisfy your own needs.

A few minutes after Ben left the office, he returned, excitedly saying that he had no pain in his hip or leg. I replied noncommittally and told him I looked forward to seeing him in a few days. I also suggested that he begin using a cane.

When he returned for his second treatment appointment, Ben reported that he had felt pain-free from the moment he'd left my office, even driving home (and driving was normally quite painful); and, although some pain had returned later in the evening, he had generally felt much better throughout the day. The pain had returned the next morning, however, and had remained unabated until this morning. Forcing himself to mow his yard (another painful activity), he suddenly noticed that he was entirely pain-free. And he had remained pain-free throughout the morning and was still so now in the early afternoon. "But how can that be," he asked, "since I wasn't hypnotized last week?"

I responded by asking how he would determine if he was hypnotized or not. He replied that arm levitation (an ideomotor phenomenon that can be evoked hypnotically) would be sufficient. I then showed him how really simple it was to accomplish arm levitation and (using a post-hypnotic suggestion I had given at the previous appointment), suggested that he could develop a very absorbing and pleasant hypnotic state even though he was already feeling quite comfortable.

From that time on, Ben felt increasingly confident in his hypnotic abilities and was increasingly able to control his pain. However, at that appointment, I revived the discussion of an issue we'd had at the first appointment: If his hip joint was becoming increasingly deteriorated with use, so that movement was causing injury, wouldn't it make sense, now that he'd shown his ability to cope with the pain, to have the surgery his rheumatologist suggested? Ben's answer was a definite "No." He did not want surgery; he wanted to perfect his hypnotic abilities. I suggested that he might not be able to continue to control his pain if he was contributing to his injury. Curiously enough, although Ben proved to be hypnotically quite able, he began to be less and less able to control his pain. Within a week it was clear to him that he could be hypnotized, but that he could not relieve his hip pain. Over a month of determined effort went by before Ben decided to discuss surgery with an orthopedic surgeon.

After Ben had made plans for surgery (which was to take place a month later), he again became able to control his hip pain. This fact was understood by him to mean that he was unconsciously controlling his analgesic ability so that he did not contribute to further injury of his hip joint. Now, however, that he was going to get proper treatment, he was again able to reduce his pain. Ben underwent hip joint replacement surgery a month later and, following suggestions from me in this regard, was pleasantly surprised that he did not have significant post-operative pain. Ben is now back at work walking comfortably with the aid of his "high-tech hip," as he calls it.

Ben's case is an important example of the power of *meaning* in pain control. When his pain meant injury (and further injury without treatment), Ben was unable to control it. However, when his pain became an irrelevant signal (now that he had decided to have surgical treatment), his pain was controllable. Although this issue has never been experimentally verified, anecdotal accounts (Erickson, personal communication, 1976; London, personal communication, 1975) suggest that the signal value of pain is an important determiner of its hypnotic modification.

SUMMARY

From these case examples it is clear that hypnotic treatment of chronic pain is not a simple task, nor is it simply a matter of hypnotizing a patient and offering suggestions for analgesia. The particular way an individual patient's pain is integrated into his or her life will determine some of the twists and turns that treatment is likely to take. Isadora's distress, for instance, was primarily a function of unusually severe central pain. At certain points in treatment, however, her depression and mental confusion contributed significantly to her distress. It is important for the clinician to identify the various contributors

to the patient's distress and determine the best intervention for each. Hypnotic suggestion, for instance, was not likely to reduce Isadora's depression, and certainly was not likely to reduce her mental confusion (and, in fact, was made difficult to use because of her sometimes demented state). Ben's pain could have been best treated by surgery; however, Ben's fear of the consequences of putting himself so fully into the hands of others rendered that treatment unlikely, at least temporarily. One could conceptualize Ben's treatment as increasing his self-confidence by way of reducing his pain, so that he was able to decide on the best treatment.

Sometimes, concomitant psychological issues render the treatment of chronic pain quite puzzling and complicated. Susan, a very likeable professional writer, had endured significant pain for 58 of her 60 years. She contracted polio when she was 2, and her lower body was consequently weakened. She is now confined to a wheelchair, but nonetheless professionally and socially quite active. Largely as a consequence of aging, her upper body joints were increasingly painful, and no medical treatment was likely to make much difference. She avoided taking analgesics, but found it increasingly necessary to take oxycodone for relief. What made her case complicated was the following:

Susan was very adept at developing hypnotic analgesia. Literally within moments of beginning a hypnotic induction, Susan was totally free of pain. However, this pain-free condition was unsettling and even frightening to her. "This isn't me," she explained. Her identity is partly characterized by experiencing constant, unrelenting pain. So she finds it ego-dystonic to feel such relief. Subsequently, we have found that the best solution to this dilemma is to reduce her pain hypnotically, but only to a point that is tolerable to her. Her most comforting experience is to feel pain, but not such a high level of it that it interferes with her life.

The use of hypnosis is a vitally important adjunct in the treatment of chronic pain — but it is not itself a complete treatment. The patient's psychological and physical needs must of course be met. (e.g., as part of Susan's treatment, she is receiving Feldenkrais treatment to relieve some of the actual physical causes of her myofascial syndrome.)

The change in a patient's self-image, and the dramatic increase in confidence that a patient realizes when, for the first time, he or she experiences hypnotic analgesia, is itself salutary. Hypnosis is uniquely capable, of all psychological treatments, of bringing such dramatic relief. How that capability is channelled, and how the relief is integrated into the patient's life, is a significant clinical issue for the therapist using hypnosis.

Sometimes a patient's associated psychological difficulties render hypnosis useless, at least for a time. Linda, a 50-year-old film director, was referred for treatment of chronic pelvic pain. Linda was almost totally disabled by the pain, which had begun 3 years previously, apparently the result of chronic bladder infection, and had been certainly exacerbated by numerous invasive procedures and by 3 years of muscular contraction as a defense against the pain. Her condition was not well understood by a score of highly competent physicians who had examined and treated her. This was not an uncommon case (Reading, 1982), but was a difficult one to treat. Linda obtained temporary relief from tranquilizers, which she took sparingly, but increasingly. She also obtained temporary relief with hypnosis, sometimes, but exhibited a characteristic obsessive attentiveness to her pain, which made long-lasting relief unlikely. Because of her impatience with only temporary relief, because of unresolved issues of secondary gains, and because of her continued attentiveness to her pain, Linda is a clear example of a patient for whom hypnosis will be of limited usefulness; in effect, she is not ready to do what is necessary to obtain relief. What Linda needs is intensive behavioral management, preferably beginning with an inpatient chronic pain program.

How best to integrate hypnosis into a full treatment program is an important clinical issue and requires understanding of pain treatment in general, rather than hypnosis in particular. Given that hypnosis is such a demonstrably powerful analgesic technique, it is puzzling that it is not more widely used. Although I do not know of a systematic survey, it is my impression, based on conversations with colleagues, that the use of hypnosis in pain treatment programs is the exception rather than the rule. As we gain an understanding of how hypnosis is best used, the clinical use of hypnosis in pain management will likely become more frequent and more effective.

REFERENCES

Alman, B.M., & Carney, R.E. (1981). Consequences of direct and indirect suggestions on success of posthypnotic behavior. *American Journal of Clinical Hypnosis, 23*, 112–118.

Barber, J. (1977). Rapid induction analgesia: A clinical report. *American Journal of Clinical Hypnosis, 19*, 138–147.

Barber, J. (1980). Hypnosis and the unhypnotizable. *American Journal of Clinical Hypnosis, 23*, 4–9.

Barber, J. (1982). Incorporating hypnosis in the management of chronic pain. In J. Barber & C. Adrian (Eds.), *Psychological approaches to the management of pain* (pp. 40–59). New York: Brunner/Mazel.

Barber, J., & Adrian, C. (Eds.). (1982). *Psychological approaches to the management of pain.* New York: Brunner/Mazel.

Barber, J., & Mayer, D. (1977). Evaluation of the efficacy and neural mechanism of a hypnotic analgesia procedure in experimental and clinical dental pain. *Pain, 4*, 41–48.

Bowers, K.S. (1983). *Hypnosis for the seriously curious.* New York: Norton.

Crasilneck, H.B., & Hall, J.A. (1975). *Clinical hypnosis: Principles and applications.* New York: Grune & Stratton.

Diamond, M.J. (1984). It takes two to tango: The neglected importance of the hypnotic relationship. *American Journal of Clinical Hypnosis, 26*, 1–13.

Edelstien, M.G. (1981). *Trauma, trance, and transformation.* New York: Brunner/Mazel.

Esdaile, J. (1857). *Hypnosis in medicine and surgery. Introduction and supplementary reports by Wm.S. Kroger.* New York: Julian.

Finer, F., & Terenius, L. (1981, September). *Endorphin involvements during hypnotic analgesia in chronic pain patients.* Paper presented at the Third World Congress on Pain of the International Association for the Study of Pain, Edinburgh, Scotland.

Fordyce, W.E., Fowler, R.S., Lehmann, J.F., DeLateur, B.J., Sand, P.I., & Trieschmann,

R.B. (1983). Operant conditioning in the treatment of chronic pain. *Archives of Physical Medicine and Rehabilitation, 54,* 399–408.

Fricton, J. (1981, September). *The effects of direct and indirect hypnotic suggestions for analgesia in high and low susceptible subjects.* Paper presented at the Third World Congress on Pain of the International Association for the Study of Pain, Edinburgh, Scotland.

Gardner, G.G., & Olness, K. (1981). *Hypnosis and hypnotherapy in children.* New York: Grune & Stratton.

Gillett, P.L., & Coe, W.C. (in press). The effects of rapid induction analgesia (R.I.A.), hypnotic susceptibility, and the severity of discomfort on the reduction of dental pain. *American Journal of Clinical Hypnosis.*

Goldstein, A., & Hilgard, E.R. (1975). Lack of influence of the morphine antagonist naloxone on hypnotic analgesia. *Proceedings of the National Academy of Sciences, 72,* 2041–2043.

Haley, J. (Ed.). (1967). *Advanced techniques of hypnosis and therapy: The collected papers of Milton H. Erickson.* New York: Grune & Stratton.

Hartland, J. (1971). *Medical and dental hypnosis.* 2nd ed. Baltimore: Williams and Wilkins.

Hilgard, E.R. (1977). *Divided consciousness: Multiple controls in human thought and action.* New York: John Wiley and Sons.

Hilgard, E.R., & Hilgard, J.R. (1983). *Hypnosis in the relief of pain* (rev. ed.). Los Altos, CA: William Kaufman.

Hilgard, E.R., & Morgan, A.H. (1975). Heart rate and blood pressure in the study of laboratory pain in man under normal conditions and as influenced by hypnosis. *Acta Neurologiae Experimentalis, 35,* 741–759.

Hilgard, J.R. (1975). *Personality and hypnosis: A study of imaginative involvement.* (rev. ed.). Chicago: University of Chicago Press.

Hilgard, J.R., & LeBaron, S. (1982). Relief of anxiety and pain in children and adolescents with cancer: Quantitative measures and clinical observations. *The International Journal of Clinical and Experimental Hypnosis, 30,* 417–442.

Hilgard, J.R., & LeBaron, S. (1984). *Hypnotherapy of pain in children with cancer.* Los Altos, CA: William Kaufman.

Kellerman, J., Zeltzer, L., Ellenberg, L., & Dash, J. (1983). Adolescents with cancer. *Journal of Adolescent Health Care, 4,* 85–90.

Melzack, R., & Wall, P.D. (1973). *The puzzle of pain.* Basic Books.

McCauley, J.D., Thelan, M.H., Frank, R.G., Willard, R.R., & Callan, K.E. (1983). Hypnosis compared to relaxation in the outpatient management of chronic low back pain. *Archives of Physical Rehabilitation, 64,* 548–552.

Orne, M.T. (1976). Mechanisms of hypnotic pain control. In J.J. Bonica & D. Albe-Fessard (Eds.), *Advances in pain research and therapy* (Vol. 1, pp. 717–726). New York: Raven Press.

Orne, M.T. (1980). Hypnotic control of pain: Toward a clarification of the different psychological processes involved. In J.J. Bonica (Ed.), *Pain* (pp. 155–172). New York: Raven Press.

Price, D.D. (1983). Roles of psychophysics, neuroscience, and experiential analysis in the study of pain. In L. Kruger & J.C. Liebeskind (Eds.), *Advances in pain research and therapy* (Vol. 6, pp. 341–355). New York: Raven Press.

Price, D.D., & Barber, J. (1985). *Hypnotic alteration of pain perception in the laboratory: Implications for the clinic.* Unpublished manuscript.

Rausch, V. (1980). Cholecystectomy with self-hypnosis. *The International Journal of Clinical and Experimental Hypnosis, 22,* 124–129.

Reading, A.E. (1982). Chronic pain in gynecology: A psychological analysis. In J. Barber & C. Adrian (Eds.), *Psychological approaches to the management of pain* (pp. 137–149). New York: Brunner/Mazel.

Sachs, L.B., Feuerstein, M., & Vitale, J.H. (1977). Hypnotic self-regulation of chronic pain. *American Journal of Clinical Hypnosis, 20,* 106–113.

Schafer, D.W. (1975). Hypnosis use on a burn unit. *The International Journal of Clinical and Experimental Hypnosis, 23,* 1–14.

Shor, R.E. (1965). Hypnosis and the concept of the generalized reality-orientation. In R.E. Shor & M.T. Orne (Eds.), *The nature of hypnosis* (pp. 288–305). New York: Holt, Rinehart & Winston.

Shor, R.E., & Orne, E.C. (1962). *The Harvard group scale of hypnotic susceptibility, form A.* Palo Alto, CA: Consulting Psychologists Press.

Spiegel, D., & Albert, L.H. (1983). Naloxone fails to reverse hypnotic alleviation of chronic pain. *Psychopharmacology, 81,* 140–143.

Sternbach, R.A. (1982). On strategies for identifying neurochemical correlates of hypnotic analgesia. *International Journal of Clinical and Experimental Hypnosis, 30,* 251–256.

Turner, J.A., & Chapman, C.R. (1982). Psychological interventions for chronic pain: A critical review. II. Operant conditioning, hypnosis, and cognitive-behavioral therapy. *Pain, 1,* 23–42.

Wakeman, R.J., & Kaplan, J.Z. (1978). An experimental study of hypnosis in painful burns. *American Journal of Clinical Hypnosis, 21,* 3–12.

Weitzenhoffer, A.M., & Hilgard, E.R. (1959). *Stanford Hypnotic Susceptibility Scale, Forms A and B.* Palo Alto, CA: Consulting Psychologists Press.

Zeltzer, L., Dash, J., & Holland, J. (1979). Hypnotically induced pain control in sickle cell anemia. *Pediatrics, 64,* 533–536.

11 COGNITIVE–BEHAVIORAL ASSESSMENT AND MANAGEMENT OF PEDIATRIC PAIN

James W. Varni
Susan M. Jay
Bruce J. Masek
Karen L. Thompson

In marked contrast to the rather extensive research literature on adult chronic pain management, the systematic investigation of pediatric pain from a cognitive-behavioral perspective represents a relatively recent area of scientific inquiry (cf. Varni, 1983, for a review). In the past several years, however, a growing number of investigators have begun generating a substantial data base from which the clinical potential of cognitive-behavioral techniques in managing acute and chronic pain in children has become clear (Varni & Thompson, in press).

Pain in children represents a complex cognitive-developmental phenomenon, involving a number of biobehavioral components that synergistically interact to produce differential levels of pain perception and verbal and nonverbal manifestation. Given children's various cognitive-developmental states, then their conceptualizations of pain and discomfort must be assessed. Thus, an adequate understanding of pain in children cannot be gleaned from simply applying the knowledge of pain in adults; rather, pediatric pain assessment and management must generate a parallel data base.

In the cognitive-behavioral assessment and management of pediatric pain, it is essential to distinguish between acute and chronic pain. Acute pain serves as an adaptive biological warning signal, directing attention to an injured part or disease condition, functioning within an avoidance paradigm to encourage escape or avoidance of harmful stimuli and indicating the need for rest or treatment of an injured area. While neurophysiological processes may distinguish acute from chronic pain (Bonica, 1977; Katz, Sharp, Kellerman, Marston, Herschman, & Siegel, 1982), it is often the severe intensity of acute pain and its associated anxiety reaction that most parsimoniously differentiate acute and chronic pain expression (Varni, 1983). Particularly during painful medical procedures, the anxiety component must be taken into consideration (Katz, Varni, & Jay, 1984). Pediatric chronic pain, on the other hand, is typically characterized by the absence of an anxious component, with a constellation of reaction features such as compensating posturing, lack of developmentally appropriate behaviors, depressed mood, and inactivity or restriction in the normal activities of daily living. These chronic pain behaviors may eventually be maintained independently of the original nociceptive impulses and tissue damage, being reinforced by socioenvironmental influences (Fordyce, 1976). Acute pain, in contrast, typically occurs in temporal proximity with a pathogenic agent or noxious stimulus.

Varni (Varni, 1983; Varni, Katz, & Dash, 1982) has identified four primary categories of pediatric pain: (a) pain associated with a disease state (e.g., hemophilia, arthritis, sickle cell anemia); (b) pain associated with an observable physical injury or trauma (e.g., burns, lacerations, fractures); (c) pain not associated with a well-defined or specific disease state or identifiable physical injury (e.g., migraine and tension headaches, recurrent abdominal pain); and (d) pain associated with medical/dental procedures (e.g., lumbar punctures, bone marrow aspirations, surgery, injections, extractions).

In this chapter, we will present case studies representing each of the above four categories, specifically pain associated with hemophilia, burns, migraine headaches, and lumbar punctures/bone marrow aspirations. Before describing the cognitive-behavioral assessment and management of these four pediatric pain conditions, however, the essential issue of comprehensive pediatric pain assessment, within the considerations of each child's cognitive-developmental stage, will be presented and illustrated by a case of chronic musculoskeletal pain in juvenile rheumatoid arthritis.

PEDIATRIC PAIN ASSESSMENT

Whatever intervention methods — pharmacological, psychological, or behavioral — are used, effective and efficient management of pain in children or adults depends upon accurate assessment (Beales, 1982; Thompson & Varni, in press; Varni, 1983). Evaluation of the pain experience in adults is facilitated by an adult's knowledge and understanding of what pain means, what services are available for relief from pain, and how to communicate painful sensations to health care professionals. Pediatric pain assessment, however, can be confounded by inadequate communication between children and health care providers. Words like "pain" may be entirely absent from a child's vocabulary or given an abstract meaning quite different from that of an adult. Language and specific examples that are appropriate to a child's age and developmental stage should be used in explaining symptoms, procedures, and health instructions (Perrin & Perrin, 1983). Awareness of a child's cognitive-developmental level and cognitively related misconceptions is therefore essential when assessing and treating pediatric pain (Thompson & Varni, in press; Varni, 1983).

Several researchers have documented stages of health and illness conceptualizations that mirror Piaget's stages of cognitive development (Bibace & Walsh, 1981; Brewster, 1982; Feldman & Varni, 1985; Perrin & Gerrity, 1981; Steward & Regalbuto, 1975; Whitt, Dykstra, & Taylor, 1979). Briefly, six categories are hypothesized: phenomenism and contagion (ages 2 to 6), contamination and internalization (ages 7 to 10), and physiological and psychophysiological (ages 11 or older).

Phenomenism is the most developmentally immature explanation. The cause of illness is an external event that may co-occur with the illness but is spatially and/or temporally remote. In the stage of *contagion*, the cause of illness is located in objects or people that are proximate to but not touching the child. People get sick by magic or because they are near certain objects.

Contamination is a concrete-logical form of reasoning. The cause of illness is viewed as a person, object, or action that is external to the child and that has an aspect or quality that is bad or harmful to the body. Physical contact is necessary for illness to occur. Illness becomes located inside the body in the stage of *internalization*, even though the ultimate cause of illness may still be external. Confusion still exists about internal organs and functions, but the child can offer vague ideas about his or her internal state.

The greatest amount of understanding occurs with children who are able to comprehend *physiological* and *psychophysiological* explanations of illness. In the physiological stage, the source and nature of the illness lie in specific internal physiological structures and functions. Psychophysiological explanations, the most mature understanding of illness, still describe illness in terms of internal physiological processes; additionally, psychological causes are also delineated. The child is aware that a person's thoughts or feelings can affect the way the body functions. (See Bibace & Walsh, 1981, and Varni, 1983, for comprehensive reviews.)

The effects of cognitive-developmental level on the assessment of pediatric pain have not been empirically validated; nevertheless, the importance of considering developmental level when assessing pain in children has been proposed by several clinicians and researchers (Gildea & Quirk, 1977; Schecter, 1984; Thompson & Varni, in press; Varni, 1983). Despite these acknowledgments, developmentally appropriate assessment instruments that measure more than just pain intensity are noticeably lacking.

As stated by Melzack (1975):

> The word "pain" refers to an endless variety of qualities that are categorized under a single linguistic label, not to a specific single sensation that varies only in intensity. To describe pain solely in terms of intensity is like specifying the visual world only in terms of light flux without regard to pattern, texture, and the many other dimensions of visual experience. (p.278)

If, as hypothesized, a child's cognitive-developmental level affects his or her perception and report of pain, and we as health care providers have been neglecting to evaluate dimensions other than pain intensity, we may be unable to provide children with the most effective intervention possible because of inadequate pain assessment.

The ideal assessment of pediatric pain requires an interdisciplinary, multidimensional, and comprehensive approach, combining self-report, behavioral, cognitive, socioenvironmental, medical, and biological parameters (Varni, 1983). Rarely have pediatric pain assessments addressed all of these areas. Self-report measures of pain intensity, such as the visual analogue scale and color spectrum ratings, are two of the more commonly used methods with children (despite the drawbacks of only measuring pain intensity).

The Visual Analogue Scale (VAS) is a form of cross-modality matching, in which line length is the response continuum. The ends are marked with the two extremes for pain, such as "no pain" and "very severe pain" or "pain as bad as it could possibly be." The main advantage of the VAS is the avoidance of numbers or word descriptors and categories (Stewart, 1977). The patient is free to indicate on a continuum the intensity of the pain without relating to specific words chosen by the clinician. Typical instructions to the child would be "if this end of the line means no pain at all, and this end of the line means very severe pain, can you place a mark on the line to show how much you hurt now?" (Abu-Saad, 1984). Selection of colors to communicate pain intensity has also been used with children (Eland, 1981).

In an attempt to assess pediatric pain reliably and validly, Varni and Thompson (1985) have developed the Pediatric Pain Questionnaire (PPQ). The Varni/Thompson PPQ is a comprehensive, multidimensional assessment instrument specifically designed for the study of acute and chronic pain in children, with both parent and child forms. The PPQ-Child Form addresses the intensity of pain, the sensory, emotive, and affective qualities of pain, and the location of pain in a form comprehensible to children. The PPQ-Parent Form consists of similar components to the PPQ-Child Form to allow for cross-validation of the child's reporting of pain. A comprehensive family history section addresses the child's pain history and the family's pain history with questions pertaining to symptomatology, past and present treatments for pain, and socioenvironmental situations that may influence pain. The following case illustrates the utilization of the Varni/Thompson PPQ with a child with chronic musculoskeletal pain (see Thompson, Varni, & Hanson, 1985).

*Case Study: An 8-year old Child
With Rheumatoid Arthritis*

The child was an 8-year-old female with systemic onset juvenile rheumatoid arthritis (see Varni & Jay, 1984, for a comprehensive review of JRA). At the time of pain assessment, she had morning stiffness for approximately 1 hour each morning. Three joints exhibited active disease. A pediatric rheumatologist rated the child's overall disease activity as moderate on a 5-point scale. Aspirin and heat applied to the affected joints were reported as being used to control pain episodes.

The child's mother completed the Varni/Thompson PPQ-Parent Form and Comprehensive Family History Form. The parent form can be completed by the parent in approximately 20 minutes and reviewed by health care professionals immediately after completion. The PPQ-Parent Form documented the child's pain as adversely affecting her mobility, appetite, sleep, and schoolwork. On the 10-cm visual analogue scale, the child's mother estimated her present pain intensity at 5-cm (moderate pain). When choosing qualitative descriptions of her child's pain, the words "burning," "sore," "sharp," and "tiring" were selected. A body diagram was provided for localization of pain. The child's mother localized pain in the fingers and ankles. The Comprehensive Pain History revealed no family history of chronic pain. The child's father had chronic asthma. The information provided by the child's mother was used to provide a measure of validity for the child's self-report of pain.

The PPQ-Child Form was administered to the child by a trained child health care professional. Before beginning the assessment, care was taken to sensitize the child to the topic of pain. Questions addressing what the child thinks pain or hurt is and what words she uses to mean pain were established. A word list was then presented to the child, and words were selected to describe the pain she felt at the time of the interview. The child chose the words "tingling," "uncomfortable," "sad," "sore," "tiring," and "horrible." The 10-cm visual analogue scale was anchored by happy and sad faces with the words "no pain" and "severe pain" and related developmentally appropriate words to measure child self-report of pain intensity. The child estimated her pain at 5-cm (the same rating provided by her mother). A color spectrum similar to the procedure used by Eland (1981) provided intensity ratings for the body localization of pain. The child localized pain in her fingers and ankles, consistent with her mother's locations.

The assessment provided through use of the Varni/Thompson PPQ provides a comprehensive basis for pediatric pain management. By using a developmentally appropriate instrument, pain intensity, pain location, and the qualitative aspects of the pain experience can be obtained from the child, as well as potential socioenvironmental factors. Optimum management of pain in children requires adequate means of assessing a child's level of physical discomfort and related parameters. By combining an understanding of cognitive-developmental level and conceptualizations of health, illness, and pain within a multidimensional assessment instrument, health care professionals can better understand and manage acute and chronic pain in children.

TREATMENT

The primary cognitive-behavioral treatment techniques utilized in the management of pediatric pain may be categorized into (a) *pain perception regulation* modalities through such self-regulatory processes as guided imagery, meditation, and progressive muscle relaxation, and (b) *pain behavior regulation* which identifies and modifies the socioenvironmental factors that may influence pain expression and rehabilitation (Varni, 1983). Self-regulatory processes are the primary treatment modality in the management of pediatric acute pain, whereas self-regulation of pain and pain behavior regulation are utilized in chronic pain syndromes, depending on the particular disorder and the existing socioenvironmental influences. The self-regulation techniques share common features with self-hypnosis, autogenic therapy, meditation, progressive muscle relaxation, and biofeedback training.

Laboratory research on experimental pain has indicated the role of distraction, dissociation, or refocusing of attention from thoughts concerned with pain, anxiety reduction, suggestions of pain relief, and the imagination of past experiences that were incompatible with pain as potent cognitive variables in the reduction of pain perception (see Hilgard, 1975). On the other hand, the pain behavior regulation modality follows the socioenvironmental modification approach initially developed for adult chronic pain patients (see Fordyce, 1976).

Although similar mechanisms may be operating in both pain perception regulation and pain behavior regulation (e.g., distraction from pain perception as the patient concentrates on emitting developmentally appropriate behaviors or increases in mobility and sleep as pain perception decreases), the focus of treatment has typically identified one or the other treatment modality as the primary management strategy.

Following the four pain categories identified by Varni (1983), the next four sections will illustrate the current cognitive-behavioral treatment approaches for pediatric pain.

RECURRENT PAIN ASSOCIATED WITH HEMOPHILIA

Hemophilia represents a congenital hereditary disorder of blood coagulation, characterized by recurrent, unpredictable internal bleeding episodes affecting any body part, especially the joints and extremities. Re-

peated hemorrhages into the joint areas (hemarthroses) eventually result in a condition similar to osteoarthritis, a chronic disease characterized by destruction of articular cartilage, pathological bone formation, and impaired function (Sokoloff, 1975). Chronic degenerative arthritis represents the most frequent problem confronting the physician who manages the care of adolescent and adult hemophiliacs, with an estimated 75% of hemophilic adolescents and adults demonstrating one or more affected joints (Dietrich, 1976). Anti-inflammatory drugs may be employed but are of limited usefulness, with analgesic abuse and dependency of constant concern (Varni & Gilbert, 1982).

Whereas acute pain in the hemophiliac is associated with a specific bleeding episode, chronic arthritic pain represents a sustained condition over an extended period of time. Thus, pain perception in the hemophiliac truly represents a complex psychophysiological event, complicated by the existence of both acute bleeding pain and chronic arthritic pain, and requires differential treatment strategies (Varni, 1981a, 1981b). More specifically, acute pain of hemorrhage provides a functional signal, indicating the necessity of intravenous infusion of factor replacement which temporarily replaces the missing clotting factor, converts the clotting status to normal, and allows a functional blood clot to form. Arthritic pain, on the other hand, represents a potentially debilitating chronic condition which may result in impaired life functioning and analgesic dependence (Varni & Gilbert, 1982). Consequently, the development of an effective alternative to analgesic abuse and dependency in the reduction of perceived chronic arthritic pain that does not interfere with the essential functional signal of acute bleeding pain has been the goal of the behavioral medicine approach to hemophilia pain management (Varni, 1981a, 1981b; Varni & Gilbert, 1982).

Unfortunately, approximately 10% of hemophilic children develop an inhibitor to factor replacement, presenting a serious problem in the management of bleeding episodes. Although the bleeding frequency is not different, the neutralization of factor replacement by an inhibitor (antibody) makes the control of bleeding ineffective. The pain associated with uncontrolled hemorrhage can be extremely severe, with narcotic analgesics traditionally prescribed. Thus, although the acute pain of hemorrhage provides a functional signal indicating the necessity of factor replacement therapy, in the hemophilic child with factor replacement inhibitor, the intensity of the pain supersedes its functional intent, and analgesic dependence is of constant concern. Consequently, an effective alternative to analgesic dependence in the reduction of perceived pain in the patient with an inhibitor has been greatly needed.

Case Study: A 9-year-old Hemophilic Child

Varni, Gilbert, and Dietrich (1981) reported on a study involving a 9-year-old hemophilic child with factor replacement inhibitor. At 4 years of age, when the inhibitor developed and subsequent factor replacement therapy became impossible, the child began to require narcotics in order to tolerate the pain of each hemorrhage. Progressively, the need for pain medication increased for both bleeding pain and for arthritic pain in his left knee secondary to degenerative arthropathy. Since the arthritic pain eventually occurred almost daily, the requests for analgesics further increased so that the acute pain of hemorrhage required ever larger doses for pain relief, even though home medication and joint immobilization continued for the management of bleeding episodes. As a consequence of bleeding and arthritic pain in the lower extremities, the child was wheelchair bound nearly 50% of the time, hospitalized 16 times in the $4\frac{1}{2}$-year period prior to the study for a total of 80 days after the development of the inhibitor, and kept analgesic medication at his school for pain control. The final precipitating event in this steadily worsening cycle occurred during an evening visit to the emergency room because of a very painful and severe left knee hemorrhage that had not responded to home therapy; the administration of an adult dose of meperidine and I.V. diazepam provided no pain relief.

Training in the cognitive-behavioral self-regulation of pain perception consisted of three sequential phases. The child was first taught a 25-step progressive muscle-relaxation sequence involving the alternative tensing and relaxing of major muscle groups (see Varni, 1983). He was then taught meditative breathing exercises, consisting of medium deep breaths inhaled through the nose and slowly exhaled through the mouth. While exhaling, the child was instructed to say the word "relax" silently to himself and to initially describe aloud and subsequently visualize the word in warm colors, as if written in color chalk on a blackboard. Finally, the child was instructed on the use of guided imagery techniques, consisting of pleasant, distracting scenes selected by the child. Initially, the child was instructed to imagine himself actually in the scene, not simply to observe himself there. The scene was evoked by a detailed multisensory description by the therapist and subsequently described out loud by the child. Once the scene was clearly visualized by the child, the therapist instructed the child to experiment with other, different scenes to maintain interest and variety.

The child recorded the severity of his pain on a 10-point scale for a $2\frac{1}{2}$-week baseline prior to self-regulation training. The average score for both arthritic and bleeding pain during this period was 7, indicating rather intense pain. At a 1-year follow-up after the initiation of the self-regulation training, the child reported that both arthritic and bleeding pain were reduced to 2 on the scale when he engaged in the self-regulation techniques. In addition to this measure of pain perception, the child's evaluation at the 1-year follow-up session on a comparative assessment inventory (see Varni, 1983) indicated substantial positive changes in arthritic and bleeding pain, mobility, sleep, and general overall functioning.

As may be seen in Table 11.1, once the child began using the self-regulation techniques for pain management, there were no further requests for meperidine during the 1-year post-treatment assessment, with substantially decreased amounts of acetaminophen with

TABLE 11.1 PARAMETERS ASSOCIATED WITH PAIN INTENSITY

Parameters	1-year pre self-regulation training	1-year post self-regulation training
Pain intensity (1 = mild; 10 = severe)	7*	2**
Meperidine	74 tablets (50 mg/ea.)	0 tablets
Acetaminophen/codeine elixir	438 doses (24 mg codeine/dose)	78 doses (24 mg codeine/dose)
Physical therapy measures		
Range of motion	Normal r. knee 0°–150° Arthritic l. knee 15°–105°	R. knee 0°–150° L. knee 0°–140°
Quadricep strength (0–5 scale)	Normal r. knee 4– Arthritic l. knee 3+	R. knee 4+ L. knee 4
Girth (knee joint circumference)	Not available	R. knee 26 cm L. knee 25.8 cm
Ambulation on stairs	2–3 maximum	No limitation
School days missed	33	6
Hospitalizations		
Total days	11	0
Number admissions	3	0

Note. From "Behavioral medicine in pain and analgesia management for the hemophilic child with factor VIII inhibitor" by J.W. Varni, A. Gilbert, and S.L. Dietrich, 1981, *Pain, 11*, p. 124. Reprinted by permission.
*2.5-week pre assessment during pain episodes just prior to self-regulation training.
**1-year average rating during pain episodes when using self-regulation techniques.

codeine elixir required. Table 11.1 also shows significant improvements in other areas of functioning, including improved mobility, as evidenced by the physical therapy measures, in his arthritic left knee compared with his normal right knee on the dimensions of range of motion (0–150 = normal) and quadricep strength (1 = no joint motion, 5 = complete range of motion against gravity with full resistance). Normalization of psychosocial activities is suggested by increased school attendance and decreased hospitalizations and by parental report, which noted a distinct elevation of the child's overall mood, with considerably less depression during pain episodes because he had the skills to actively reduce his pain perception without depending on pain medication.

The analysis of the various parameters assessed in this study suggests a significant improvement across a number of areas. As envisioned by the authors, a deteriorating cycle was evident prior to the intervention, schematically represented as: hemorrhage → pain → analgesics/joint immobilization → at-rophy of muscles adjacent to the joints/joint deterioration → hemorrhage. Thus, as has been previously suggested (Dietrich, 1976), pain-induced immobilization results in muscle weakness surrounding the joints and sets the occasion for future hemorrhaging. By breaking this deteriorating cycle at the point of pain severity, the child was offered the opportunity to decrease immobilization and increase therapeutic activities such as swimming, subsequently improving the strength and range of motion in his left knee. With this improved ambulatory status, school attendance and his general activity level were consequently increased. The possibility that this early intervention may have prevented or reduced the likelihood of later drug abuse must also be considered (Varni & Gilbert, 1982). Finally it is important to reiterate that these procedures were used for a child with an inhibitor. For the hemophiliac without an inhibitor, bleeding pain serves as a functional signal and is best managed with factor replacement therapy. In the present case, however, no effective medical procedure was available to control severe bleeding pain other than powerful narcotic analgesics, clearly an undesirable therapy modality for recurrent pain.

PEDIATRIC MIGRAINE

Recurrent migraine headache is a common clinical entity in pediatrics (Prensky & Sommers, 1979). Longitudinal studies (Bille, 1962; Sillanpaa, 1976) indicate that migraine is rare before 2 years of age, and the incidence is estimated to be 2.5% at ages 7 to 9, increasing to 5.3% between ages 13 and 15. Before puberty there is no sex difference, but thereafter females outnumber males by a 3:2 ratio. Recent evidence indicates that between 40% and 60% of children continue to experience migraine into adulthood (Bille, 1981).

The chief clinical characteristic of migraine is recurrent, intermittent attacks of throbbing pain with frequency varying from several times per day to once or twice per year. Classic and common migraine are the most frequently diagnosed types in children (Shinnar & D'Sousa, 1981). Classic migraine is distinguished by the occurrence of a specific neurological disturbance known as a prodrome preceding the headache; the pain is unilateral in onset; and nausea, vomiting, or abdominal pain are associated with the headaches. Common migraine differs from the classic type in that there is a vague or undistinguishable prodrome; the pain is typically bilateral; and gastrointestinal symptoms are less prominent. Other symptoms found in both types include photophobia, sonophobia, odorophobia, and exacerbation of pain by movement.

Therapy usually beings with simple analgesics, such as aspirin and acetaminophen or a mild sedative such as Fiorinal, combined with rest. This approach, along with the reassurance that intracranial pathology or systemic illness is not involved, is sufficient for children with infrequent, less severe migraine (Newberger & Sallan, 1981). In children with classic migraine, who are at least 10 years of age, ergotamine preparations taken during the prodrome can be effective in aborting

the headache. Because ergotamine is a powerful vasoconstrictor, however, only a limited amount can be taken in a week; and the wisdom of allowing children to carry the medicine around with them is questionable (Barlow, in press). In frequent severe migraine, prophylactic therapy can be effective in reducing the number of attacks but has increased risk of side-effects. Propranolol is usually the drug of first choice because there is a low incidence of side-effects in children, notably fatigue and nausea (Artman, Grayson, & Boerth, 1982). It is contraindicated in asthma and heart disease. For some patients the antidepressant amyitriptyline can act prophylactically in low doses. Side-effects include drowsiness, dry mouth, dizziness, and urinary retention. Occasionally, phenobarbital and Dilantin are used when minor EEG abnormalities are present. Sedation limits the usefulness of phenobarbital (Shinnar & D'Sousa, 1981).

Until recently, if medications were ineffective, caused side effects, were contraindicated, or were not acceptable to patients (or parents), there were few treatment alternatives. In the past 4 years, however, a number of case reports and small-scale retrospective studies have been published indicating the effectiveness of biofeedback (Werder & Sargent, 1984), biofeedback and relaxation (Andrasik, Blanchard, Edlund, & Rosenblum, 1983; Houts, 1982; Labbe & Williamson, 1983; Olness & MacDonald, 1981; Waranch & Keenan, in press), and behavior modification (Ramsden, Friedman, & Williamson, 1983) in the treatment of pediatric migraine. Additionally, two small-scale prospective studies have recently been completed documenting the effectiveness of biofeedback, relaxation, and pain behavior management (Fentress, Masek, Mehegan, & Benson, 1984; Mehegan, Masek, Harrison, Russo, & Leviton, 1984).

Thermal biofeedback training has been extensively investigated as a treatment for migraine. The usual procedure is to record surface skin temperature from the index finger and display this information continuously in the form of an analogous signal. The patient is instructed to increase hand temperature using the feedback display to guide performance. How and why thermal biofeedback acts as a treatment for migraine remains controversial. Current thinking favors the hypothesis that vasomotor instability of cerebral and peripheral vasculature is the heritable condition responsible for migraine (Olton & Noonberg, 1980). Learning to increase hand temperature has the effect of stabilizing peripheral (perhaps cerebral) vasculature which, if practiced regularly, reduces occurrence (Dalessio, Kunzel, Sternbach, & Sorak, 1979). The implicit assumption is that learning to increase hand temperature can be done without the aid of biofeedback in the natural environment, possibly even to abort an attack in its early stages. However, virtually no experimental evidence exists in support of this fundamental assumption (Johansson & Ost, 1982; Pikoff, 1984). Despite the apparent lack of a solid theoretical foundation, biofeedback training continues to be widely used in the treatment of migraine and other types of headache.

Relaxation training is also of proven efficacy as a treatment for migraine (Blanchard & Andrasik, 1982). The physiology of the relaxation response is reasonably well understood. Regular practice of any number of relaxation techniques (Masek, Spirito, & Fentress, 1984) is associated with a reliable pattern of lowered heart rate and blood pressure, decreased skeletal muscle and vasomotor tone, changes in the EEG, and increased oxygen perfusion to peripheral tissue (Benson, 1975). It may well be that a more general effect of relaxation, which acts to prevent migraine, is the attenuation of sympathetic (Hoffman et al., 1982) and skeletal muscle responsivity to emotional and physical stressors. It has also been hypothesized that relaxation represents the "final common pathway" by which biofeedback and other self-regulation procedures work in the treatment of headache (Blanchard, Andrasik, Ahles, Teders, & O'Keefe, 1980). The following case study exemplifies the current cognitive-behavioral treatment of pediatric migraine.

Case Study: A 13-year-old Child With Migraine

The child was a 13-year-old male suffering from classic migraine which began when he was 7 years old. He was referred by a pediatric neurologist after neurological evaluation. The pain was localized in his left temple and eye and was accompanied by nausea and vomiting. His mother, maternal grandmother, and younger brother also had migraine headaches. Aspirin and rest controlled mild to moderate attacks, but Caffergot PB (ergotamine, belladonna, and pentobarbital) and bed rest for the remainder of the day were necessary for severe attacks. The child documented in a headache diary two mild, two moderate, and two severe migraines in the month preceding the start of treatment. Lack of sleep, arguments with his brother, and pressures associated with school were identified as possible precipitants of headache. During allergy seasons his headaches were sometimes worse. He was an honors student, was active in sports, and described himself as a perfectionist. No significant family or psychosocial problems were identified.

Treatment consisted of biofeedback and relaxation training provided in five 1-hour sessions over a period of 9 weeks. Two follow-up appointments 3 months apart were completed after treatment. He kept a headache diary throughout treatment which provided information about the intensity, duration, medication use, antecedents, and consequences of each migraine attack. During the first session he was taught meditative relaxation (Benson, 1975). While seated in a comfortable chair, he was instructed to: (a) close his eyes, (b) breathe slowly and more deeply, and (c) subvocally repeat a prearranged word (e.g., calm or quiet) and notice the sensations of relaxation. The entire procedure took about 10 minutes the first time through. He was instructed to practice for 5 to 10 minutes twice each day at home at agreed upon times. In subsequent sessions, he practiced this procedure for 4 minutes twice during biofeedback training, primarily to assess his performance in terms of frontal EMG muscle activity and finger temperature. Also, the results of a relaxation practice trial could be displayed on a television monitor for instructional purposes or to reinforce a good performance. It was suggested that he begin to use his relaxation skill to calm down after a stressful interaction with his younger brother or in response to increased tension experienced a day or two before an exam in school. The school was contacted so that he could use the nurse's office to practice relaxation if an attack occurred there.

EMG biofeedback of frontal muscle activity was provided during each session. A disposable-type surface electrode was placed on his forehead with the explanation that persons with migraine often develop excessive facial muscle activity before an attack that they must learn to control. The purpose of the biofeedback training was to teach him to relax his facial muscles as much as possible. Feedback in the form of a line-graph tracing of integrated EMG activity was displayed on a color television monitor. Each session he received three consecutive 4-minute training trials in which he was instructed to relax his facial muscles, as indicated by a downward slope of the line graph. Resting baseline trials 4 minutes in length preceded and followed feedback training. Meditative relaxation assessments were conducted at the beginning and end of biofeedback training. Skin temperature was recorded from the index finger of the dominate hand using a thermistor taped to the volar surface. It was explained that the relaxation response involved many organs and physiological processes and that increased temperature at the surface of the skin was another good indication that he was learning the response. Finger temperature was not displayed during feedback trials, but the results were available at the end of a trial for review.

During the first month of treatment, the child experienced two severe and two moderate migraines, all of which developed in school. The severe attacks forced him to leave school for the day. Towards the end of the month, his mother reported that he was much more relaxed in the face of his younger broth-

er's provocations. During the second month of treatment, he experienced one mild and one severe attack and was able to abort another attack as it was starting by using relaxation techniques. Again, these headaches began in school, but he only missed a few classes as a result. Corresponding to the decrease in headache occurrence was a reliable decrease in EMG of 3 to 4 microvolts and an increase in finger temperature of approximately 2°F during meditative relaxation assessments. During the next 3 months, he experienced one moderate to severe attack per month and had three more experiences aborting attacks using relaxation. At the final follow-up appointment near the end of the school year, he reported only one severe headache in 3 months. He practiced relaxation daily when he was tense, felt angry, or felt a headache coming on, or for a few minutes near bedtime if no occasion arose to use his skill. His relaxation performance in the biofeedback laboratory was on a par with end-of-treatment performance. He attributed the decrease in headache activity to the sense of control he had developed with the relaxation techniques which, in turn, reduced his fear of migraine and panic during the initial stages of an attack. As a result of keeping a headache diary, he also felt better equipped to identify stressors that could potentially trigger attacks.

This case is fairly representative of a typical pediatric headache patient, that is, a bright, achievement-oriented individual with a strong family history of migraine. Decreased functioning during attacks and lack of control over their occurrence is a very frustrating set of circumstances for the child. Increased irritability, withdrawal, and lowered self-confidence are common responses to the onset of migraine. During biofeedback and relaxation training, the emphasis is on the child assuming control over the headaches by using skills acquired in treatment. Rarely does the environment play a role in maintaining headache by reinforcing pain behavior in these patients (Masek, Russo, & Varni, 1984). Not surprisingly, most of these patients do very well with the combination of biofeedback, which appeals to their achievement orientation, and relaxation techniques, because it provides them with a practical method to limit the tension they feel in stressful situations and controls the anxiety and pain associated with headache.

Not all children are as cooperative or as motivated to learn to control headache. Engaging these children in treatment is often difficult. They may not share the same concern that their parents do regarding the severity of their headache and do not see the need for treatment. Some never overcome their initial feeling that the treatment is silly or could not possibly work. The presence of significant emotional disturbance or family problems usually results in less than adequate cooperation with treatment recommendations. Also quite difficult are those children (along with their parents) who view "biofeedback" as a means to effect a quick cure and are disappointed to learn that treatment requires weeks of participation, data collection, skills acquisition, and behavior change; and that most probably a gradual reduction in headache will occur. Nevertheless, with education, additional clinical intervention, or the continued encouragement of the referring physician, many of these children can be effectively treated. Treatment is usually longer (8 to 12 sessions), and procedures to increase cooperation with treatment recommendations are usually needed to be successful.

Biofeedback and relaxation training continue to be employed in the treatment of migraine for the simple reason that they are effective treatments for a considerable number of children. There are no known side effects to either procedure and both have the advantage of being short-term treatments. Some progress has been made in the search for understanding how and why these procedures are effective, what their limitations are, and who is likely to benefit most from them. Our understanding is far from complete, however, despite burgeoning literature, because the more critical research efforts lie ahead (Blanchard & Andrasik, 1982).

CHRONIC PAIN ASSOCIATED WITH A BURN INJURY

An important consideration of the following case study was the rationale developed for the treatment program, which was essential in presenting the behavioral program to the medical and professional staff managing the child and enlisting their cooperation in implementing the program. The treatment rationale entailed the proposition that attending to pain complaints in attempts to comfort the child may not always be in the child's long-term best interest, but that demonstrations of affection, concern, and comfort may be rearranged to maximize rehabilitation and improve the child's psychological status by increasing the probability of "well" behaviors. Thus, the study was designed to test empirically the observation that pediatric chronic pain behaviors may be influenced by the child's social environment. The objectives of the investigation were to: (a) identify the influences of adult attention and demand situations on the emission of chronic pain behaviors, (b) devise a treatment strategy useful in decreasing chronic pain behaviors and increasing the child's rehabilitative or "well" behaviors, and (c) assess the practical efficacy of the procedures by training the nursing staff and the physical therapist to carry on the behavioral treatment.

Case Study: A 3-year-old Child With Burn Injury

The patient was a 3-year-old child who had been hospitalized for 10 months for the treatment of second and third degree burns to her buttocks, legs, and perineum as the result of immersion in hot water, with the circumstances surrounding the burn incident indicating the possibility of child abuse (Varni, Bessman, Russo, & Cataldo, 1980). The child's development had been normal previous to the injury; afterward, however, skills were lost and further development was slightly delayed. Secondary complications to the burn condition included heart murmur, sepsis, and ulcerative lesions that required extensive intravenous therapy. Scar contractures and subsequent decreased range of motion in both knees made it necessary for the child to wear Jobst stockings and knee-extension splints to prevent contractures while undergoing a series of operations for plastic surgery.

At the time of the initiation of the behavioral program, the child was exhibiting an array of chronic pain behaviors that interfered significantly with her rehabilitation and with constructive patient-caregiver interactions. Furthermore, these pain responses appeared to increase in both intensity and frequency in attention-seeking and demand-avoidance situations. Data were obtained in three different settings: (a) clinic room where the child wore the knee extension splints in a contrived setting, (b) bedroom where the child wore the splints in the natural hospital environment, and (c) physical therapy situation during which the physical therapist focused on improved range of motion and independent ambulation.

Three categories of chronic pain behaviors were recorded: (a) crying, which ranged in intensity from sobbing to screaming; (b) verbal pain behaviors, which consisted of such statements as "My leg/ankle/foot/stomach hurts," "Ouch," or "I can't stand up"; and (c) nonverbal pain behaviors consisting of any gestural response expressing pain or discomfort such as facial grimaces, rubbing her legs or buttocks, or not standing. In addition, a rehabilitative activity measure, number of steps descended, was measured in physical therapy, because it was essential for improving the child's range of motion and independent ambulation.

During the baseline assessment, it became evident that the child's pain behaviors were a function of adult attention and demand situations. (See Figures 11.1 and 11.2.) In the absence of adult presence, chronic pain behaviors were noticeably infrequent. In fact, the data for crying in the clinic no-adult-present condition are very similar to those that occur during programmed extinction; that is, the behavior initially occurred at a very high rate, gradually decreased, increased

to a high rate, and then decreased to 0% for the majority of the remaining sessions. Perhaps more importantly, it was observed that when the child was engaged in interesting activities with accompanying staff attention for these appropriate behaviors, pain complaints were reciprocally low.

Specifically, two types of baseline sessions were conducted in the clinic. In one, an adult was present in the room with the child and interacted with her. These baseline sessions were arranged so as to be analogous to the contingencies occurring during the patient's naptime in her bedroom, which had been identified by the nursing staff as a time of high-frequency pain occurrence. Thus, the adult's attention in this condition was contingent upon the occurrence of the patient's pain behaviors. In the clinic, the adult attended to the child's pain responses saying, "I'm sorry it hurts. Show me where it hurts," and other such comforting statements. In the other type of baseline sessions, no adult was present with the child. At the beginning of this condition, the adult would leave the room, saying, "I'll be back in a few minutes. Why don't you rest awhile?" The child would then remain alone in the room for 5 minutes.

During baseline sessions in the child's bedroom just prior to naptime, no instructions were given to the nursing staff except that they should put on the patient's knee extension splints in the usual manner and place the patient in her crib. Baseline sessions in the physical therapy setting during the demand condition consisted of placing the child on a small four-step wooden staircase asking her to descend the steps. If she did not respond, the child was prompted with such statements as, "It's time to start down the steps. Come on now." If she refused to stand by herself, the therapist helped her up and continued to encourage her. In the no-demand condition, the therapist simply played with the child with her favorite toy.

Since the baseline assessment demonstrated that the chronic pain behaviors were influenced by socioenvironmental factors, treatment focused on rearranging the existing

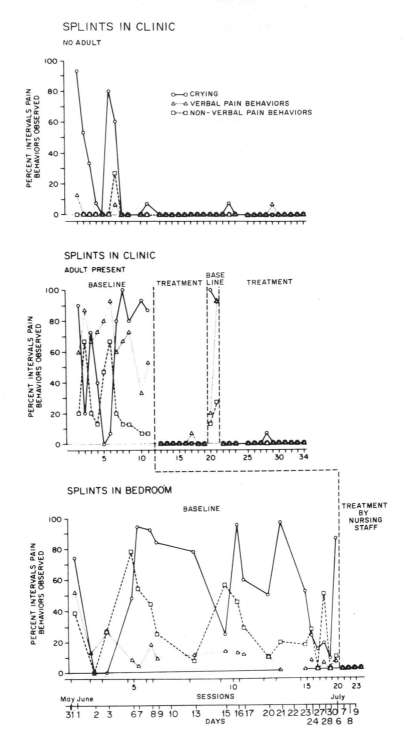

Figure 11.1. Percent of Observation Intervals in which Chronic Pain Behaviors Were Noted in Each of Three Situations. From "Behavioral management of chronic pain in children" by J.W. Varni, C.A. Bessman, D.C. Russo, and M.F. Cataldo, 1980, *Archives of Physical Medicine and Rehabilitation*, *61*, p. 377. Reprinted by permission.

STEPS IN PHYSICAL THERAPY

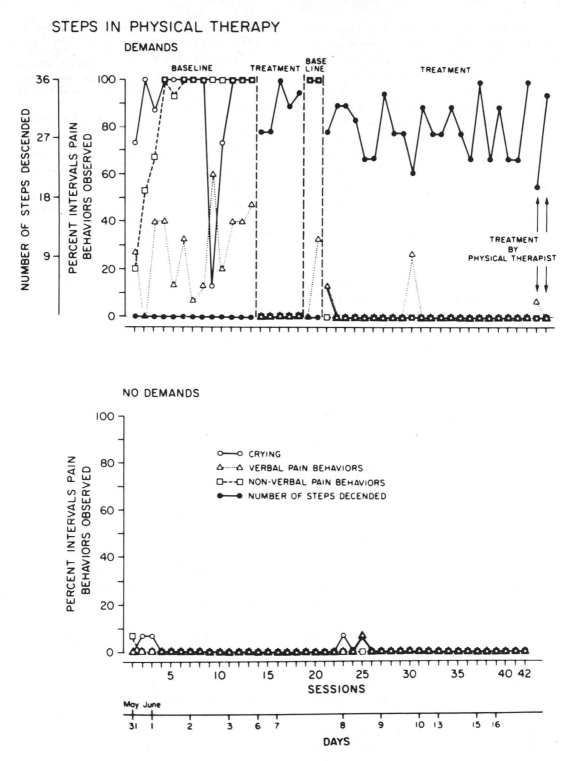

Figure 11.2. Number of Steps Descended and Percent of Observation Intervals in which Chronic Pain Behaviors Were Noted. From "Behavioral management of chronic pain in children" by J.W. Varni, C.A. Bessman, D.C. Russo, and M.F. Cataldo, 1980, *Archives of Physical Medicine and Rehabilitation*, *61*, p. 377. Reprinted by permission.

contingencies. A combination of an intrasubject multiple-baseline design across settings and a reversal design was employed to determine the functional effects of the behavioral program on the patient's pain behaviors. Multiple baselines were begun simultaneously in all three settings, with treatment implemented first in the physical therapy department, while baseline assessment continued in the clinic and bedroom. Shortly afterward, treatment began in the clinic setting and subsequently in the bedroom. Brief reversals back to baseline conditions were conducted in the clinic and physical therapy setting to further test the significance of the intervention.

In the clinic, treatment began with the adult verbalizing the following contingency to the child: "I'm going to put your splints on. If you don't cry, we can play for a while and I'll give you some ice cream (cookies, etc.)." At the end of each minute in which no pain behaviors occurred, the adult reinforced the child with praise and a treat. Throughout the session, praise was given for periods of such "well" behaviors as helping to put on the splints, positive verbalizations, smiling, and the like, as well as the lack of pain behaviors (DRO schedule). Emission of pain behavior was placed on extinction (ignored), while the schedule of reinforcement was gradually changed so that the treat was offered at the end of the 5-minute session if no pain responses had been observed during that period (DRL schedule).

At the beginning of treatment in the bedroom, the nursing staff was instructed to verbalize the contingency, "If you don't cry while I put your splints on, you can have some ice cream (cookies, etc.) when I'm finished." The nurse then placed the splints on the child while giving praise for "well" behaviors, such as, "You're being so good. What a big girl you are. Don't you look so nice." After the splints were secured, the nurse verbalized a secondary contingency: "If you don' cry during naptime, when you wake up you can have some more ice cream." The nurse then returned to her other duties, periodically

checking for the emission of pain behaviors. At the end of the hour-long naptime, the nurse returned, praised the child, and gave her a treat if no pain behaviors had occurred. Any pain responses made during naptime were ignored by the nursing staff, and no reinforcers were provided at the end of the hour.

Finally, the treatment in physical therapy began with the therapist verbalizing the contingency to the child, "I want you to go down the steps by yourself. If you do, I'll give you an M&M." Praise was given continuously for each step taken, and any instance of pain behavior was ignored. The schedule of reinforcement was gradually changed so that the child was reinforced with a treat for descending the entire four-step sequence every third time, while social reinforcement continued on a continuous schedule.

The objective data on chronic pain and rehabilitative behaviors obtained throughout baseline and treatment conditions demonstrated the therapeutic effectiveness of the behavioral program (Figures 11.1 and 11.2). In addition, other clinically significant changes were observed. At the beginning of the study, the child's behaviors had severely disrupted her physical as well as emotional rehabilitation. Physical therapy was essentially terminated because of the patient's interfering pain behaviors. Two patterns emerged in her bedroom when the patient was placed in her crib with the knee extension splints on. First, the child would struggle until she had removed the splints, resulting in further contractures and the need for additional plastic surgery. Second, if she failed to remove the splints, her crying would intensify to the point of screaming. At times she would fall asleep exhausted and continue sobbing well into the naptime hour. Other times, she would continue screaming until the nursing staff removed her to a separate room for the remainder of the hour in consideration of the other children. Thus, pain behaviors during the pretreatment period resulted in the child being separated from the other children, interfering with the normalization and socialization processes important for a child with a history of prolonged hospitalization and suspected previous abuse.

Following the behavioral intervention, a number of concomitant responses were noted. Whereas the child initially resisted splinting attempts, she subsequently began requesting to assist, saying for example, "I'll do it. I want to help you." She began to make positive statements about her accomplishments instead of statements of pain and resistance to rehabilitation. Rather than seeking attention from her caregivers for pain behaviors, there was a shift to the utilization of "well" behaviors to attract social attention and praise.

Fordyce (1976), in his extensive work with adult chronic pain, has suggested that during periods of initial trauma and its resultant pain, the patient has many opportunities for the pairing of environmental stimuli to feelings of pain. Whether or not the subjective experience of pain abates over the course of time may be independent of the pain behaviors that the patient displays. While it is not possible to determine if the patient actually feels pain or simply displays the associated behaviors, in the present case no further pain displays were observed in the treatment environments after the onset of the behavioral program. As further suggested by Fordyce (1976), through learning the patient may actually come to experience pain in certain circumstances in excess of the accompanying physical basis for such pain, or even in the absence of a physical basis for perceived pain. In such cases, or in cases like the present one in which the pain behavior served the patient's immediate needs while hindering long-term rehabilitation, the behavioral program provides an essential component in the comprehensive management of pediatric chronic pain.

In acute cases, pain is an important symptom of underlying distress, requiring sympathy, empathy, and a detailed search for the sources of the pain and appropriate therapies. Continued expression of pain in chronic cases, however, may serve as a signal to investigate more closely the conditions of the child's daily care and therapy environment. In pediatric chronic pain, therefore, attempts should be made not only to determine the possible underlying physical distress causing pain, but also the potential socioenvironmental influences on pain expression for the patient. Considerations should be given to the secondary gains of pain behavior, particularly if the result is to increase the attention of staff and to avoid rehabilitation. Such an analysis can serve as the basis for therapeutic strategies to decrease the use of pain expression as manipulative behavior.

As a cautionary note, it is essential to point out that this approach to chronic pain would not contraindicate empathy and concern expressed to the child by staff and parents, but would examine the extent of empathetic attention and its contingent relationship to chronic pain behaviors. Contingent empathy for all pain expression runs the risk of reinforcing and maintaining the pain expression to the detriment of the child. Health care staff should delineate when and where contingencies for pain behavior are in the therapeutic interests of the patient. Particular situations where pain expression occurs should result in empathy, while others should result in alternative consequences, including ignoring pain behavior and providing attention (and other reinforcers if necessary) for adhering to rehabilitation programs. Thus, as in the present case, the aim is not the total suppression of pain expression, since such communication often serves an essential personal and societal function, but rather the relatively greater expression or 'well" behaviors in those situations where chronic pain behaviors interfere with the child's long-term rehabilitation and psychosocial adjustment. Such differential expression of emotion represents both a normal and adaptive developmental process.

INVASIVE MEDICAL PROCEDURES

Invasive medical procedures constitute a significant threat to children as well as adults. Most children respond to any kind of invasive procedure with trepidation. Acute conditioned anxiety and pain responses may develop, particularly in chronically or terminally ill children who are forced to endure numerous painful procedures on a routine basis. Although injections and venipunctures are the most common procedures children must undergo, a review of the literature on psychological intervention and assessment indicates little attention has been addressed to these procedures. Instead, most of the work has been done in the area of childhood cancer.

Children with cancer, particularly leukemia, must undergo painful procedures called bone marrow aspirations (BMAs) and lumbar punctures (spinal taps). These procedures involve the insertion of a needle into the marrow of the bone or the spinal column, respectively, and fluid is withdrawn to be examined for the presence or absence of cancer cells. The procedures are painful and very anxiety-provoking; studies have indicated that distress related to BMAs and spinal taps is a virtually ubiquitous phenomenon in samples of pediatric cancer patients (Jay, Ozolins, Elliott, & Caldwell, 1983; Katz, Kellerman, & Siegel, 1980).

Since most of the work on procedure-related pain and anxiety in children has been related to bone marrow aspirations and spinal taps, this section will focus on intervention and assessment approaches developed for these particular procedures. The intervention and measurement approaches reviewed, however, are certainly applicable to other invasive procedures. For a more extensive review of other invasive medical procedures in pediatrics, see Jay (in press).

Hypnosis has been the most frequently reported intervention for acute procedure-related distress and pain in pediatric cancer patients. Hilgard and Morgan (1976) reported that formal hypnotic procedures were not effective with children under the age of 6 years who were undergoing bone marrow aspirations and lumbar punctures. Other studies, however, have reported the efficacy of hypnosis in reducing procedure-related distress of children 6 years and older (Kellerman, Zeltzer, Ellenberg, & Dash, 1983; Zeltzer & LeBaron, 1982).

Kellerman et al. (1983) reported that for 16 adolescents, hypnosis was effective in ameliorating discomfort and anxiety associated with bone marrow aspirations, spinal taps, and chemotherapeutic injections. Patients were taught an initial induction technique such as eye fixation or hand levitation. They were then given suggestions for progressive muscle relaxation, slow rhythmic breathing, and increasing sense of well-being until they were able to "visualize" or "experience" being in a "favorite" or "special" place. Once patients achieved observable deep relaxation (slow regular breathing, immobility, narrowed attention), posthypnotic suggestions for increased well-being, reduced discomfort, and greater mastery during the procedure were given. The intervention was given in a multiple-baseline design across subjects. Postintervention reductions were found in self-reported ratings of anxiety and discomfort and in trait anxiety scores.

Hilgard and LeBaron (1982) reported that hypnosis was effective in reducing self-reported pain in 27 children undergoing bone marrow aspirations. Hypnotic procedures were individualized for each child, but generally involved an induction, imaginative involvement and imagery, and posthypnotic suggestions. The authors failed to specify the age classifications of children who were treated, although there were no subjects below the age of 6 years in the study.

Case studies and nondata-based reports suggest further support for the efficacy of hypnosis in reducing treatment-related anxiety and pain in pediatric cancer patients (Ellenberg, Kellerman, Dash, Higgins, & Zeltzer, 1980; Gardner, 1976; LaBaw, Holtin, Tewell, & Eccles, 1975; Olness, 1981; Zeltzer, 1980). The major methodological shortcomings of the majority of reports on hypnosis include the following: (a) objective measures of distress, such as behavioral observations or physiological indices of distress, are rarely used as dependent measures;

(b) control groups are rarely used; and (c) hypnotic procedures are vaguely specified. Furthermore, few studies have reported the use of hypnosis for children under the age of 6 years, which is unfortunate because children under the age of 6 or 7 years have been documented as being most in need of intervention (Jay et al., 1983).

One study stands out in the hypnosis literature in that it is a controlled outcome study with objective dependent measures. Zeltzer and LeBaron (1982) compared the efficacy of hypnotic techniques with a supportive counseling and distraction intervention, using a sample of 33 cancer patients (ages 6–17 years) undergoing bone marrow aspirations and spinal taps. Patient self-reports and observer ratings were used as dependent measures. The hypnosis intervention consisted of imagery and fantasy designed according to the individual characteristics of the patient, parents, and environment. Exciting or funny stories were told to patients, with the therapist asking the child questions requiring imagination. For example, a child might be asked to "notice the elephant about to squirt water on us," and to "describe what he or she sees" (p. 1033). Patients were also helped to take deep breaths while using the imagery techniques. The nonhypnotic condition included a combination of deep breathing, distraction, and practice sessions aimed at decreasing fear. Distraction involved asking the child to focus on objects in the room rather than on fantasy. For example, a child might be asked to squeeze her mother's hands, take a few deep breaths, or count the stripes or flowers on her blouse during the needle insertion.

The results of this investigation indicated that hypnotic techniques were consistently more effective than supportive counseling, although nonhypnotic techniques were very useful for some patients. The authors proposed that the generally superior efficacy of hypnotic techniques may be due to an ability of imagery techniques to hold a child's attention longer than techniques that do not involve imagery. Gardner and Olness' (1981) book on hypnosis and hypnotherapy with

children is the most comprehensive compilation of information concerning application of hypnosis to pediatric problems and is recommended for practitioners interested in applying hypnotic techniques with children.

Jay and colleagues (Jay, Elliott, Katz, & Siegel, 1984; Jay, Elliott, Ozolins, Olson, & Pruitt, in press) developed a multicomponent cognitive-behavioral intervention "package" designed to teach effective coping skills and to reduce children's distress during bone marrow aspirations and spinal taps. The treatment package is based, in part, on a stress-inoculation model described by Meichenbaum (1976). In this stress-inoculation approach, the subject is first provided with information concerning the nature of the stressful situation. In the second phase, the subject is taught a number of coping skills or techniques, such as distraction, relaxation, altering attributions, imagery, and these coping skills are rehearsed. Finally, the subject is given the opportunity to practice his or her coping skills during exposure to relevant stressors.

The intervention package developed by Jay et al. (in press) consists of five primary components: filmed modeling, reinforcement, breathing exercises, emotive imagery/distraction, and behavioral rehearsal. The exact procedures of this intervention package will be discussed in the case illustration. Studies have suggested that this intervention package is quite effective in reducing children's distress during bone marrow aspirations and spinal taps, even for children as young as 3 years of age.

A pilot study conducted with 10 pediatric cancer patients, ages 3 to 10 years, who were referred for intense procedure-related distress, indicated dramatic postintervention decreases in behavioral distress. Preliminary results of an ongoing 3-year treatment-outcome study (1982–85) at Children's Hospital of Los Angeles also support the efficacy of the intervention package in reducing the distress of 30 leukemic patients (ages 4 to 14) undergoing bone marrow aspirations. Reductions in distress (as compared to a control condition) were observed across a variety of response systems, including behavioral distress, self-reported pain, and physiological arousal (Jay, Elliott, Katz, & Siegel, 1984a). The following case presentation illustrates the use of the cognitive-behavioral intervention package developed by Jay et al. (in press) with a pediatric cancer patient referred for procedure-related distress.

Case Study: A 7-year-old Child With Leukemia

Sharon was a 7-year-old child who was diagnosed with leukemia $3\frac{1}{2}$ years prior to the intervention and had remained in remission since diagnosis. Despite the fact that she had had numerous previous bone marrow aspirations (at least 16), she had continued to exhibit significant anxiety and fear related to the procedures prior to referral for psychological intervention. Nurses who had observed her during the procedures noted her as needing intervention for her procedure-related distress, and she was referred to the ongoing treatment outcome study at Children's Hospital of Los Angeles.

Sharon was entered on the intervention study which is designed to evaluate the efficacy of (a) cognitive-behavioral techniques and (b) Valium as compared to (c) a minimal-treatment control condition. The design of the study was a counterbalance design (every patient receives all three intervention conditions in a randomized sequence), and Sharon was randomly assigned to the following sequence of intervention: control condition, Valium condition, and cognitive-behavior therapy condition. She received these interventions 3 months apart on consecutive bone marrow aspiration procedures. The procedures for each intervention condition are as follows:

Minimal Treatment Attention Control. In this condition, Sharon was shown cartoons 30 minutes prior to the bone marrow aspiration.

Valium Condition. For her next bone marrow aspiration 3 months later, Sharon was ad-ministered 0.3 mg/kg of oral Valium 30 minutes prior to her bone marrow aspiration.

Cognitive-Behavioral Condition. For her next bone marrow aspiration 3 months later, Sharon received the cognitive-behavioral intervention package 30 minutes prior to the procedure. This package involved the five components described in the following paragraphs:

1. *Filmed Modeling.* Sharon was first shown a 12-minute video presentation entitled "Getting Bone Marrows and Spinal Taps: A Child's View".[1] This videotape is about a 6-year-old leukemic patient, Danielle, who comes to the oncology clinic for her routine bone marrow aspiration and spinal tap. Danielle describes her thoughts and feelings and models positive coping behaviors throughout the procedures. The film is based on a "coping" rather than a "mastery" model, since coping models have been found to facilitate identification with the model more easily and have been more effective in reducing anxiety (Meichenbaum, 1975). As a "coping" model, Danielle admits she is scared about the procedures, exhibits some signs of distress, but then copes effectively with the stressor. The film is also intended to provide information as the model explains *why* she has to have the procedures and illustrates *what* happens at each point in the procedures. The film shows the model going through a treatment session with the psychologist (practicing her breathing, role-playing, etc.), the rationale being that modeling of the intervention process might also facilitate response to the intervention.

2. *Breathing Exercises.* After viewing the film, Sharon was taught a simple breathing exercise which provided her with an active attention-diversion strategy to use during the procedure. She was taught to "pump herself up like a big tire and then let the air out very slowly, making a hissing sound." This tech-

---

[1]Videotapes for filmed modeling purposes for children ages 4 to 14 are available for rental or purchase. For further information, write Susan Jay, PhD, Psychosocial Program, Hematology-Oncology, Children's Hospital of Los Angeles, 4650 Sunset Blvd., Los Angeles, CA 90027.

nique was practiced with Sharon until she demonstrated it with ease.

3. *Positive Reinforcement*. Sharon was shown a small trophy and was told that trophies are given to children who "do the very best that they can" during the medical procedures. To obtain the trophy, Sharon was encouraged to lie still during the procedure and do the breathing exercises she was taught. These contingencies were based upon two rationales: (a) lying still makes it much easier for the nurse/physician to conduct the procedures as quickly as possible without complications and (b) the breathing exercises distract the child and generally preclude severe behavioral distress (screaming, kicking, and fighting).

4. *Imagery*. "Emotive" imagery was used with Sharon as a cognitive coping strategy. Sharon was asked about her favorite super-hero who turned out to be Wonderwoman. The psychologist and Sharon then discussed how Sharon could use her imagination about Wonderwoman to help her with the bone marrow aspiration and spinal tap. For example, they discussed the following scenario:

> Wonderwoman invited Sharon to be on her Superpower Team and Wonderwoman gave Sharon special powers, which made her very strong and tough so that she could stand almost anything. Wonderwoman asked Sharon to take some tests to try out these superpowers. These tests were called bone marrow aspirations. These tests hurt, but with her new superpowers, she could take deep breaths and could lie very still and then it would be over soon.

The psychologists also discussed with Sharon another technique, that of pretending to be in a favorite, fun place. Sharon was given a choice of which imagery technique she thought would be most helpful to her, and during the procedure the psychologist cued her and reminded her of the agreed-upon imagery.

5. *Behavioral Rehearsal*. During the behavioral rehearsal, the procedure was practiced twice with Sharon. First, Sharon was allowed to play doctor and to give a doll the bone marrow aspiration or spinal tap with real medical equipment. As Sharon administered the procedure, the doll was coached to stay still and do her breathing exercises. Then, the psychologist had the child practice actually undergoing the procedure. The child was coached to lie still and to do the breathing exercises while the psychologist pretended to administer the procedure. The psychologist accompanied Sharon into the treatment room and reminded her to do her breathing exercises and imagery-distraction during the bone marrow aspiration. After the procedure, Sharon received the trophy and was very pleased with herself.

Sharon's level of procedure-related distress was measured via three response systems: self-report, behavioral, and physiological. She was asked, after the procedure, to rate "how much the bone marrow hurt" on a Pain Thermometer (0 to 100). An observer coded her behavior prior to and during the procedure using the Observation Scale of Behavioral Distress (OSBD) (Jay et al, 1983; Jay & Elliott, 1984).[2] Sharon's blood pressure and heart rate were taken upon arrival in the clinic, just before the bone marrow, and after the bone marrow. Nurse ratings of observed distress were also obtained.

Figure 11.3 illustrates Sharon's behavioral, physiological, and affective responses to each of the intervention conditions. As indicated, Sharon's behavioral distress was markedly less when she received the behavior therapy intervention as compared to the control and Valium conditions. Nurse ratings were consistent with observer scores except for the Valium condition. The fact that the nurse rated her behavioral distress lower may reflect an expectancy effect since nurses are always aware when Valium is administered, but they are usually blind to the other two intervention conditions. Sharon's self-reported pain scores are the most dramatic indication of the efficacy of behavior therapy for her as

[2]The OSBD and information concerning development, scoring, reliability, and validity can be obtained from the author: Susan Jay, PhD, Psychosocial Program, Hematology-Oncology, Childrens Hospital of Los Angeles, 4650 Sunset Boulevard, Los Angeles, CA 90027.

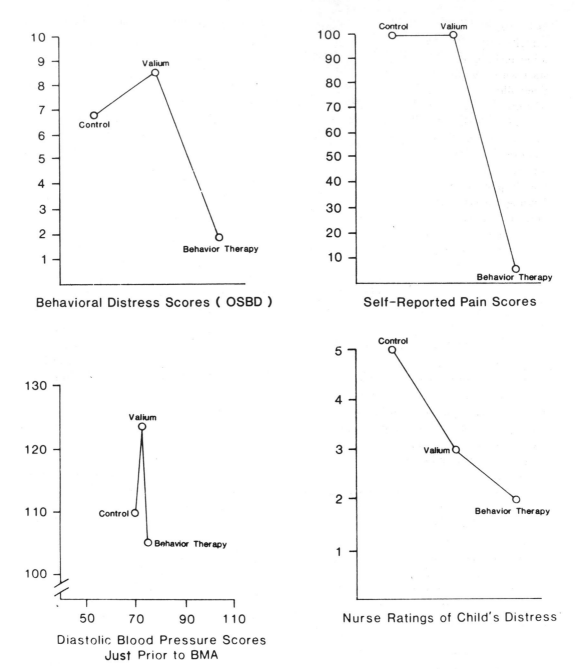

Figure 11.3. Dependent Scores According to Intervention Condition.

compared to the other conditions. During the control and Valium conditions, she rated her pain at the top of the Pain Thermometer (100 – "the most it could possibly hurt"), whereas after the behavior therapy interven-tion she rated her pain as "5" on a 0 to 100 scale. Finally, Sharon's blood pressure scores were lowest after receiving behavior therapy, although the differences are minimal when compared to the control condition.

For this particular child, behavior therapy appeared to be most effective in reducing behavioral distress and self-reported pain during bone marrow aspirations. She reported that, of the components in the intervention package, the breathing exercises and the trophy helped her the most. Her father reported that Sharon coped "the best she ever had" in her $3\frac{1}{2}$ years of treatment for leukemia. Furthermore, the behavior therapy intervention program provided her with coping skills that she could use during future procedures.

Individual children differ in the type of intervention that they find most helpful. Research on individual coping styles suggests that some children benefit from prior information and preparation whereas others might find less informative approaches, such as medication-sedation, more helpful (Jay, in press). Preliminary data from 30 subjects who completed the aforementioned treatment outcome study indicated that both Valium and behavior therapy were more effective in reducing distress than the minimal treatment control condition (Jay et al., 1984b). Further research must be conducted in order to determine what type of intervention is most effective for individual children with varying styles of coping, so that optimal intervention programs are developed for each child.

CONCLUSION

As suggested by the case studies in this chapter, the potential of cognitive-behavioral assessment and management techniques in making a significant clinical contribution to pediatric pain comprehensive care appears to be as great as that experienced during the past 15 years for adult chronic pain management. What clearly needs to be avoided, however, is the mere application of techniques developed for adult patients. Children are not "little adults," and as such, more clinical research into children's cognitive-developmental stages and their conceptualizations of pain and discomfort must be conducted to ensure that assessment and management techniques are utilized appropriately. Thus, research

and clinical practice in pediatric pain must assume a separate, if not parallel, status from the adult pain field. The development of interdisciplinary pediatric pain clinics is an example of such a parallel development. While advances in adult pain management will continue to provide useful information, advances in pediatric pain assessment and management will depend on clinical research sensitive to the unique characteristics of children.

REFERENCES

Abu-Saad, H. (1984). Assessing children's responses to pain. *Pain, 19*, 163–171.

Andrasik, F., Blanchard, E.B., Edlund, S.R., & Rosenblum, E.L. (1983). Autogenic feedback in the treatment of two children with migraine headache. *Child & Family Behavior Therapy, 4*, 13–23.

Artman, M., Grayson, M., & Boerth, R.C. (1982). Propranolol in children: Safety-toxicity. *Pediatrics, 70*, 30–31.

Barlow, C.H. (in press). *Migraine and other headaches in childhood.* London: Spastics International.

Beales, J.G. (1982). The assessment and management of pain in children. In P. Karoly, J.J. Steffen, & D.J. O'Grady (Eds.), *Child health psychology: Concepts and issues* (pp. 154–179). New York: Pergamon Press.

Benson, H. (1975). *The relaxation response.* New York: William Morrow.

Bibace, R., & Walsh, M.E. (1982). Children's conceptions of illness. In R. Bibace & M.E. Walsh (Eds.), *Children's conceptions of health, illness and bodily functions* (pp. 31–48). San Francisco: Jossey-Bass.

Bille, B. (1981). Migraine in childhood and its prognosis. *Cephalalgia, 1*, 71–75.

Bille, B.S. (1962). Migraine in school children. *Acta Pediatrics Scandanavia, 51* (Suppl), 1–151.

Blanchard, E.B., & Andrasik, F. (1982). Psychological assessment and treatment of headache: Recent developments and emerging issues. *Journal of Consulting and Clinical Psychology, 50*, 859–879.

Blanchard, E.B., Andrasik, F., Ahles, T.A., Teders, S.J., & O'Keefe, D. (1980). Migraine and tension headache: A meta-analytic review. *Behavior Therapy, 11*, 613–631.

Bonica, J.J. (1977). Neurophysiologic and pathologic aspects of acute and chronic pain. *Archives of Surgery, 112*, 750–761.

Brewster, A.B. (1982). Chronically ill hospitalized children's concepts of their illness. *Pediatrics, 69*, 355–362.

Dalessio, D.J., Kunzel, M., Sternbach, R., & Sorak, M. (1979). Conditioned adaptation-relaxation in migraine therapy. *Journal of American Medical Association, 242*, 2102–2104.

Dietrich, S.L. (1976). Medical management of hemophilia. In D.C. Boone (Ed.), *Comprehensive management of hemophilia*. Philadelphia: F.A. Davis.

Eland, J.M. (1981). Minimizing pain associated with prekindergarten intramuscular injections. *Issues in Comprehensive Pediatric Nursing, 5*, 361–372.

Ellenberg, L., Kellerman, J., Dash, J., Higgins, J., & Zeltzer, L. (1980). Use of hypnosis for multiple symptoms in an adolescent girl with leukemia. *Journal of Adolescent Health Care, 1*, 132–136.

Feldman, W.S., & Varni, J.W. (1985). Conceptualizations of health and illness by children with spina bifida. *Children's Health Care, 13*, 102–108.

Fentress, D.W., Masek, B.J., Mehegan, J.E., & Benson, H. (1984). *Behavioral treatment of childhood migraine*. Unpublished manuscript.

Fordyce, W.E. *Behavioral methods for chronic pain and illness*. St. Louis: Mosby, 1976.

Garden, G.G. (1976). Childhood, death, and human dignity: Hypnosis for David. *International Journal of Clinical and Experimental Hypnosis, 24*, 122.

Gardner, G.G., & Olness, K. (1981). *Hypnosis and hypnotherapy with children*. New York: Grune & Stratton. 1981.

Gildea, J.H. & Quirk, T.R. (1977). Assessing the pain experience in children. *Nursing Clinics of North America, 12*, 631–637.

Hassett, J. (1978). *A primer of psychophysiology*. San Francisco: W.H. Freeman.

Hilgard, E.R. (1975). The alleviation of pain by hypnosis. *Pain, 1*, 213–231.

Hilgard, J.R., & LeBaron, S. (1982). Relief of anxiety and pain in children and adolescents with cancer: Quantitative measures and clinical observations. *International Journal of Clinical and Experimental Hypnosis, 30*, 417–442.

Hilgard, J.R. & Morgan, A.H. (1976). *Treatment of anxiety and pain in childhood cancer through hypnosis*. Paper presented to the 7th International Congress of Hypnosis and Psychosomatic Medicine, Philadelphia.

Hoffman, J.W., Benson, H., Arns, P.A., et al. (1982). Reduced sympathetic nervous system responsivity associated with the relaxation response. *Science, 215*, 190–192.

Houts, A.C. (1982). Relaxation and thermal feedback treatment of child migraine headache: A case study. *American Journal of Clinical Biofeedback, 5*, 154–157.

Jay, S.M. (in press). Invasive medical procedures. In D. Routh (Ed.), *Handbook of pediatric psychology*. New York: Guilford.

Jay, S.M., & Elliott, C.M. (1980). *The observation scale of behavioral distress*. Unpublished scale.

Jay, S.M., & Elliott, C.M. (1984). Behavioral observation scales for measuring children's distress: Effects of increased methodological rigor. *Journal of Consulting and Clinical Psychology, 52*, 1106–1107.

Jay, S.M., Elliott, C.M., Katz, E.R., & Siegel, S.E. (1984a, August). *Stress reduction on children undergoing painful medical procedures*. Paper presented at American Psychological Association, Annual Convention, Toronto.

Jay, S., Elliott, C., Katz, E., & Siegel, S.E. (1984b, May). *Assessment of children's distress during painful medical procedures*. Paper presented at Society of Behavioral Medicine, Philadelphia.

Jay, S.M., Elliott, C.M., Ozolins, M., Olson, R., & Pruitt, S. (in press). Behavioral management of children's distress during painful medical procedures. *Behaviour Research and Therapy*.

Jay, S.M., Ozolins, M., Elliott, C.M., & Caldwell, S. (1983). Assessment of children's distress during painful medical procedures. *Health Psychology, 2*, 133–147.

Johansson, J., & Ost, L. (1982). Self-control procedures in biofeedback: A review of temperature biofeedback in the treatment of migraine. *Biofeedback and Self-regulation, 7*, 437–442.

Katz, E.R., Kellerman, J., & Siegel, S.E. (1980). Behavioral distress in children with cancer undergoing medical procedures: Developmental considerations. *Journal of Consulting and Clinical Psychology, 48*, 356–365.

Katz, E.R., Kellerman, J., & Siegel, S.E. (1981). Anxiety as an affective focus in the clinical study of acute behavioral distress: A reply to Shacham and Daut. *Journal of Consulting and Clinical Psychology, 49*(3), 470–471.

Katz, E.R., Varni, J.W., & Jay, S.M. (1984). Behavioral assessment and management of pediatric pain. In M. Hersen, R.M. Esler, & P.M. Miller (Eds.), *Progress in behavior modification* (Vol. 18). Orlando, FL: Academic Press.

Kellerman, J., Zeltzer, L., Ellenberg, L., & Dash, J. (1983). Adolescents with cancer: Hypnosis for the reduction of the acute pain and anxiety associated with medical procedures. *Journal of Adolescent Health Care, 4*, 85–90.

Labbe, E.E., & Williamson, D. A. (1983). Temperature biofeedback in the treatment of children with migraine headaches. *Journal of Pediatric Psychology, 8*, 317–326.

LaBaw, W., Holton, C., Jewell, K., & Eccles, D. (1975). The use of self-hypnosis by children with cancer. *American Journal of Clinical Hypnosis, 17*, 233–238.

Masek, B.J., Russo, D.C., & Varni, J.W. (1984). Behavioral approaches to the management of chronic pain in children. *Pediatric Clinics of North America, 31*, 1113–1131.

Masek, B.J., Spirito, A., & Fentress, D.W. (1984). Behavioral treatment of symptoms of childhood illness. *Clinical Psychology Review, 4*, 561–570.

Mehegan, J.E., Masek, B.J., Harrison, R.H., Russo, D.C., & Leviton, A. (1984). *Behavioral medicine treatment of pediatric migraine.* Unpublished manuscript.

Meichenbaum, D. (1976). A self-instructional approach to stress management. A proposal for stress inoculation training. In C. Spielberger & I. Sarason (Eds.), *Stress and anxiety in modern life.* New York: Winston and Sons.

Melzack, R. (1975). The McGill Pain Questionnaire: Major properties and scoring methods. *Pain, 1*, 277–299.

Newburger, P.E., & Sallan, S.E. (1981). Chronic pain: Principles of management. *Journal of Pediatrics, 98*, 180–189.

Olness, K. (1981). Imagery (self-hypnosis) as adjunct therapy in childhood cancer. *American Journal of Pediatric Hematology/Oncology, 3*, 313–321.

Olness, K., & MacDonald, J. (1981). Self-hypnosis and biofeedback in the management of juvenile migraine. *Journal of Developmental and Behavioral Pediatrics, 2*, 168-170.

Olton, D.S., & Noonberg, A.R. (1980). *Biofeedback: Clinical applications in behavioral medicine.* Englewood Cliffs, NJ: Prentice-Hall.

Perrin, E.C., & Gerrity, P.S. (1981). There's a demon in your belly: Children's understanding of illness. *Pediatrics, 67*, 841–849.

Perrin, E.C., & Perrin, J.M. (1983). Clinician's assessments of childrens' understanding of illness. *American Journal of Diseases of Children, 137*, 874–878.

Pikoff, H. (1984),. Is the muscular model of headache still viable? A review of conflicting data. *Headache, 24*, 186–198.

Prensky, A.L. & Sommers, D. (1979). Diagnosis and treatment of migraine in children. *Neurology, 29*, 506–510.

Ramsden, R., Friedman, B., & Williamson, D. (1983). Treatment of childhood headache reports with contingency management procedures. *Journal of Clinical Child Psychology, 12*, 202–206.

Schechter, N.L. (1984). Recurrent pains in children: An overview and an approach. *Pediatric Clinics of North America, 31*, 949–968.

Shinnar, S., & D'Souza, B.U. (1981). The diagnosis and management of headaches in childhood. *Pediatric Clinics of North America, 29*, 79–94.

Sillanpaa, M. (1976). Prevalence of migraine and other headache in Finnish children starting school. *Headache, 15*, 288–290.

Sokoloff, L. (1975). Biochemical and physiological aspects of degenerative joint diseases with special reference to hemophilic arthropathy. *Annals of New York Academy of Science, 240*, 285–290.

Steward, R., & Regalbuto, G. (1975). Do doctors know what children know? *American Journal of Orthopsychiatry, 45*, 146–149.

Stewart, M.L. (1977). Measurement of clinical pain. In A. Jacox (Ed.), *Pain: A sourcebook for nurses and other health professionals* (pp. 107–137). Boston, MA: Little, Brown.

Thompson, K.L., & Varni, J.W. (in press). A developmental cognitive-biobehavioral model for pediatric pain assessment. *Pain.*

Thompson, K.L., Varni, J.W., & Hanson, V. (1985). *Comprehensive assessment of chronic musculoskeletal pain in juvenile rheumatoid arthritis.* Unpublished manuscript.

Varni, J.W. (1981a). Behavioral medicine in hemophilia arthritic pain management. *Archives of Physical Medicine and Rehabilitation, 62*, 183–187.

Varni, J.W. (1981b). Self-regulation techniques in the management of chronic arthritic pain in hemophilia. *Behavior Therapy, 12*, 185–194.

Varni, J.W. (1983). *Clinical behavioral pediatrics: An interdisciplinary biobehavioral approach.* New York: Pergamon Press.

Varni, J.W., Bessman, C.A., Russo, D.C., & Cataldo, M.F. (1980). Behavioral management of chronic pain in children. *Archives of Physical Medicine and Rehabilitation, 61*, 375–379.

Varni, J.W., & Gilbert, A. (1982). Self-regulation of chronic arthritic pain and long-term analgesic dependence in a hemophiliac. *Rheumatology and Rehabilitation, 22*, 171–174.

Varni, J.W., Gilbert, A., & Dietrich, S.L. (1981). Behavioral medicine in pain and analgesia management for the hemophilic child with factor VIII inhibitor. *Pain, 11*, 121–126.

Varni, J.W., & Jay, S.M. (1984). Biobehavioral factors in juvenile rheumatoid arthritis: Implications for research and practice. *Clinical Psychology Review, 4*, 543–560.

Varni, J.W., Katz, E.R., & Dash, J. (1982). Behavioral and neurochemical aspects of pediatric pain. In D.C. Russo & J.W. Varni (Eds.), *Behavioral pediatrics: Research and practice* (pp. 177–224). New York: Plenum Press.

Varni, J.W., & Thompson, K. L. (1985). *The Varni/Thompson Pediatric Pain Questionnaire.* Unpublished manuscript.

Varni, J.W., & Thompson, K.L. (in press). Biobehavioral assessment and management of pediatric pain. In N.A. Krasnegor, J.D. Arasteh, & M.F. Cataldo (Eds.), *Child health behavior.* New York: Wiley.

Waranch, H.R., & Keenan, D.M. (in press). Behavioral treatment of children with recurrent headaches: A report of clinical outcomes. *Journal of Behavior Therapy and Experimental Psychiatry.*

Werder, D.S., & Sargent, J.D. (1984). A study of childhood headache using biofeedback as a treatment alternative. *Headache, 24,* 122–126.

Whitt, J.K., Dykstra, W., & Taylor, C.A. (1979). Children's conception of illness and cognitive development. Implications for pediatric practitioners. *Clinical Pediatrics, 18,* 327–335.

Zeltzer, L. (1980). The adolescent with cancer. In J. Kellerman. (Ed.), *Psychological aspects of cancer in children.* Springfield, IL.: C.C. Thomas.

Zeltzer, L., & LeBaron, S. (1982). Hypnosis and nonhypnotic techniques for reduction of pain and anxiety during painful procedures in children and adolescents with cancer. *Journal of Pediatrics, 101,* 1032–1035.

12 BEHAVIORAL CONTROL OF CANCER PAIN*

Charles S. Cleeland
Blake H. Tearnan

The use of suggestion, support, distraction, and exhortation as methods of helping the cancer patient cope with pain is no doubt as old as history and certainly antedates the use of opium and other analgesics. While hypnosis has been the prototypic behavioral method for reducing pain due to cancer, newer techniques such as biofeedback, relaxation, and variants of cognitive control have been advocated more recently in the management of pain due to a variety of diseases, including cancer. This advocacy has been supported by accumulating laboratory and clinical-outcome research that suggests the effectiveness of these techniques for pain reduction.

Pain caused by cancer and its treatment has been designated a national health problem of the first priority (National Institute of Health, 1979). It has been estimated that hundreds of thousands are affected nationally, and, by extension, millions worldwide. Most of us think of cancer as a very painful disease, and survey data suggests that a significant minority of the public report that they would

*The preparation of this chapter was supported by grant CA26582 from the National Cancer Institute and by a grant from the Robert Wood Johnson Foundation's program "New Applications in Medical Practice."

delay or avoid treatment for cancer because of the expected pain (Levin, Cleeland, & Dar, 1985). A majority of persons surveyed think that persistent cancer pain would be a sufficient reason to discontinue cancer treatment or even to actively end one's life. Depending on the type of cancer, as many as one third of patients with metastatic cancer will report pain at a level of severity that interferes with their social and physical activity and enjoyment of life (Daut & Cleeland, 1982). In the terminal stages of most cancers, the majority of patients will report significant pain. Pain can interfere with sleep, appetite, and physical exercise, producing adverse effects on health status. On the other hand, reduction in pain is associated with improvement in appetite and activity (Cleeland, 1984).

Comprehensive medical management of pain can often dramatically reduce the suffering experienced by cancer patients. The integration of systemic analgesics, anti-inflammatory drugs, antidepressant medications, palliative radiotherapy and chemotherapy, and destruction of pain pathways by surgery and destructive nerve blocks can often provide significant pain relief. The expertise necessary for this type of pain management, however, is rarely available outside of comprehensive cancer centers. The majority of patients with cancer pain are managed with systemic analgesics alone. Unfortunately, our data indicate that only about 50% of patients report good to excellent relief from these medications (Cleeland, 1984).

The behavioral management of cancer pain might provide relief for patients not responding favorably to traditional medical management or to comprehensive medical pain treatment. This approach has several desirable features: It has few known side effects, it can be applied to several areas of patient distress, and it can be taught by persons from a wide variety of professional backgrounds who have secured the proper training. If behavioral techniques could produce even a modest reduction in the pain experienced by cancer patients, the aggregate effect would be enormously valuable.

BACKGROUND

The behavioral clinician working with cancer pain needs to have some understanding of cancer, the physical basis of pain caused by cancer, and the impact of pain on the cancer patient. The assumptions and goals of behavioral therapy for cancer also need to be reviewed in light of the specific requirements of cancer patients. Cancer is a generic term that is applied to a variety of different diseases that have as their common basis distortion of cell development leading to invasion and metastases. The primary site of cancer dictates many of its features including rate of development, response to anticancer therapies, metastatic spread of disease, and the course, severity, and quality of pain.

In contrast to other painful conditions, pain in cancer can be due to diverse causes because of its multiple primary and metastatic sites. Of hospitalized patients who have pain, Foley (1979) reported that 78% of cancer patients in one study had pain due to direct tumor involvement, with 50% due to bone disease, 25% due to nerve compression, and 3% due to invasion of hollow viscus. Challenging a widely held notion, she found

only 19% had post-therapy pain. We have reported very similar results in patients with advanced cancer (Schwettmann, Shacham, & Cleeland, 1983), with the additional finding that the majority of patients had multiple mechanisms for their pain. Pain due to nerve involvement is often similar in characteristic and distribution to other types of nerve-related pain that may be seen in a multidisciplinary pain clinic. Treatment-related pain may resemble the neuropathic pain associated with diabetes or the diffuse muscle-type pain sometimes called myofascial. Pain caused by invasion of bone shows less in common with the noncancerous pain syndromes more familiar to behavioral clinicians. It is often described by patients as severe and throbbing in character. Unfortunately, pain due to this most-common cancer pain mechanism appears the most difficult to treat, even with multimodal medical pain therapy.

While pain can signal the presence of malignant growth to the patient, it is rarely a management problem early in the course of the disease. Immediate postoperative pain is generally well managed by systemic analgesics. Many cancers that were painless at onset, however, will have a relatively high prevalence of pain as the disease progresses. Using requirements for analgesics while hospitalized as a criterion, Foley (1984) found that 85% of patients with primary bone tumors and 52% of patients with breast cancer had pain, in contrast to 20% with lymphomas and only 5% with leukemias. Studying both inpatients and outpatients with cancer, we found that only 6% of patients with nonmetastatic, but fully 33% of patients with metastatic, disease had pain due to their cancer (Daut & Cleeland, 1982). Additional patients will have pain due to treatment-related causes.

Many health care providers share with the general public the view that cancer pain is very severe. Our survey data indicate that the public thinks of cancer as extremely painful, causing pain of a severity equal to that of a myocardial infarction (Levin et al., 1985). Many terminal patients experience severe pain, but the pain reported by the majority of patients, even those with advanced disease, is more moderate in severity. The majority of patients surveyed rate their pain at its worst close to the midpoint or lower on conventional pain ratings scales (Daut & Cleeland, 1982). Comparing the severity of pain across different diseases, patients with metastatic cancer rated their worst pain at about the same level as patients with rheumatoid arthritis. Both the cancer and arthritis groups rated their worst pain at a significantly lower level than patients with chronic, stable pain seen in a multidisciplinary pain clinic. Although most of the patients in our sample were on narcotic or nonnarcotic analgesics at the time they made their ratings, the behavioral clinician should realize that the majority of cancer patients referred for behavioral pain intervention will have pain of a severity similar to other patients they have worked with.

Those patients who have pain that is adequately controlled by analgesics with few side effects are poor candidates for behavioral treatment. Few of them are motivated to expend the time and effort to learn behavioral methods. At the other extreme, patients with severe pain will be limited in their capacity to learn new skills. The best candidates are patients with moderate pain not completely controlled by appropriately prescribed analgesics.

The behavioral clinician who is new to working with cancer patients often has his or her own doubts about the potency of behavioral treatments. These doubts are often reinforced by the skepticism of some members of the medical staff. Patients who are unaware of the potential of behavioral pain control may also question how effective self-control techniques can be against the pain caused by a powerful and fatal disease. Unfortunately, the behavioral clinician does not have a strong research base demonstrating that behavioral control is effective with cancer pain. Most of the studies that do exist report outcome data on small numbers of patients, and they lack the requisite control groups to eliminate assessment and nonspecific effects. Fortunately, there is strong evidence that behavioral control methods are effective with pain due to other clinical conditions where

both the severity of pain and the physical basis of the pain are similar.

Those who have experience working with patients who have chronic stable pain have come to expect that the typical patient with persistent pain has major life adjustment problems. Many of those patients are depressed, and it is easy to see how depressed mood may perpetuate their pain. However, a reorientation of these expectations is necessary when working with cancer patients in pain. Only a minority of them will report significantly depressed mood. In addition, relatively few patients will have operant-based pain.

We have had a major interest in investigating the relationship between pain and mood in cancer patients. In one study (Shacham, Reinhard, Raubertas, & Cleeland, 1983), patients with advanced disease and moderate to severe pain at initial contact were interviewed and completed ratings of pain severity, mood, and activity. Surviving patients completed the same scales for 5 months thereafter. The relationship between pain ratings and mood measures was examined using both individual (cross-sectional) and intra-individual (within subject) methods of correlational analyses. Both types of analyses demonstrated small but significant relationships between pain severity and measures of negative mood and inverse correlations with positive mood. A more compelling finding was that those patients with end-stage disease and poorly controlled pain reported little mood disturbance on any assessment occasion. We considered several interpretations of this finding, including artifacts of methodology, presentational style, and denial of emotional disturbance; but this finding has been robust in studies using alternative designs and examining other groups of cancer patients. For example, a composite measure of mood disturbance and both clinical and psychometric measures of depression were not predictive of cancer patients' response to medical treatment for pain (Cleeland, 1984).

The absence of significant emotional disturbance in the majority of cancer patients with pain is a distinct advantage for using behavioral pain control techniques. As a group, these patients are highly motivated to learn, practice, and accurately report whether or not the techniques are effective. Most find that success in pain reduction achieved through their own effort is highly reinforcing. The cancer patient can often feel helpless, caught between the power of the disease on one hand, and the powerful treatment forces used against the disease on the other. Self-control measures can help restore a sense of personal efficacy. Finally, behavioral treatments always remain elective. Patients have the option to terminate them at any time, which can serve to strengthen their commitment to utilize them well. Few other aspects of cancer therapy offer this option without fatal consequences.

Almost every behavioral treatment for pain control has been developed for the patient with chronic, stable pain, where there is absence of progressive disease. As we shall see, some of the features of these therapies may be helpful for the cancer patient without active disease but who now has persistent pain due to the treatment for the disease (postsurgical, postchemotherapy, or postradiation pain). The chronic pain treatment model, however, implies certain goals that do not apply, or at least have to be qualified, in the management of pain due to active cancer: (a) the reduction or elimination of the monitoring and reporting of pain, (b) an increase in physical activity, and (c) the elimination of analgesic and other palliative medications.

When pain is persistent but stable, it can be argued that the patient's continued reporting of pain to whomever will listen produces undesirable consequences including social and family alienation. It is also obvious that continual reporting of pain that is stable contributes little information that is diagnostically useful or that can serve to redirect treatment efforts. With pain due to malignancy, however, it is important to *encourage* patients to report their pain to medical staff, as well as to report the effectiveness of therapies directed at pain reduction. New pain can signal a change in disease status. Accurate reporting is also a prerequisite for adequate titration of analgesic medication.

In the presence of progressive malignant disease, encouraging increased physical activity can be counterproductive. Some patients experience pain only when active. With patients who have vertebrae compromised by metastatic disease, increased physical activity can be dangerous. When physical activity is contraindicated, the behavioral clinician may be able to suggest other activities that may serve as distractions for the patient.

The most significant difference between the management of pain of malignant disease and that of stable, non-life-threatening disease is in the use of analgesic medications, including narcotics. Elimination of analgesic medications has been advocated as an appropriate treatment goal for chronic pain patients. This goal is motivated by concern about psychological addiction, physical dependence, and the depressant and mental blurring effects of narcotics. While it is beyond the scope of this chapter to examine the use of analgesics in chronic pain, we must underline that reduction of analgesics is rarely a reasonable goal for the patient with progressive malignant disease—quite the opposite. We teach patients to recognize the role that analgesics play in pain control, and, with the cooperation of medical staff, ensure that the patient has an understanding of how to take them. We teach patients how to request needed analgesics so that they are most likely to receive them.

It is now being recognized that many cancer patients are undermedicated for pain (Bonica, 1978; Marks & Sacher, 1973). Physicians have often been reluctant to prescribe analgesics in effective doses because of concerns about addiction and the rapid development of narcotic tolerance and respiratory depression. Much of the problem of undermedication, however, has its basis in patients' beliefs and attitudes. Patients don't want to think of themselves as addicts. They may refuse to follow a medication schedule carefully designed to maintain effective blood levels of analgesics, instead taking medications only when pain is unbearable. They may not wish to report that the medications they are taking are not effective. To do so would "bother the doctor." Some patients may wish to avoid taking narcotics because to do so would be to acknowledge that their disease is beyond hope (Twycross & Lacks, 1983).

Behavioral control techniques should never be used as a substitute for appropriate analgesic management of cancer pain. Their use to ease staff's concern about narcotic addiction is rarely in the patient's best interest. If patients volunteer that they wish to reduce their analgesics after some success with behavioral control, this can be tried on an experimental basis after appropriate medical consultation.

ASSESSMENT OF THE PAIN PROBLEM

The overall aim of the behavioral assessment is to conduct a functional analysis in order to pinpoint the specific person–environment interactions and events related to the patient's pain. The clinician should be guided by his or her sensitivity to the multitude of variables that can affect the assessment process such as setting and factors that influence a patient's report of pain. The clinician also needs to have a knowledge of frequently recurring controlling variables unique to each pain problem. This is particularly important for understanding cancer vs. chronic benign pain. There are many factors unique to cancer pain that do not apply to other other pain problems.

Functional Analysis

The basis of pain assessment and treatment planning is a functional analysis. This includes a detailed evaluation of the pain complaint across cognitive, behavioral, and physiological response dimensions.

Cognitive Responses

The assessment of the patient's cognitions includes an analysis of cognitive errors and self-statements. Cognitive errors refer to maladaptive patterns of thinking that are unrealistic and distorted. They are assumed to

be causally related to the maintenance and exacerbation of the pain complaint and can interfere with treatment. Cancer pain patients can present several different types of cognitive errors, but among the most frequently observed are thoughts that they can do nothing to reduce their pain, that they should have better control over their pain problem than they do, and that pain in cancer is inevitable and should be tolerated.

Self-statements are thoughts cancer patients may have regarding their pain such as "the pain is frightening," or "it hurts so bad." Self-statements are internal dialogues patients have that reflect the cognitive appraisal of their pain state. They differ from cognitive errors in that they have not been analyzed to represent some underlying belief system or faulty logic such as "I will never be able to overcome this problem."

Both cognitive errors and self-statements can be assessed during the interview by direct questioning, but often the most reliable method is to have patients self-monitor their pain and report their experiences.

Overt Behavioral Responses

The assessment of cancer pain behavior can include the verbal and nonverbal behaviors patients use to communicate the experience of pain, such as facial grimacing, limping, bracing, and groans. Other measures of pain behaviors are also useful. For example, estimates of physical activity have been used in pain assessment. Time spent in bed, physical exercise, amount of housework, etc., have all been used with chronic pain patients (Keefe, Brown, Scott, & Ziesat, 1982). Because cancer patients are frequently physically disabled as a result of their disease or the effects of treatment, the use of activity measures should be limited to the range of behaviors that patients are physically capable of engaging in but that are restricted because of pain.

The amount and type of pain medication usage is another behavioral measure of pain that is frequently reported. Records should include the milligram dosage per day and the specific type of palliative drug prescribed or taken. Because analgesic orders vary with practice setting and patients may not accurately report levels of pain to their physicians prescribing the drugs, the reliability of medication usage as a measure of the pain experience is questionable. In addition, patients may not take the medication as prescribed.

Some of the most useful information regarding pain behavior can be collected through direct observation by others such as nursing personnel, other therapists, and significant others. Simple rating sheets can be constructed for use on a time-sampling basis, or the behaviors can be recorded at the end of a specific time period such as the end of the day. Unfortunately, systematic ratings can be costly, in terms of observation time, interference with other procedures, and training observers to an acceptable reliability criterion. Although recording sheets used once daily are inexpensive, there is some loss of reliability due to memory interference.

The self-report of pain behaviors can also be collected. This includes self-monitoring of target behaviors or information obtained from pain behavior inventories or by interview. The loss of reliability and validity with any self-report is well known, but these measures are easily obtainable, and are sometimes the only information available, especially with cancer patients. A very useful self-report measure of pain behavior is patients' ratings of pain interference for activity. It is easily obtainable and has been shown to be significantly correlated with mood, pain intensity, and physical disability in cancer patients (Cleeland, 1984).

Any self-report measure used with cancer patients should be kept simple and not too time-consuming. Many patients are quite ill and obtunded because of high narcotic doses and will not be able to follow complicated instructions, or will be too fatigued to complete anything but the simplest of tasks. An additional reason for simplicity that applies to chronic pain patients equally well is patient compliance. Patients do not always share the clinician's enthusiasm for comprehensive data bases.

Sensory-Physiological Responses

The final response system is physiological. Measures of heart rate, muscular activity, respiration, and other responses have been used to estimate autonomic arousal and pain severity. However, the usefulness of these measures, with the possible exception of muscular activity, is of questionable value, especially in chronic pain. Most reports have not shown a clear relationship between physiological measures and degree of pain (Hilgard, 1969).

Instead, most clinicians have relied upon patients' descriptions of the sensory-physiological aspects of their pain including intensity, temporal aspects, location and quality (see Melzack, 1983). Intensity measures are usually simple numeric rating scales of subjective pain intensity. They normally require the patient to rate his or her average, worst, least, and present pain on a 10-point scale or an equivalent visual analogue scale without numerical anchors for a specific time period such as the past week or month. The temporal aspects of the patient's pain should be assessed for frequency and duration. Most cancer patients will complain of constant, daily pain. However, fluctuations in the pain most likely occur and should be documented. Location parameters of the pain are also collected by having patients shade the location of their pain on the front and back of human figures, or simply by describing where the affected area is located. The patient is also asked to indicate if the pain is deep or shallow. Finally, the measure of pain quality is obtained by asking patients to describe their pain using words such as burning, stabbing, and cramping.

The use of pain quality ratings has been shown to be a useful alternative to assessing pain intensity with cancer patients. Tearnan and Cleeland (1984) found that cancer patients who reported high levels of pain intensity tended to use certain sensory words such as sharp, gnawing, and pressing more frequently than patients who rated their pain intensity lower. In addition, it was found without the aid of word lists as prompts, patients' word usage overall was limited to a few sensory descriptions. Very few evaluative words and virtually no affective descriptors were used.

Physiological data can be obtained with the use of sophisticated instrumentation such as electromyographic recordings. Usually, however, patients are simply asked to describe their pain and its location or they are instructed in self-monitoring. Again, the use of some procedures is limited with cancer patients. A great deal depends on the physical status of the patient, as well as what is permissible and appropriate in the setting where the cancer patient is being treated. One method of collecting ongoing pain intensity ratings, as well as other measures of pain by nursing and additional health care staff, is to place a recording sheet directly in the patient's chart with clear instructions (see McCaffrey, 1979).

Pain Precipitators

One of the most important aspects of the functional analysis is defining the relationship between the exacerbation of pain and various cognitive, behavioral, physiological, emotional, and environmental stimuli. Cognitive stimuli can include any thoughts, beliefs, or images cancer patients have that appear to aggravate or trigger their pain state. The clinician should use numerous examples of whatever verbal or imaginal prompts are necessary to systematically explore potential cognitive antecedents. The question "Are there any thoughts or images that seem to make your pain worse?" will not produce many affirmative responses. Most patients do not carefully monitor their thinking. Examples of cognitive antecedents cancer patients have identified include images of fire, a red hot poker or a sharp knife, thoughts that the pain is all consuming and out of control and nothing can be done to control it, as well as "I must be weak-minded because I can not tolerate the pain." Many cognitive antecedents will also be useful in defining the cognitive response of pain. Whether they should be

included as antecedent stimuli is based on the presumption that they may also exacerbate or trigger the pain state.

By far the largest category of antecedent stimuli are behaviors cancer patients engage in that contribute to the onset or worsening of pain. These behaviors can include certain bodily movements such as bending, twisting, coughing, and reaching as well as activities such as walking, getting out of bed, eating, standing, and sitting. Most cancer patients with vertebral metastases will experience pain with any movement and are usually advised to confine themselves to bed because of the dangers of fracture, whereas patients with prostatic disease may experience pain whenever they stress the pelvic region with certain activities. Each cancer patient and cancer type will differ, and only a thorough assessment will uncover the particular behaviors that contribute to the experience of pain.

Physiological precipitants of the pain response include the disease, but also disease- and treatment-related adverse effects that make patients more vulnerable or intolerant to pain sensation. Fatigue, nausea, weakness, and dry mouth are commonly observed. These can sometimes produce an exacerbation of the pain experience. In addition to treatment- and disease-related sources, the ingestion of stimulants or other substances needs to be assessed because they can substantially alter the biochemistry of the patients and modify the pain response.

Emotional upset can also be related to the patient's pain complaint. It is well understood that anxiety and depression can alter the experience of pain. The cancer patient who has just been informed that his or her disease has progressed and metastasized to the lung will undoubtedly be anxious and report higher levels of pain, especially since the pain can serve as a constant reminder of the disease. Questions that elicit from patients information that the pain is less, the same, or worse when they are relaxed or in a good mood should be a standard part of the assessment inquiry.

Environmental factors can often precipitate

pain, and many are unique to the hospital setting. For example, patients may complain that their pain seems to worsen when they are alone or when the doctors are making their rounds. Frequently, patients will state that their pain is hardest to cope with when they are not comfortable because their bed is cold or too hard or there is too much noise in the hallways for them to rest properly (McCaffery, 1979). Certain staff or family behaviors can also be environmental stimuli that are associated with pain.

It is important that antecedent events be operationally defined and reliability understood between clinician and patient and/or staff. Simplicity and specificity are the rules of a good behavioral description. Too often patients and staff are asked to monitor pain and note the presence or absence of previously identified antecedent events without being sure what to look for.

Pain Diminishers

The next aspect of the assessment strategy should be a focus on factors that help reduce the patients' pain severity. A thorough coverage of pain diminishers should include the same general categories used to systematically explore pain antecedents. Namely, the clinician should first examine cognitive coping strategies that the patient may engage in to help lessen the pain. These include self-statements, ignoring the pain, reinterpreting the pain, praying, and distraction (Keefe et al., 1982). Cancer patients, like chronic pain patients, will differ in their use of strategies that they find helpful. Common behavioral pain diminishers include bed rest, physical or social activity as distractors, use of heating pads and warm baths. The range of behavioral distractors will be restricted in cancer patients confined to bed. Medication and alcohol ingestion are common physiological pain reducers. The type and amount of medication and degree of pain relief should be assessed. Lastly, environmental events that can diminish pain will vary with the setting and resources the patient is exposed to. For instance, some hospital staff provide cancer information-support groups that many patients find useful in helping to cope with their pain.

Consequences

The immediate consequences of the patient's pain behavior should be assessed in order to determine if environmental supports are operating in any way to maintain or exacerbate the pain complaint. The most common reinforcers include social attention for the pain complaint from the medical staff or significant others. The evaluation of pain operants should be focused on cancer patients who show no evidence of disease and whose pain has persisted for more than 6 weeks (Foley, 1984). Here, the assessment protocol is similar to that for the patient with chronic stable pain where the pain behavior may be a function of pain-contingent reinforcement.

Onset, History, and Development

The next step in the assessment strategy should be an examination of the onset, history, and development of the pain complaint. This information is of primary importance because it helps the clinician put the problem in perspective and may lead to the discovery of antecedent stimuli that were overlooked in the initial part of the assessment. Additionally, the knowledge of previous therapy attempts is vital since steps must be taken to correct the inadequacies of past failures and build on previous successes. The development of the patient's pain problem will provide clues as to how the patient has coped in the past and over what time frame changes occurred.

Other Complications

Cancer pain inevitably produces adverse changes in mood, work, physical activity, and interpersonal relationships. These are areas that need to be routinely evaluated in any pain assessment to determine the overall impact of the pain problem on the patient's life. These changes, if pronounced, can compromise the patient's response to medical treatment and interfere significantly with the quality of life. They can also amplify the pain experience. Ratings of pain interference in mood, pleasant activities, and overall enjoyment of life can be used in addition to more traditional assessment tools to help plan treatment and provide a more thorough understanding of the pain problem. Interviews with significant others can also provide worthwhile information regarding the impact pain has had on the family and marriage.

Formulation

The final step in the assessment strategy is to formulate a treatment plan and to make predictions regarding the patient's response to intervention. This is accomplished by proposing several hypotheses regarding the onset, development, and maintenance of the patient's pain complaint and justifying particular treatment interventions based on these conclusions. For instance, the cancer patient who reports anxiety as one antecedent consistently associated with the exacerbation of his or her pain, and who reports less pain after taking diazepam, might be a good candidate for relaxation therapy.

Assessment Instruments

There are many instruments available that can assist the clinician in the assessment process. Some have been designed specially for pain assessment, and others are used primarily for determining the patient's level of mood and personality disturbance. Most are self-report measures. Cancer patients are often unable to complete a comprehensive test battery or lengthy test such as the Minnesota Multiphasic Personality Inventory (MMPI) because of their physical status. The best assessment tool for this population is one that can be easily understood with minimal instructions and is relatively short. It should also require little administrative supervision by psychological staff. Additionally, nurses

and other health care staff should find the instrument useful and easily interpretable. Finally, it should include items that sample pain behaviors as well as mood disturbance.

The Pain Research Group at the University of Wisconsin Medical School developed the Wisconsin Brief Pain Inventory (BPI) for the specific purpose of administration to cancer pain patients (Daut, Cleeland, & Flannery, 1983). It is a short questionnaire that normally requires only 10 minutes for the patient to complete. It includes several types of questions such as: (a) whether or not the patient has had any surgery in the past month; (b) front and back human figures with instructions for the patient in pain to shade the painful area; (c) numeric ratings of worst, average, least, and present pain intensity; (d) requests for the patient to describe any pain diminishers or antecedents that have been associated with pain relief or exacerbation; (e) requests to list current pain treatments; and (f) questions regarding response to treatment. In addition, the patient is instructed to rate several pain adjectives such as throbbing and burning on a scale of 0 to 10. Another section of the questionnaire includes several items that ask patients how their pain has interfered with their mood, general activity, walking ability, normal work, relations with other people, sleep, and enjoyment of life. Finally, the questionnaire contains a short version of the Profile of Mood States (POMS) that has shown to be statistically equivalent to the full version (Shacham, 1983). The POMS is included to screen for mood disturbance. The BPI has demonstrated respectable validity and reliability and is a useful pre- and posttreatment measure (Daut et al., 1983).

General Assessment Issues

Several general issues need to be addressed when assessing the cancer pain patient. These matters can significantly affect an evaluation, and unless the clinician is cognizant of their presence they can lead to spurious conclusions or disrupt the assessment process.

Setting

One factor every clinician encounters is the unique setting of the cancer patient. Most cancer patients in pain are inpatients or outpatients at medical centers. They are receiving ongoing cancer therapy, palliative care, or are being evaluated periodically for reoccurrence of their disease. In most cases when conventional therapy fails to relieve pain, a member of a liason service specializing in pain is requested to consult. The role of a consultant in a medical setting is that of an expert who is expected to render an opinion quickly without consuming too much of the patient's time. Under these circumstances, lengthy procedures are unsuitable since the consultant often has to present recommendations after only one session. This necessitates a streamlined version of an ideal assessment. If the consultant is expected to treat the patient, he or she can afford more elaborate procedures but is still limited by the brief residence of inpatients and by the physical and mental incapacitation of many patients.

The behavioral clinician should be sensitive to the patient's primary care providers who may not share the clinician's enthusiasm for behavioral control and may see the intervention as an interference. Unfortunately, these negative opinions can sometimes be communicated to the patient and compliance reduced. Frequent physician updates on the patient's progress and rationale for particular assessment and treatment protocols can help eliminate most obstacles.

Overcoming a Reluctance to Participate

Cancer pain patients are medical patients. Often patients' beliefs about the role of a psychologist or other behavioral clinician run counter to their expectations for being treated for medical problems. As a result, some patients are reluctant to participate in assessment or treatment. DeGood (1983) does a commendable job discussing practical ways in which to overcome this barrier and increase compliance with chronic pain patients. His suggestions can also be applied to cancer patients in pain. In brief, he first explains to

patients that he is a psychologist and reassures them that often pain produces changes in one's life that can affect work, mood, etc. According to DeGood, this usually helps to de-escalate the implicit message that "the referral was because the doctor thinks the pain is all in my head." Although most cancer patients are believed regarding the organic basis of their pain complaints, they may have a history of diagnostic procedures in which nothing was discovered and may feel that the severity of the pain and their inability to tolerate it is related to psychological weaknesses. DeGood mentions that this initial explanation also helps challenge the belief that because psychological variables may be correlated with the exacerbation of pain, this in some way makes the physical problem less legitimate.

DeGood recommends that the interview initially focus on physical symptoms. This helps to reduce patients' defensiveness and to establish the credibility of the behavioral clinician. He also advises that, when assessing other aspects of the pain complaint such as depression, these topics should be introduced with a statement to the effect that "pain often makes us feel. . . ." Patients are reluctant to admit to emotional problems since doing so confirms the belief that something is wrong mentally. Lastly, we have found that cancer patients need be assured that their participation in no way indicates that their medical therapy, including the use of analgesic medications, will be jeopardized.

Factors Affecting the Report of Pain

Numerous factors can influence a patient's report of pain. The clinician should be familiar with the more frequently occurring since they can significantly affect how cancer patients communicate their pain experience. For instance, the patient's history can determine how pain is reported. Patients who have received support in the past from health care professionals for their pain problem and for requesting medication will be more inclined to admit to pain.

Frequently cancer patients are reluctant to

report pain because of beliefs that discourage disclosure. One study found that many cancer patients do not complain of pain because they feel there is a social stigma attached to people who do (Jacox & Stewart, 1973). Other patients admit that they do not want to bother their doctor or detract him or her from their medical treatment. Our society also reinforces the notions that a good patient does not complain when in pain and that a complainer is one who has lost self-control. Unfortunately, health care professionals sometimes directly reinforce these beliefs (McCaffery, 1979).

The nature of the pain itself can also influence a patient's report. Patients who have severe pain may be more motivated to admit to pain and to request medications than patients experiencing mild or moderate pain levels. Certain pain locations such as rectal or genital discourage reports of pain because of personal embarrassment (Hardy, 1956). Patients will also acknowledge pain more readily if it is constant as opposed to episodic. The expectation of pain-free periods can increase the patient's tolerance level (McCaffery, 1979). Finally, patients experiencing significant interferences in mood and physical activity due to their pain may be more likely to communicate their experience.

The stage of disease is another factor that may affect the report of pain. Abrams (1966) wrote an intriguing paper in which she observed that cancer patients are less likely to communicate to others as their disease progresses. She found that initially patients are optimistic and hopeful concerning treatment and that anxiety is lessened by direct answers to questions. As the disease advances, there is a change in what patients desire to know and to whom they direct their questions. Patients also develop a fear of abandonment by their physician which they manage by becoming compliant and uncomplaining. In the terminal stages, communication becomes minimal and support from others is more important. Although Abrams did not address the issue of pain communication specifically, the points she raised certainly have many implications for pain assessment.

Other variables influencing the pain report of cancer and chronic pain patients that have been mentioned in the literature include neuroticism (Bond, 1976), level of awareness and education (Moses & Cividoli, 1966), depression and chronicity (Kremer, Block, & Gaylor, 1981), use of certain medications (Kremer, Block, & Atkinson, 1983), desire to manipulate treatment (Ignelzi, Kremer, Atkinson, 1980), and staff support of pain complaints (Kremer et al., 1983). Each of these factors should be carefully considered in the assessment process.

General Treatment Methods

The behavioral control techniques that are of use in the management of pain due to cancer are not unique, and it is not the purpose of this chapter to describe them in detail. It is the selection and combination of these techniques for the specific characteristics of cancer pain that are of interest to us. We regard what we can offer as skills training and describe these methods to patients as such. In the context of presenting this training, we expect to do more such as providing support, acknowledging distress, and discussing issues relating to the termination of life. Our focus of intervention, however, remains the learning of specific methods of self care, and we often make referrals for other types of psychological interventions. Recognizing the interaction between pain and its personal context, it is difficult to challenge the idea that dealing with critical intra- and interpersonal issues might not reduce the impact of pain. But our contract with the patient is limited to the teaching of those skills our assessment indicates are appropriate for that patient.

It is important that both patient and therapist acknowledge that behavioral skills will not control all pain all of the time. A sense of failure can be viewed as the most noxious potential side effect of behavioral intervention. It can be helpful if the patient is encouraged to adopt an experimental attitude—"Let's see how well some of these methods might work in reducing some of your pain." We teach several self-control techniques to each patient, which reinforces this experimental attitude and the expectation that no one measure will be effective in all situations.

Our "menu" of behavioral control techniques includes biofeedback-assisted muscle relaxation (using surface electomyography) and autonomic relaxation (using feedback of skin temperature), as well as progressive relaxation (using surface electromyography) Bernstein and Borkovec (1973), training in rhythmic breathing, and cognitive control techniques (see Turk, Meichenbaum, & Genest, 1983). The cognitive control techniques can be tailored for episodic or tonic pain and include diversion of attention, sensory transformation (for example, from "pain" to "numb"), emotional response control, self-reinforcement for having mastered peak periods of pain, and memory control to avoid rehearsing these same periods. In contrast to our use of cognitive control techniques with chronic pain, these procedures are often taught to cancer patients with the aide of hypnotic induction and self-hypnosis to enhance their use of cognitive control. Even with patients who are not particularly suggestible, we feel that hypnotic induction enhances the importance of the time to be devoted to cognitive manipulation of the pain. Hypnotic induction may also serve to increase the patient's perception of the potency of the behavioral intervention because of the widely accepted notion that hypnosis is powerful treatment. This is important for patients who feel that they are victims of their disease.

It is important to add a word about the level of training of persons teaching behavioral pain control techniques. We strongly feel that most of these techniques can be taught by persons with a wide variety of professional backgrounds who have a core of interpersonal skills typically associated with successful behavioral change (Kendall & Norton-Ford, 1982). We have trained numerous oncology nurses in the majority of techniques outlined and have been impressed with their effectiveness. We have reserved hypnotic induction for professional psychological staff, but this restriction is based more on caution

than common sense. We doubt that self-hypnosis taught by persons with limited hypnotic training presents major problems when restricted to relaxation and pain control.

We next describe the treatments for four groups of patients that differ in their requirements for behavioral pain management. These examples have been selected because they present the most common pain-control problems that the behavioral clinician will encounter. As we have stated before, an adequate assessment of the patient is the most critical determinant of a successful intervention. In many instances the behavioral clinician will see the patient for assessment only, depending on other professional staff to provide elements of the treatment package. If this is the case, it is important that follow-up consultation be planned so that treatment effectiveness can be measured and necessary adjustments in the treatment plan can be recommended.

The patient with no active disease but persistent post-treatment pain. In this patient group the treatment plan will most closely parallel the approach to patients with chronic, stable pain. Pain may be due to postsurgical scarring, neuropathy induced by chemotherapy, or postirradiation myleopathy or fibrosis. Phantom limb pain may follow amputation for osteosarcoma. Destruction of nerve is the most common basis for the majority of these pain syndromes, causing a burning pain as well as dysesthesias which are extremely unpleasant but difficult to describe. These patients are free of their disease, at least for the forseeable future, but have to anticipate pain that may last indefinitely. The pain may have its onset weeks or months after the termination of treatment. Because the disease has been arrested, most would agree that these patients are not candidates for continued narcotic medications. Narcotic use may become an issue in treatment, however. We have seen patients with long histories (one to two decades) of narcotic analgesic use, initially started for treatment of pain due to malignancy.

Specific applications of behavioral techniques should become apparent during the assessment. If sustained muscle contraction is contributing to the pain, muscle-based relaxation techniques are indicated. We prefer to start with EMG biofeedback because it effectively illustrates to the patient abnormal levels of muscle contraction that are associated with the area of primary pathology. As indicated previously, we also train patients in other relaxation techniques to promote generalization and to demonstrate the multiplicity of ways that deep muscle relaxation might be achieved. Damage to sympathetic nerves may be present, causing pain due to sympathetic dysregulation. In this instance it is possible to provide pain control by training patients to increase their skin temperature using a thermistor-based biofeedback. This training has been most frequently described in its application for migraine headache (Turin & Johnson, 1976) and Raynaud's phenomenon and disease (Surwit, Pilon, & Fenten, 1978). Patients who learn this type of physiological control may find that they experience pain relief only when they are actively practicing the technique with little carry-over to nonpractice time. This happens frequently enough that it is important to forewarn patients of this possibility before they undertake training.

Cognitive control techniques can be used for the majority of patients in this group. They can benefit from coping strategies designed to minimize the functional impairment caused by their pain. We have found that these patients are highly motivated to deal with their pain strategically. As with other cancer patients, the prevalence of emotional disturbance appears to be significantly lower for this group than for patients with chronic, stable pain. Perhaps as a result, they readily accept the notion of self-control and are highly motivated to learn the requisite skills. The specific elements of cognitive control techniques are treated elsewhere in this volume. (See chapter 3.)

A small minority of this group will face major problems as cancer survivors because of preexisting personal-situational difficulties. The assessment may reveal that persistent pain has come to play a role in these problems Having a life-threatening disease may produce reinforcement in terms of increased attention and forgiveness of responsibility that is diminished when their cancer is cured. Some patients may then develop operant pain-related behavior that appears to have as its function the reestablishment of this reinforcement. They may profit from brief, highly structured, and cognitively oriented therapy which emphasizes reappraisal of their situation and their objectives, coupled with training in social skills for attaining their objectives. On occasion, such patients may need to consider an operantly based pain management program. (See chapter 2.)

Case Study 1: A 33-year-old Woman With Shoulder Pain

Approximately 9 months after radiation to the thoracic area, a 33-year-old divorced woman developed pain in a cape-like distribution across both shoulders due to radiation fibrosis of both trapezius muscles. She also had probable fibrosis about the right bracial plexus causing pain in the right arm. She rated her worst pain at a level of 7 on a 0–10 scale. She was felt to be in remission at the time of the consultation. The patient was the mother of two children, ages 8 and 10, who were now living with her ex-husband because of her extended illness. After the onset of her disease, the patient had become very isolated socially. Her only consistent social contacts were occasional visits from her mother and her visits to the cancer center. Despite the reassurance that there was no current progression of her disease, she was preoccupied with thoughts of dying. She expressed the particular fear of dying in a public place while out with her friends who then would have to take care of the body. Personality measures indicated high levels of tension and anxiety but only mild depression. Laboratory assessment demonstrated high levels of sustained muscle contraction in the muscles of the neck and shoulders. Muscle contraction and reported pain increased when she imagined herself in social situations.

Behavioral treatment followed the model outlined above. She first received four sessions of biofeedback-assisted muscle relaxation and PRT. She was able to achieve lowered levels of muscle contraction and associated reduction in pain in the laboratory and after scheduled practice sessions at home. She began to make the connection between stress, muscle contraction, and her pain. At this point, however, she continued to have pain of approximately pretreatment severity at other times, and she remained seclusive. She was eager, however, to learn to use relaxation skills to resume contact with her friends whom she missed. She was next seen for three sessions of behaviorally oriented therapy that used desensitization. After relaxing deeply, she imagined increasingly socially demanding situations, again relaxing when tension or an increase in pain was reported. She was encouraged to begin brief social contacts of circumscribed and preplanned duration. These contacts proved to be extremely reinforcing for her, and she soon was as active socially as she had been before the onset of her disease. Her pain was absent much of the time and was mild when it was present. Her reduction in pain and restored social activity remained at 6- and 24-month follow-up assessments.

The rather profound effect of a relatively simple combination of behavioral interventions in this case is worthy of comment. First, her motivation to change was high. She had been relatively outgoing and social before the diagnosis and extended treatment of her cancer. Her pain and isolation were negatively reinforcing. Second, her history of social isolation was relatively brief and was reactive to her disease. Finally, her success in pain control through relaxation increased her belief that she could change other negative aspects of her life through her own efforts.

The patient preparing for intensive anti-cancer therapy which will produce pain. Most treatment-related pain can be adequately controlled by properly prescribed analgesics (Foley, 1984). Some patients, however, will face prolonged pain as a result of heroic therapies for their disease. Examples include extensive surgical procedures (such as hemipelvectomy), bone marrow transplantation, and hyperthermia. If there is sufficient time, patients can be taught pain control skills that they can practice before the onset of pain. At a minimum, our behavioral approach to working with these patients consists of three elements: (a) providing the patient with information about the pain of the procedure, (b) training the patient to be assertive in asking for pain relief, and (c) training the patient in specific pain-related coping skills, namely, relaxation and self-hypnosis.

Providing the patient with information needs to be coordinated with the nursing staff. Our particular interest is determining when the patient is expected to have pain and the characteristics and severity of that pain. This information can provide the patient with a type of cognitive map of the territory. If possible, we have the patient practice his or her coping strategies in the physical surroundings where they will be needed.

As stated before, we never minimize the relief that can be provided by analgesics and train patients in assertively requesting pain medication as needed. This training includes a review of the characteristics of analgesics including their duration of effect, the negligible risk of addiction to properly administered narcotics, and the necessity of maintaining a given plasma level for analgesics to be effective. We also train patients how to ask for pain medications. It is our impression that patients are more successful if they request analgesics in a serious, matter-of-fact style that is not overly dramatic, or, on the other hand, too cheerful. Either extreme may foster the judgment that the patient doesn't "need' the medication. We find it helpful if patients and staff can communicate about the severity of pain and the effectiveness of pain medications by using some type of rating scale.

If there is sufficient time before the patient undergoes the painful procedure, we train him or her in both relaxation and self-hypnosis. Three or four training sessions in EMG biofeedback-assisted relaxation training are planned. During these sessions, patients are taught rhythmic breathing and PRT. The instructions for PRT are recorded on a cassette for review by the patient during subsequent painful episodes. Training in self-hypnosis follows relaxation training. Two or three sessions are scheduled, depending on the needs of the patient. The first session is used to explore hypnosis as a phenomenon, deal with misconceptions, and, if the patient wishes to proceed, investigate the type of induction that will be most effective. A cassette of the induction is also made for use during painful episodes. Since patients in this group have yet to experience the pain they are preparing for, the focus of hypnosis is on the development of a pleasant image, often of a "special place," a place of deep relaxation and retreat. This image is built with the help of the patient's recall or fantasy.

Case Study 2: A 39-year-old Man Preparing For Bone Marrow Transplant

A 39-year-old health care professional sought training in behavioral control techniques prior to bone marrow transplantation for acute lymphoblastic leukemia. He was concerned about painful oral mucocitis, which can occur with preparatory chemo- and radiotherapy. He felt that the chances of successful transplantation would be increased if he could minimize his requirement for narcotic analgesics during this period. He was also concerned that he would not be able to complete the extended isolation in the hospital that this procedure requires. He had become quite fearful during previous hospitalizations for chemotherapy and left before the course was completed.

He was divorced and had two children under 12 whom he visited frequently. His sister had died of the same disease 2 years before. Her disease also began after she was divorced. He was particularly attuned to coping with his disease himself. He was very careful with his diet and, with his physician's supervision, exercised to tolerance three to five times a week. He was a keen observer of

his personality style and his reactions to situations. He described himself as a highly competitive, highly competent, and hard-working individual who could rarely recall feeling relaxed. Fear was even more foreign to him. He was quite self-critical about the previous episode of leaving the hospital. While motivated to learn behavioral control, he was rightfully skeptical of any possible changes in his personality pattern, even though he felt his behavior was responsible for many personal sadnesses and may have contributed to the onset of his disease.

Following four sessions of PRT and biofeedback-assisted relaxation training, he reported a profound sense of relaxation and calm which, much to his surprise, he liked very much. He found time in his overcommitted day to practice relaxation once or twice and, without specific prompting from our therapy group, began to cut back on his scheduled work and to plan for more things that he enjoyed. Training in behavioral control was then presented in the context of hypnosis, and he also received training in self-hypnosis. He easily formed a pleasant image of a lake in the woods of New England where he had spent a great deal of time as a boy and young man. He proved particularly adept at forming a very detailed image, complete with sounds, smells, and tactile features. With the help of unit personnel, we arranged for him to practice his skills on the unit where he was to undergo transplantation. He was also introduced to glove anesthesia, which he learned to transfer to his mouth in anticipation of treatment-related oral pain. Finally, he was urged to discuss the possible negative effects of narcotic medications on his treatment with his physician and to use them as needed if there was little evidence that they would impede his progress.

Following the transplantation, he reported that he had used the full range of techniques he had been taught and had found some quite helpful. He relied heavily on the audio cassettes of both relaxation and hypnosis during episodes of pain and other discomforts. He rarely felt panic during the hospitalization and never felt compelled to leave. Glove anesthesia was minimally effective, if at all, in contrast to the pleasant imagery in dealing with acute pain. Although he used narcotic analgesics and had been reassured that this was appropriate, he expressed satisfaction that he had required less medication than others undergoing the same procedure.

The patient with pain due to active disease with a prognosis of several months. Patients with an indefinite prognosis are often excellent candidates for behavioral pain-control methods. Most individuals in this group are on narcotic and other analgesic drugs. They may wish to continue to work or manage their households, continue with avocational activities, and have an active family life. In order to stay active they may elect to reduce analgesic medications to minimize side-effects, primarily mental blurring. Many will want to learn behavioral control techniques to increase their sense of control over some aspects of their disease. Some patients will want to manage other areas of disease-related discomforts such as nausea, sleep disturbance, and procedurally related anxiety.

A few patients will have the open or hidden agenda of using these skills to retard or stop the progress of their disease itself. If this goal is preeminent, we counsel patients that research in the area of behavioral control of disease is too experimental for us to make a judgment about its effectiveness. Our main goal is to enhance their control of symptoms. Nonetheless, we never challenge a patient's belief in the curative effects of personal effort. Some patients may wish to develop images of their body fighting their disease and we support them in this attempt. We would never initiate that kind of image, however, preferring instead to work with images of symptom control.

The behavioral treatment approach with these patients has many features in common with what is offered to the previous two groups. Patients are taught a combination of relaxation techniques with the set of skills to be learned based on the physical basis of their pain. Considerable time is spent in exploring the type of functional impairment caused by pain. Following relaxation training, cognitive control techniques for episodic and tonic pain are reviewed, and appropriate ones are taught to the patient. Reappraisal is especially important. Some patients will set unrealistically high goals for themselves in the face of the limitation caused by their pain and other aspects of their disease. Self-reinforcement is tied to reappraisal. Patients need to tell themselves when they have been heroic. Cognitive manipulation of pain, such as sensory transformation, may provide periods of helpful distraction from pain as well.

Unlike the patient with arrested disease, but like the patient preparing for painful treatment procedures, the appropriate use of narcotic medication is reviewed. Issues of addiction, tolerance, dependence, and sufficient plasma levels are reviewed with the patient with the cooperation of medical staff. Again, the clinical pharmacist can provide this type of information. As with the previous group, effective ways of requesting needed pain medications are examined.

We offer to teach techniques of self-hypnosis to this group. We find the technique effective in producing deep relaxation and in helping focus attention on distraction strategies. Hypnosis is useful in developing the pleasant image for use as a respite and in developing an image of the pain to be used with sensory transformation.

Case Study 3: A 37-year-old Woman With Colon Cancer

A 37-year-old woman was experiencing severe back pain and pain in the right inguinal area and right leg felt to be due to retroperitoneal invasion by tumor. Her primary disease was colon cancer, and pain was the first symptom of her disease. She initially attributed the pain to tension and anxiety due to visiting her father who also had cancer. Her cancer was first diagnosed when the pain became more constant. She rated her pain as 9 on a 0–10 scale. Narcotic medication reduced the pain to a level of 3.

At the time of consultation, she was working half-time. She was married and had two young children, ages 5 and 8. By this time, she was taking methadone for pain control and claimed that the medication made her feel confused, disoriented, and "foggy." She was concerned that she have quality time with her children and was hopeful that behavioral control techniques might help her reduce her medication. Although aware that her prognosis was poor, she reported only mild depression but did admit moderate levels of tension. She was psychologically oriented and, if anything, tended to attribute her discomfort to psychological rather than physical mechanisms.

Training in relaxation techniques was effective in diminishing her anxiety but was associated with only nominal reductions in her pain. The remaining sessions were conducted using hypnosis. She was able to use pleasant imagery in distracting herself when confronted with acute episodes of pain and was able to titrate the medications to her satisfaction. We found that she was also quite adept at transforming the pain. She was able to develop an image of the sensation she described as black, heavy, about the size and shape of a softball, and covered with extremely rough edges. After she formed this image, she found she could alter it and its location. She was able to change its color, hardness, and shape, making it a smooth, soft yellow ball that she could squeeze and compress. Finally, she could move the image, at first within her body and then later to a position outside her body where she could study it with some degree of abstraction.

She reported that she derived the greatest benefit from pain control using the distraction provided by pleasant imagery and by transformation of her pain. Although the relaxation techniques were helpful for reducing her anxiety and she used them frequently, they provided little pain relief.

The patient in the terminal stages of illness. The majority of patients with solid tumors will face moderate to severe pain in the last few weeks of their life. It is important that all available medical pain management techniques, including destructive surgical procedures and nerve blocks, be reviewed for their potential benefit to the individual.

Pain will become a primary focus for family members once hope for a cure has been abandoned. Family members need to be encouraged to keep track of the severity of pain by using the same rating scale that has been taught to the patient. In this way, they can provide useful information to staff about the effectiveness of behavioral treatments. As obvious as it sounds, families need to be reassured that it is appropriate to be concerned about how much pain the patient is having and to demand reasonable control.

Families are rightfully protective of patients and may be suspicious of behavioral interventions. It is necessary to describe behavioral control methods in a circumspect fashion, indicating that they are effective for some, but not for all who use them. Neither patients nor families should be made to feel guilty by a refusal to accept them. With the patients' permission, family members can be encouraged to stay during the sessions. Some family members benefit themselves from sharing suggestions for deep relaxation and calm.

We usually offer pain control techniques in the context of hypnotic induction. This is rarely refused. The public image of hypnosis is one of a powerful procedure potent enough to be of use with profound pain. A standard assessment of suggestibility is frequently too difficult to administer under the circumstances, although patients report varying depths of hypnotic trance.

The patient's ability to concentrate and to remember are often limited by palliative medications and by fatigue. Cognitive functions may be additionally impaired if brain metastases are present. Because of these factors, we rely more heavily on direct suggestion and on cassette recordings of those suggestions. Structured relaxation and other behavioral pain control training are rarely possible. We may only be able to schedule two sessions with a patient.

During the first session the patient is taught hypnotic induction and methods of deepening. If the patient is too impaired to learn self-hypnosis, the instructions can be recorded on cassette and used as needed. The majority of time is spent helping the patient develop a pleasant image so that he or she can feel relaxed, calm, and secure. These images can be ones that are recalled or that exist only in fantasy. The patient is encouraged to use the images as often as he or she feels the need. We attempt to clarify the image as much as possible, suggesting various sensory attributes including sights, sounds, and smells.

During the second session, the patient's use of the induction tape and pleasant imagery are reviewed. If the patient wishes, training can continue with suggested glove analgesia and transfer of analgesia to painful areas of the body. Transformation of the pain is also explored. He or she is encouraged to develop an image of the pain — reporting its size, color, texture, temperature, and shape. If the patient is able to do this, he or she is encouraged to manipulate the components of the image. It can be suggested that the image of the pain be changed, perhaps even moved outside of the body.

Case Study 4: A 54-year-old Woman With Terminal Cancer

A 54-year-old married woman with breast cancer and disseminated metastases involving the skull, femur, spine, liver, and other multiple boney sites requested training in behavioral control for management of pain. She rated her pain at 10 on a 0–10 scale before medications were started. She obtained relatively good pain control with Levorphanol with bed rest. She was hopeful of regaining some freedom of movement through the use of behavioral control techniques. She was a health professional who had witnessed the effective use of hypnosis. Part of her motivation for better control of pain was to be able to spend her final days at home.

Her husband was initially skeptical about the use of hypnosis but did not share his doubts with the patient. He requested that he be present during the sessions. Despite high doses of narcotics, she was a good hypnotic subject and readily achieved a profound state of relaxation and suggestibility. We first worked with pleasant imagery, which for her was a creation of fantasy. She found that she could use the tape-recorded induction to create other images that provided a sense of deep calm and relaxation for her. Some of these were from the past and some were of a more beneficient future. Her husband became a participant in the sessions as well, achieving at least a moderate stage of relaxation and reporting that he felt a decrease in tension for the first time in several weeks. Both the patient and her husband continued to use the techniques effectively while she was in the hospital, although we have no information about her success when she returned home.

Several points are worth making about this case. First, the patient was an adept hypnotic subject who had a high level of confidence in the technique. Second, once he had experienced the effects of hypnosis, her husband strongly encouraged her use of the procedure. Third, the hypnotic suggestions used were simple. Much more detailed hypnotic suggestions for pain in the terminally ill have been offered by Sacerdote (1983) and others.

CONCLUSIONS

We have reviewed the diverse expressions of pain associated with cancer and have seen how the behavioral assessment and resulting behavioral treatment plan must be based not only in a thorough understanding of the pain complaint but also in an adequate knowledge of the disease itself and its stages of progression. We have also emphasized the importance of simultaneous and comprehensive medical antipain therapies. We have underscored the need for behavioral clinicians with previous experience in the management of chronic pain to reorient themselves to the specific needs of cancer patients.

The very lack of controlled outcome studies examining the effectiveness of behavioral methods for cancer pain underlines the critical need for such studies. Those who undertake such studies should be aware of the enormous difficulties that they face. The effect of behavioral interventions can never be studied in a vacuum. Multiple medical therapies for pain must be used simultaneously. Differences in cancer site, stage of the disease, physical basis of pain, and concurrent medical therapies will make equivalent group composition difficult. The effectiveness of behavioral pain control for the dying patient may never be studied to everyone's satisfaction.

Despite the complexity of the issues, we hope that by sharing our clinical impressions we have made a case for concluding that behavioral control techniques have a place in the comprehensive management of pain due to cancer. We suggest that relatively simple behavioral skills training can be surprisingly effective in pain reduction, that a package of different behavioral techniques appropriately selected for the individual has distinct advantages over any skill presented in isolation, and that cancer patients, as a group, are extremely well motivated to learn and practice these skills.

REFERENCES

Abrams, R.D. (1966). The patient with cancer—his changing pattern of communication. *New England Journal of Medicine, 274*, 317–322.

Bernstein, D.A., & Borkovec, T.D. (1973). *Progressive relocation training: A manual for the helping professions.* Champaign, IL: Research Press.

Bond, M.R. (1976). Pain and personality in cancer patients. In J.J. Bonica & D. Albe-Fessard (Eds.), *Advances in pain research and therapy* (Vol. 1). New York: Raven Press.

Bonica, J.J. (1978). Cancer pain: A major national health problem. *Cancer Nursing, 1*, 313–316.

Cleeland, C.S. (in press). The impact of pain on the patient with cancer. *Cancer.*

Daut, R.L., & Cleeland, C.S. (1982). The prevalence and severity of pain in cancer. *Cancer, 50*(9): 1903–1918.

Daut, R.L., Cleeland, C.S., & Flanery, R.C. (1983). Development of the Wisconsin brief pain questionnaire to assess pain in cancer and other diseases. *Pain, 17*, 197–210.

DeGood, D.E. (1983). Reducing medical patients' reluctance to participate in psychological therapies: The initial session. *Professional Psychology: Research and Practice, 14*, 570–579.

Foley, K.M. (1979). Pain syndromes in patients with cancer. In J.J. Bonica & V. Ventafredda (Eds.), *Advances in pain research and therapy* (Vol. 2). New York: Raven Press.

Foley, K.M. (1984). Assessment of pain. *Clinics in Oncology, 3*, 17–31.

Hardy, J.D. (1956). The nature of pain, *Journal of Chronic Disorders, 7*, 22–51.

Hilgard, E.R. (1969). Pain as a puzzle for psychology and physiology. *American Journal of Psychology, 24*, 103–113.

Ignelzi, R.J., Kremer, E.F., & Atkinson, J.H. (1980, November). *Patient pain intensity report to different health professionals.* Paper presented at Association for Advancement of Behavior Therapy, New York.

Jacox, A., & Stewart, M. (1973). *Psychosocial contingencies of the pain experience.* Iowa City: The University of Iowa Press.

Keefe, F.J., Brown, C., Scott, D.S., & Ziesat, H. (1982). The behavioral assessment of chronic pain. In F.J. Keefe & J.A. Blumenthal (Eds.), *Assessment strategies in behavioral medicine.* New York: Grune & Stratton.

Kendall, P.C., & Norton-Ford, J.D. (1982). *Clinical psychology: Scientific & professional dimensions.* New York: John Wiley & Sons.

Kremer, E.F., Block, A., & Atkinson, J.H. (1983). Assessment of pain behavior: Factors that distort self-report. In R. Melzack (Ed.), *Pain measurement & assessment.* New York: Raven Press.

Kremer, E.F., Block, A., & Gaylor, M. (1981). Behavioral approaches to treatment of chronic pain: The inaccuracy of patient self-report measures. *Arch. Phys. Med. Rehabil., 62*, 188–191.

Levin, C.N., Cleeland, C.S., & Dar, R. (1985). Public attitudes towards cancer pain. *Cancer,* in press.

McCaffery, M. (1979). *Nursing management of the patient with pain.* (2nd ed.) Philadelphia: J.B. Lippincott.

Marks, R.M., & Sacher, E.J. (1973). Undertreatment of medical inpatients with narcotic analgesics. *Annals of Internal Medicine, 78*, 173–181.

Melzack, R. (Ed.) (1983). *Pain measurement and assessment.* New York: Raven Press.

Moses, R., & Cividoli, N. (1966). Differential levels of awareness of illness: Their relation to some salient features in cancer patients. *Ann. N.Y. Acad. Sci., 125*, 884.

National Institute of Health (1979). Report of the Panel on Pain to the National Advisory NINDS Council (NIH 79-1912). Washington, DC: Government Printing Office.

Sacerdote, P. (1982). Techniques of hypnotic intervention with pain patients. In J. Barber & C. Adrian (Eds.), *Psychological approaches to the management of pain*. New York: Brunner/Mazel.

Schwettmann, R.S., Shacham, S., & Cleeland, C.S. (1983). *Relating cancer pain to its physical basis*. Presented at the American Pain Society, Chicago, Illinois.

Shacham, S. (1983). A shortened version of the Profile of Mood States. *Journal of Personality Assessment, 47*, 305–306.

Shacham, S., Reinhardt, L.C., Raubertas, R.F., & Cleeland, C.S. (1983). Emotional state and pain: Intraindividual and interindividual measures of association. *Journal of Behavioral Medicine, 6*: 405–419.

Surwit, R.S., Pilon, R.N., & Fenten, C.H. (1978). Behavioral treatment of Raynaud's disease. *Journal of Behavioral Medicine, 1*, 323–335.

Tearnan, B.H., & Cleeland, C.S. (1984). *The use of pain descriptors by patients with cancer pain*. Unpublished manuscript, The University of Wisconsin, Madison.

Turin, A., & Johnson, N.G. (1976). Biofeedback therapy for migraine headaches. *Archives of General Psychiatry, 33*, 517–519.

Turk, D., Meichenbaum, D., & Genest, M. (1983). *Pain and behavioral medicine*. New York: Guilford Press.

Twycross, R.G., & Lacks, S.A. (1985). *Symptom control in advanced cancer: Pain relief*. London: Pitman.

13 RELAXATION AND BIOFEEDBACK FOR CHRONIC HEADACHES*

Frank Andrasik

Headache is one of the top complaints of patients seeking treatment in medical settings (Leviton, 1978). Although as many as 15 separate types of headache have been identified (Ad Hoc Committee on the Classification of Headache, 1962), the overwhelming majority can be diagnosed as either migraine or tension. Examination of patient files at a well-known headache specialty clinic revealed 94% of the patients received one of these two diagnoses (Lance, Curran, & Anthony, 1965); these same two headache types have been shown to be amenable to relaxation and biofeedback treatment approaches and are the focus of this chapter.

A migraine (or vascular) headache has a sudden onset, most often affects only one side of the head, builds quickly to an intense throbbing, pounding, or pulsating sensation at its peak, and lasts approximately 8 hours, although it can range from a few hours to several continuous days. Frequent accompaniments are anorexia, nausea, and fatigue; features less frequent are vomiting, pallor, diarrhea, dizziness, parathesias, hypersensitivity to sound and light, and cold in the

extremities. A small percentage of migraineurs (approximately 10%) experience conspicuous neurological symptoms, most commonly visual in nature, during the prodromal phase. Migraineurs experiencing such prodromes are termed "classic," whereas migraines occurring in the absence of prodromes are termed "common" (Diamond & Dalessio, 1982). This distinction appears to have little value for predicting treatment response, however, so most investigators ignore it.

Migraine is attributed to a two-phase vascular process: intra- and extra-cranial vasoconstriction prior to the headache (which in its severe form produces the neurological prodromes), followed by a reactive vasodilitation which produces the throbbing headache pain. A number of biochemical events accompany these changes in peripheral vascular tone, and it is unclear whether these biochemical changes are primary or secondary to the disorder (Kudrow, 1983).

In contrast to migraine, tension (or muscle contraction, psychogenic, or depressive) headache has a more insidious onset and resolution and is experienced as a dull, steady bilateral or band-like pain or ache. The pain is less intense than that of a migraine, but many individuals experience this type of headache on a daily basis. Pain presumably results

*Preparation of this chapter was supported by Research Career Development Award 1 K04 NS00818 from the National Institute of Neurological and Communicative Disorders and Stroke (NINCDS).

from sustained contractions of skeletal muscles occurring as a response to life stress (Ad Hoc Committee on the Classification of Headache, 1962) and is attributed to stimulation of pain receptors in the contracted muscles and ischemia produced by compression of intramuscular arterioles (Haynes, 1980). One fifth to one third of all headache sufferers may experience both types of headache. These mixed or combined headache types are assumed to result from both vascular and musculoskeletal aberrations.

The above accounts, however, are not universally accepted and are the source of two controversies at present. The first concerns whether migraine is more correctly viewed as a central rather than a peripheral disorder (Olesen, Lauritzen, Tfelt-Hansen, Henriksen, & Larsen, 1982; Sicuteri, 1982). The second questions whether the etiologies of migraine and tension headaches are really qualitatively different. Symptom overlap and commonalities among certain biochemical and psychophysiological events have led some to speculate that migraine and tension headaches may both result from the same underlying cause. This view places tension and migraine on the same etiological continuum and attributes all differences merely to severity of involvement (e.g., Bakal, 1982). Lacking definitive data, most researchers continue to distinguish between these two headache types and to tailor their treatments accordingly.

Until the mid 1960s, pharmacological and related medical procedures were the only legitimate forms of treatment available to the recurrent headache sufferer. Around this time it was discovered at the Menninger Clinic in Topeka, Kansas, that a marked increase in hand temperature accompanied cessation of migraine headache. Researchers at this clinic then began to pilot-test ways to teach individuals to increase their hand temperatures as a method for combating migraine. They added certain features of autogenic therapy (Schultz & Luthe, 1969) and referred to this combination of thermal biofeedback and autogenic therapy as "autogenic feedback" (Sargent, Green, & Walters, 1972, 1973; Sargent, Walters, & Green, 1973).

A continuing puzzle for researchers is how this handwarming leads to improvement in migraine activity. Blood flow through the peripheral vasculature of the hands and fingers is the major means by which these structures become warmed. Blood flow may be increased, and the skin surface become warmer, either by the heart beating faster or the tiny arterioles and capillaries becoming dilated. Tentative evidence suggests the latter may be the chief mechanism of action (Sovak, Kunzel, Sternbach, & Dalessio, 1981). Constriction of the peripheral blood vessels is under control of the sympathetic nervous system, and a decrease in sympathetic tone is necessary for peripheral dilitation to occur. Thus, it is speculated that thermal biofeedback may be an indirect way to teach patients to reduce "sympathetic outflow" and, as such, may be useful both for prophylaxis and for abortion of migraine. This interpretation suggests further that thermal biofeedback may be a multipurpose relaxation procedure with application to any disorder linked to increased arousal of the sympathetic nervous system.

In the late 60s and early 70s another group of researchers was developing a biofeedback treatment for tension headache. Here, the treatment application evolved from a more logical theoretical rationale. Budzynski, Stoyva, and colleagues (1970, 1973) reasoned that if sustained contractions of scalp and skeletal muscles produced tension headache, then teaching individuals ways directly to reduce or prevent these contractions would result in alleviation of headache symptoms. The procedure they developed, which involves monitoring tension levels in forehead muscles and providing feedback to enable patients to lower these tension levels (via a tone that decreases in rate or pitch as the muscles relax), has become what many term the biofeedback treatment of choice for tension headache. Stoyva and Budzynski (1974) speculate that frontal/forehead EMG biofeedback produces an overall state of relaxation, which they term "cultivated low arousal," but research suggests that this type of generalized relaxation is unlikely to occur (Thompson, Haber, & Tearnan, 1981).

Publication of these early successful reports of biofeedback subsequently led researchers to speculate that relaxation training might serve similar treatment functions. Preliminary studies concerning several different relaxation treatments (both active forms, such as progressive muscle relaxation training, and passive forms, such as meditation and autogenic therapy by itself) reported similar positive results. In contrast to biofeedback treatments, which sought to produce changes in specific response system, relaxation therapies sought to produce changes in overall physiological arousal. It was not long before researchers began to pit biofeedback and relaxation procedures against one another.

An extensive body of literature now exists on the outcome effectiveness of these two types of treatments, but space limitations preclude a detailed examination of this literature. However, a "meta-analysis" of this literature does allow a quick statistical comparison across studies. In a meta-analysis, the outcome for an entire group of patients receiving a common treatment becomes the unit of analysis. Hence, it is an analysis of results from studies rather than from individual subjects.

Outcomes averaged across available studies employing relaxation, biofeedback, combinations of both, and various psychological and pharmacological placebos are summarized in Table 13.1 (Blanchard & Andrasik, 1982). For tension headache, biofeedback, relaxation, and the combination of both yielded significant improvements for nearly two thirds of the patients studied, which was double the rate for placebo treatments, which were in turn superior to symptom monitoring alone. For migraine headache, autogenic feedback and relaxation treatment produced the superior outcomes; although not statistically significant, the arithmetic difference between these two procedures is sizeable (17%). Thermal biofeedback by itself was not all that efficacious; the augmenting effects of autogenic therapy seem especially helpful. Table 13.1 references an additional biofeedback treatment procedure for migraine headache, vasomotor biofeedback. In this procedure individuals are taught to constrict blood flow in the temporal

artery so they can use this skill as a means for aborting migraine. This treatment remains somewhat experimental, and the instrumentation for its use is rather complex; it will not be discussed further.

With this serving in the way of an introduction, let us turn to assessment of the headache patient.

ASSESSMENT OF THE HEADACHE PATIENT

You open your practice for psychological treatment of headache, and on the first day, four different patients contact you for treatment.

The first patient is 60 years old and reports experiencing rather intense headaches over the past few months. The headaches are unilateral, always occurring on the same side. The patient reports that a tingling sensation and possibly a slight weakness in the extremities precede the onset of most headaches. The patient reports a marked increase in stress factors in her life, noting in particular an increase in the number of arguments with her children about the need for her to move to a more supervised living arrangement, increased concerns about her ability to pay several bills, and increased "upset" as she approaches the third anniversary of the loss of her husband. The patient reports headaches have always been "a part of my life," but previously she did not view them as warranting any type of treatment other than occasional over-the-counter preparations. A friend of hers speculated the headaches were a result of increased stress and suggested she see you.

The second patient is a 52-year-old male who first began to experience severe headaches approximately 6 years ago. He reports a somewhat peculiar pattern to his headaches. They come in bouts lasting 5 to 6 weeks, on roughly an annual basis, and within a bout the headaches are quite frequent, of excruciating intensity, but of brief duration. For most of the year, the patient reports that he is essentially headache-free. He has just entered what he terms his "terrible headache period."

The third patient is a young female who

TABLE 13.1. META-ANALYSES OF NONPHARMACOLOGICAL TREATMENTS AND NONPHARMACOLOGICAL AND PHARMACOLOGICAL PLACEBOS

Tension Headache

Frontal EMG Biofeedback Alone (N = 12)	Relaxation Training Alone (N = 9)	Biofeedback and Relaxation (N = 6)	Nonpharmacological Placebo (N = 7)	Pharmacological Placebo (N = 8)	Symptom Monitoring Only (N = 6)
60.9%	59.2%	58.8%	35.3%	34.8%	−4.5%

Migraine Headache

Autogenic Feedback (N = 11)	Relaxation Training Alone (N = 7)	Vasomotor Biofeedback Alone (N = 4)	Thermal Biofeedback Alone (N = 7)	Nonpharmacological Placebo (N = 5)	Symptom Monitoring Only (N = 6)	Pharmacological Placebo (N = 6)
64.9%	47.9%	42.3%	34.6%	27.6%	17.2%	16.5%

Note. Groups that share an underline do not differ at the .05 level.

began to experience what she terms "sick" headaches in high school. At first her headaches occurred infrequently (one to two times per month), but typically lasted an entire day and often continued into the next day. During the headaches she became very nauseated and often vomited. The headaches interfered with her ability to work, so she would stay home and retire to her bedroom, being careful to avoid any bright lights. Her physician prescribed ergotamine tartrate, a potent vasoconstrictor, for her to use in aborting her headaches. She also found it necessary to consume large quantities of Tylenol to combat her pain. Her headaches typically came during the weekend, which resulted in her missing valued social functions. Her headaches have gradually been increasing in frequency, and at the time of her appointment headaches were a near daily phenomenon for her. At this point ergotamine and Tylenol were being taken on a daily basis, with Fiorinal taken "as needed."

The fourth patient presenting to your practice struck you from the start as being rather lethargic and unmotivated. This person suffers from chronic, low-grade, continuous headache.

Let's review each patient in further detail as each illustrates an important point you need to be aware of when conducting your assessment.

Importance of Medical Consultation and Collaboration

It is rare for organic pathology to produce symptoms consistent in appearance to migraine or tension headache, but no nonmedical professional wants to be administering relaxation treatment to a patient who, for example, has a brain tumor. We require every headache sufferer to be evaluated by a physician who has special expertise in the area of headache, even though the base rates for underlying organic or other medical problems have been low in our research setting (1 to 2%). It goes beyond the scope of this chapter to discuss the types of evaluations that are necessary and the types of complicating medical factors. As a way of brief illustration, the first patient you saw in your office may have had a stroke, possess a vascular malformation or vascular insufficiency, or have a condition known as temporal arteritis. The nonmedical professional needs to remain continuously alert for any dramatic change in the presentation of the patient's headache and to treat this as cause for a repeat medical consultation. A neurologist working in our setting (Lawrence D. Rodichok, M.D.) has prepared a list of danger signs and symptoms that are indicative of the need for an immediate medical referral. These are contained in Table 13.2.

Diagnosis of Headache Type

Most researchers and practitioners base their selection of biofeedback treatment on the particular diagnosis of headache type. Results from three investigations of the efficacy of EMG biofeedback for migraine revealed improvements ranging only from 26% to 36%, which supports this practice. A recent investigation (Daly, Donn, Galliher, & Zimmerman, 1983), however, found EMG and thermal biofeedback to be highly effective and equivalent for both types of headaches. The notion that one needs a specific biofeedback treatment for a specific headache type may be modified in the future.

Diamond and Dalessio (1982) and Lance (1978) provide comprehensive descriptions of how one should conduct a headache history, which is all-important to diagnosis. Their presentations include frameworks for organizing the information obtained and illustrative examples, which are especially helpful to the practitioner just becoming familiar with headache assessment. Features critical to the diagnosis concern mode of onset and termination of headache, laterality of symptoms, nature of the pain, prodromal features, and accompanying symptoms. In our research, we have used the criteria provided in Table 13.3 for arriving at a specific diagnosis. Employing these criteria, we have found a perfect agreement rate of approximately 85% when comparing independent diagnoses made by doctoral students working in our laboratory and by consulting board certified neurol-

TABLE 13.2. "DANGER SIGNS" FOR HEADACHE PATIENTS REQUIRING IMMEDIATE REFERRAL

1. Headache is a new symptom for the individual in the past 3 months or the nature of the headache has changed markedly in the past 3 months.
2. There are sensory or motor deficits preceding or accompanying the headache other than the typical visual prodromata of classic migraine (e.g., weakness or numbness in an extremity, twitching of the hands or feet, aphasia, or slurred speech).
3. Headache is one-sided and has always been on the same side of the head.
4. Headache is due to trauma, especially if it followed a period of unconsciousness (even if only momentary).
5. Headache is constant and unremitting.
6. For a patient reporting tension headache-like symptoms:
   a. Pain intensity has been steadily increasing over a period of weeks to months with little or no relief.
   b. Headache is worse in the morning and becomes less severe during the day.
   c. Headache is accompanied by vomiting.
7. Patient has been treated for any kind of cancer and now has a complaint of headache.
8. Patient or significant other reports a noticeable change in personality or behavior or a notable decrease in memory or other intellectual functioning.
9. The patient is over 60 years of age, and the headache is a relatively new complaint.
10. Pain onset is sudden and occurs during conditions of exertion such as lifting heavy objects, sexual intercourse, or "heated" interpersonal situations.
11. Patient's family has a history of cerebral aneurysm, other vascular anomalies, or polycystic kidneys.

ogists (Blanchard, O'Keefe, Neff, Jurish, & Andrasik, 1981).

Let's return to Patient 2. Inspection of the criteria listed in Table 13.3 reveals that Patient 2 is experiencing a migraine variant known as cluster headache. Cluster headache is extremely rare and is the only functional headache with a greater prevalence among males (males outnumber females in this case approximately 4 to 1; with other forms of headache the ratio is 2 or 3 to 1 in favor of females). Cluster headache may be the most painful of all types of headaches. Patients have been known to become extremely agitated during cluster bouts and to beat upon

TABLE 13.3 CRITERIA FOR DIAGNOSING HEADACHE

Headache Type	Key Symptoms	Number Required for Definite Diagnosis
Migraine	1. Headache onset usually unilateral 2. Headache usually accompanied by nausea and vomiting 3. Headache usually described as throbbing or pulsating 4. Photophobia during headache 5. One or more first-degree relatives diagnosed as migraine 6. Independent diagnosis of migraine 7. Headache usually preceded by (a) visual changes, (b) hemiparesthesias, (c) transient hemiparesis, or (d) noticeable speech difficulty	Presence of 3 of the 7 Presence of item 7 denotes classic migraine
Cluster	1. Headaches occur in bouts that last several weeks and are separated by 3 or more months 2. During a bout headaches are of brief duration (less than 2 hours) and are present at least once every 2 days	Presence of 3 of the above 7 for migraine plus presence of both items 1 and 2
Tension	1. Headache usually described as bilateral and beginning in the occipital, suboccipital, or back of the neck region 2. Headache described as usually feeling like a tightness or external pressure on head and/or like a "cap" or "band" around the head 3. Headache usually described as a continuing "dull ache" 4. Independent diagnosis of muscle contraction headache	Presence of 2 of the 4
Combined Migraine and Tension	1. Patient clearly identifies that he or she has two distinct types of headache 2. Subject meets criteria for both migraine and tension headache	Presence of both items

Adapted from "Psychological functioning in headache sufferers" by F. Andrasik, E.B. Blanchard, J.G. Arena, S.J. Teders, R.C. Teevan, and L.D. Rodichok, *Psychosomatic Medicine*, *44*, pp. 172–173.

their heads; some suicides have even been attributed to cluster headache.

There is disagreement among medical authorities whether cluster is in fact a variant of migraine or whether it represents an independent primary headache disorder (Kudrow, 1980). Although the "garden variety" cluster headache occurs in bouts of brief duration, individuals can experience "chronic" cluster headache wherein bouts continue for a full year or so.

In our early work we treated 11 patients with episodic cluster headaches by a combination of progressive relaxation training and thermal biofeedback (Blanchard, Andrasik, Jurish, & Teders, 1982). Four patients were early dropouts. Of the seven completing treatment, only three reported any improvement when their next cluster bout occurred, and these improvements were slight. No patient reported marked improvement, and one deteriorated during treatment. Until our technologies improve, the practitioner is advised to have cluster headache ruled out and to refer these patients to a physician for planning the first line of treatment. The nonmedical practitioner, however, may be able to fulfill an adjunctive role by helping the patient to cope better with headache-related distress and by possibly administering relaxation or biofeedback as a palliative procedure.

There is one other type of headache the practitioner should seek to rule out—menstrual migraine headache. Solbach, Sargent, and Coyne (1984) carefully evaluated the efficacy of biofeedback and relaxation treatments for women experiencing menstrual migraine, defined as a migraine occurring any time during menstrual flow or within 3 days prior to or 3 days following cessation of flow. None of the behavioral treatments led to improvement that exceeded a no-treatment control condition. These authors (and others) argued that menstrual migraine, just like cluster headache, should be recognized and treated as a distinct migraine entity. Medical practitioners again should have responsibility for designing the treatment of choice; any effort of yours should be secondary or adjunctive.

When assessing the female patient it is also important to inquire about use of oral contraceptives and to see if headache onset is correlated with initiation or changing dosage of oral contraceptives. Estimates of oral contraceptive-induced headache vary from 29% to 60% depending on the proportion and type of estrogen and progesterone used in the preparation. The author's wife, an individual who previously was essentially headache-free, began to experience intense migraine headaches shortly after beginning oral contraceptives; the headaches presented in a textbook form of migraine. Her headaches stopped completely by switching to a different concentration of oral contraceptives.

A host of other substances that people in-

gest or encounter in their environment have been identified as precipitants of migraine. The interested reader is referred to Raskin and Appenzeller (1980) for further discussion of this point and to Diamond and Dalessio (1982) for a listing of foods likely to trigger migraine.

Medication Abuse

Emerging evidence suggests that some of the medications routinely taken by headache patients can, if taken in sufficient dosages for extended periods of time, actually begin to induce headaches, termed "rebound" headaches. Uncontrolled use of analgesics, for example, can even compromise outcome of what would otherwise have been an effective treatment (Kudrow, 1982). Patient 3 is fairly prototypical of the medication abuser. These individuals typically start out having infrequent but very intense migraine headaches. Over time, they begin to anticipate headache onset and self-administer medications in an attempt to prevent these suspected attacks. It is not too long before these individuals are consuming high levels of medication on a daily basis.

Kudrow (1982) speculates that frequent use of analgesics, for example, may sustain pain by suppressing central serotonergic pathways concerned with the regulation of dull pain. With such cases, treatment of choice would involve elimination of all analgesics. This request is easily made, but not easily followed. The analgesic abuser has often exhausted all other medical treatments and may be reluctant to give up the current medication, even though the individual realizes it is not optimal for him or her. One approach is to have the patient eliminate analgesics in a gradual manner while you provide a concurrent course of relaxation or biofeedback. This approach was used by the author (Andrasik, in press) in treating a tension headache patient who regularly consumed 40+ extra-strength Tylenol and 20+ Coricidine-D tablets each week. Kudrow's preliminary data suggest that a sizeable number of patients may become markedly improved following withdrawal from analgesics alone. Such was the case for Patient 3 described earlier; no further treatment was needed.

Patients undergoing analgesic withdrawal may experience an intense rebound headache later on. They need to be advised of this possibility so they won't falsely interpret this as indicating their medication needs to be resumed. Some patients find it impossible to be detoxified as an outpatient and may require a brief inpatient stay to accomplish this goal.

In a related fashion, Ala-Hurula, Myllyla, and Hokkanen (1982) report that overusage of the abortive treatment of choice for migraine, ergotamine tartrate, can also serve to maintain headache. These authors reported ergotamine-rebound headache occurred in patients taking dosages as small as 0.5 to 1.0 mg per day. Again, relatively severe withdrawal symptoms similar to migraine occurred upon discontinuation of daily use. All of this again points to the importance of a close working relationship with physicians when seeing individuals with chronic headache.

Preliminary evidence suggests that two other medications commonly administered to headache patients can be disruptive to biofeedback therapy. Jay, Renelli, and Mead (1984) report that regular use of propranolol impeded the progress of patients undergoing thermal biofeedback while amitriptyline impeded the progress of patients receiving EMG biofeedback. All patients were able to reach the established training criteria, but with significantly greater difficulty and increased frustration. Informing patients about the potential interference effects of these medications may minimize frustration and patient lapses in motivation.

Psychological Factors

Depression and headache have a strong association. Not only are chronic headache sufferers frequently depressed, but headache is the most frequent somatic symptom of depression occurring in over 50% of depressed patients (Davis, Wetzel, Kashiwagi, & McClure, 1976; Diamond, 1983; Kudrow, 1976; Ziegler, Rhodes, & Hassanein, 1978). One assessment task for the practitioner is to determine whether the depression preceded the headache and is thus causing or increasing the patient's vulnerability to headache (Luborsky, Docherty, & Penick, 1973) or is more a result of living with chronic pain. We routinely conduct a mental status exam with headache patients to rule out preexisting psychopathology, which may compromise behavioral self-regulatory treatments, and delay or adjust the behavioral treatment as necessary. Preliminary evidence suggests that behavioral treatments can result in concomitant decreases in depression (Cox & Thomas, 1981), but increased scores on measures of depression have also been prognostic of a poor response to behavioral treatment. (See Blanchard & Andrasik, 1982.) The practitioner is advised to proceed cautiously with patients in this category; Patient 4 is a case in point.

EVALUATION OF RESPONSE TO TREATMENT

Regardless of the particular treatment, the therapist will want the patient to collect some type of data that will permit an evaluation of treatment. Daily recordings of pain intensity have become the "gold standard," and the practitioner is advised to incorporate a similar type measure. Early investigations required patients to make hourly ratings of headache, but most investigators now shy away from this effort-intensive procedure, believing it occasions excessive noncompliance. Most investigators now ask subjects to rate their headache intensities at four highly discriminable times during the day: at the three mealtimes plus immediately prior to bedtime. Ratings are made on a 6-point intensity scale that ranges from 0, which represents no headache, to 5, which represents a headache of extreme pain, such that it clearly interferes with the individual's ability to work or recreate and may even require confinement to bed. Data collected in this manner can be summarized in a variety of ways including (a) a weekly sum of the 28 separate ratings (4 ratings per day times 7 days); (b) a recording of the peak intensity rating for a given week (to determine whether "the edge" is being taken off of the headaches); or (c) the number of recording periods the individual indicated a headache of any intensity (which is similar to a frequency measure).

Although this type of diary recording procedure has reduced demands for subjects, it does not enable the therapist to obtain a true measure of frequency or duration of headache activity. If either of these are of prime interest to the therapist, then the diary recording format will have to be altered. Chronic, near daily headache lends itself quite nicely to the four ratings per day format, whereas the clinician might want to make alterations for individuals with infrequent but intense, prolonged migraine headache. In the latter case the therapist may want the patient to make ratings repeatedly throughout an attack or, alternatively, to note the time of onset and offset and then perform a single rating of peak headache intensity. This would allow the therapist to keep track of frequency as well as duration and to monitor headache intensity as well. We are using this latter procedure in an investigation of self-regulatory treatments for children who have migraine.

It may be sufficient for the practitioner to have the patient perform only one rating of headache activity per day. The question then becomes when is the best time for collecting this measure. Intuitively, it may seem that the end of the day would be the best. Data we collected from individuals working in our laboratory, however, revealed that ratings made at bedtime were the ones most often forgot, while ratings made upon awakening were performed most consistently.

A number of alternative measurement procedures are being pilot-tested in the experimental literature at present, and two may be of value to the practitioner. The first concerns what has been termed "social validation" of response to treatment. In one investigation (Blanchard, Andrasik, Neff, Jurish, &

O'Keefe, 1981), significant others were asked to provide an independent estimate of a patient's improvement by placing a mark on a 100-mm "visual analog scale" anchored at one end, "the patient is unchanged," and at the other, "the patient is extremely improved/completely cured." Data obtained in this manner correlated modestly ($r = .44$) with actual diary measures, suggesting some usefulness to this procedure. When the line of best fit was plotted for the data, it was noted to intercept the y axis somewhat above the 0 value. We interpreted this to indicate that the significant other report has a slight positive bias or tends to overestimate patient improvement by as much as 30%. Practitioners using this type of assessment device need to be mindful of this point.

Second, most investigators note that headache pain (and other pain as well) is experienced in multidimensional fashion. The diary procedure mentioned earlier seems to assess only one of these dimensions, that termed the intensity or sensory dimension (Andrasik, Blanchard, Ahles, Pallmeyer, & Rodichok, 1982). The diary does not appear to be well suited for assessing the reactive or affective dimension of pain or how the pain affects the patient psychologically or emotionally. It is not uncommon for a patient whose diary reports of pain intensity reveal essentially no improvement later to report great satisfaction with treatment: "My headache hurts about as much as it used to, but I don't let it bother me as much anymore. I feel like I'm better able to cope with it or put it out of my mind since treatment." What seems to be happening in this case is that the reactivity/affectivity dimension is changing, in a manner that does not correspond to the sensory/intensity dimension.

We piloted a procedure for assessing both dimensions with headache patients (Andrasik et al., 1982), but this particular procedure is too involved to be of ready use to the busy practitioner. (The procedure involves an elaborate cross-modality psychophysical scaling procedure.) In research with chronic pain patients, Price, McGrath, Rafii, and Buckingham (1983) have pilot-tested a visual analog procedure for assessing these two separate aspects of pain. This could be adapted to headache patients and could be completed fairly easily at various times during the day. In this procedure the two scales are anchored as follows: "no sensation" and "the most intense sensation imaginable" for the sensory aspect of pain and "not bad at all" and "the most intense bad feeling possible for me" for the affective dimension of pain.

TREATMENT OF THE HEADACHE PATIENT

You have learned from a consulting physician that the patient's headaches are devoid of an organic component, completed your assessment, arrived at a diagnosis, and are now ready to begin treatment. How do you decide whether to use biofeedback or relaxation? Here, unfortunately, the empirical literature is unhelpful. Researchers have speculated that certain psychophysiological and psychological profiles might be predictive of response to a particular treatment, but none of the available evidence clearly supports these claims.

Psychophysiological profiling has a great deal of face validity and appeal. Essentially, this involves recording multiple psychophysiological modalities (in this case, forehead or neck muscle tension and hand temperature) and studying these parameters under various conditions of rest and simulated stress. The practitioner identifies the response system that is the most reactive and targets it for treatment. The problem with this approach is that there is, as yet, no clear psychophysiological marker of either type of headache that we can detect with available equipment. Reports on psychological variables predicting response to specific treatment modalities are few in number, and all lack cross-validation, rendering their utility uncertain.

Another view considers this question rather trivial and argues that the two procedures may only be different means to the same end; relaxation and biofeedback are simply just two different ways to achieve relaxation, with relaxation being the "shot gun" approach and biofeedback being the "rifle" approach. Some adherents of this view have gone so far as to conclude that biofeedback machines can be "thrown away"—If relaxation and biofeedback are one and the same, why not use the least expensive, least technological treatment?

The conclusion about equivalence of outcome for relaxation and biofeedback therapy is based on faulty logic. Equivalent outcomes can occur for two very different reasons. The treatments can be truly equivalent, meaning a given patient would respond equally well to either. Alternatively, patients of one type could be responding successfully to relaxation, patients of a second type could be responding successfully to biofeedback, and it could just happen that the response rates are nearly equivalent. In other words, group comparison studies have failed to take into account individual differences in responsiveness to the treatments.

A study conducted in our laboratory attempted to address the issue of differential responsiveness to treatment by first giving all headache subjects, regardless of diagnosis, a course of relaxation training, with biofeedback provided as a second treatment for any individual who failed to respond to relaxation. If the procedures were indeed truly equivalent, then no additional benefit would be expected from biofeedback. If the treatments operated in a different manner for certain people, then one might expect a certain proportion of the relaxation failures to respond to biofeedback; and that is what was found. Thirty-six percent of tension headache sufferers and 44% of vascular headache sufferers who were unresponsive to relaxation therapy became treatment successes after biofeedback treatment (Blanchard, Andrasik, Neff et al., 1982). Heightened levels of baseline headache activity and increased scores on scales measuring depression and anxiety were associated with continued failure to respond to treatment. We thought it unwise to continue a subset of the patients in relaxation therapy after they had failed initially, even though this is important from an experimental perspective. While this decision places certain limitations on this study, the data suggest that relaxation and biofeedback may not be interchangeable, but rather may offer different advantages for different subsets of patients.

The above findings suggest three things for the practitioner. First, choice of initial treatment probably still defaults to issues of practicality, patient preference, and/or therapist preference. Relaxation procedures probably win out due to their greater versatility, absence of additional costs for equipment, and amenability to group administration; some believe they may facilitate transfer to the natural environment more readily because they do not rely on external equipment. Also, relaxation is efficacious for a large proportion of individuals. Second, the practitioner should not give up on the patient who has failed to respond to a "good shot" of relaxation therapy; additional treatment in the form of biofeedback may well be worthwhile. Third, if feasible, the practitioner might want to offer patients the combination of both treatments. In our research laboratory, treatments are administered sequentially in order to minimize confusing patients and to permit us to evaluate issues related to process and outcome in a somewhat uncontaminated fashion. There is no evidence to suggest that a sequential administration is any different or more effective than a concurrent administration. One could just as readily follow a concurrent course of relaxation and biofeedback, seeking to optimize advantages of each.

Patient Education

As in all forms of therapy, treatment begins with an educational component designed to: (a) provide information about the etiology of headache (some of which will already have been discussed with your patient); (b) combat the demoralization and depression frequently associated with chronic headache; (c) convey to the patient that the self-regulatory nature of your treatment requires him or her to take an active role in managing headaches; and (d) explain what is involved in treatment. Many patients will arrive at your doorstep as a "last resort" and may possess a number of dysfunctional beliefs, such as their headache is due to some global personal inadequacy of theirs or is an inevitable response to overwhelming stress. A nontechnical discussion of etiology and precipitants of headache, which emphasizes features that can be controlled by the patient, is often helpful in combating feelings of helplessness and remobilizing or enhancing the patient's expectancies for improvement. Patients seeking medical care for their headaches claim their major aim is to receive an explanation for what is causing their headaches (Packard, 1979). In some cases, enhanced understanding of headache may itself lead to measurable improvement.

Holroyd and Andrasik (1982) describe a case wherein education alone led to significant improvement because it disconfirmed some long-held beliefs of the patient:

> Prior to seeking help for her headaches Ms. B had received 3 years of psychoanalytic psychotherapy for other adjustment problems. For 12 years she had monthly migraine attacks that appeared to be associated with menstruation, as well as less regular attacks she said occurred when she was pressured or depressed. During the presentation of didactic information about headache she responded with obvious relief. When she was questioned . . . she reported she had regarded the continued occurrence of headache as a sign that she had failed to manage her life differently than her mother who also suffered from migraine. She experienced relief when she realized her susceptibility to migraine might be genetic and not an indication that she had failed in her efforts at personal growth. Following this interview she recorded no headaches for 6 months. At the 6-month follow-up she attributed the relief of her headache symptoms entirely to the increased sense of well being and confidence this information about headaches had provided. (p. 301)

Education is an integral part of treatment, beginning at the start and essentially continuing throughout treatment as the patient

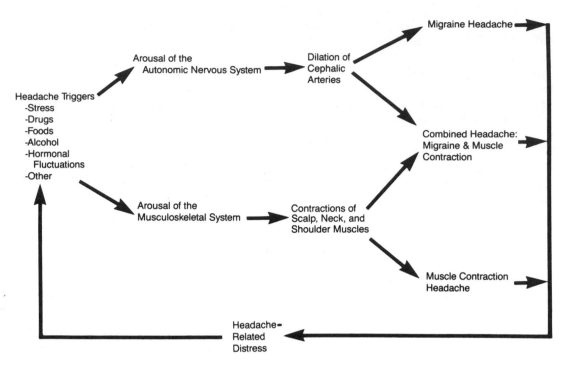

Figure 13.1. Factors Causing Headache.

begins to discover more about causes of headache and learn more about ways to manage symptoms.

In the didactic presentation, particular emphasis is placed on headache as a response to stress. Individuals who are "less psychologically minded" sometimes have difficulty accepting this model; and for these individuals it is emphasized that the experience of chronic, unremitting headache often becomes a source of stress itself and thus serves to exacerbate or maintain headache. In either case, it is explained that relaxation and biofeedback treatments are physical procedures designed to reduce the stress response and to short-circuit the physiological arousal producing headache. Reviewing a diagram like the one in Figure 13.1 can be helpful during the educational phase. It is helpful as well for the therapist to divulge his or her own "stress response" and to point out ways that he or she uses acquired relaxation skills as a means of coping with stress.

Having explained the etiology of headache, it is time to review what treatment entails.

Relaxation Treatment Procedure

The following is a verbatim transcript of what is typically said to patients at the start of relaxation treatment:

Therapist: Relaxation training consists of the systematic tensing and relaxing of the major muscle groups of the whole body. After going through this series of tension-release exercises or cycles, most people feel relaxed. With practice, one can learn to become deeply relaxed fairly rapidly.

It has been shown in numerous clinics and laboratories that teaching people to relax in general can have a very beneficial effect on headaches like yours.

Achieving a state of deep relaxation is a learned skill, somewhat like learning to ride a bicycle. To be really effective, one must practice regularly. Also, as you practice, you should begin to be more aware of the tension in your body, to be able to recognize it earlier, and to localize it so that it becomes something you can more readily cope with.

For this training to be of the most benefit

TABLE 13.4. OUTLINE OF RELAXATION TRAINING PROGRAM

		Content						
Week	Session	Introduction & Treatment Rationale	Number of Muscle Groups	Deepening Exercises	Breathing Exercises	Relaxing Imagery	Muscle Discrim- ination Training	Relaxation by Recall	Cue- Controlled Relaxation
1	1	X	14	X	X				
	2		14	X	X	X			
2	3		14	X	X	X	X		
	4		14	X	X	X	X		
3	5		8	X	X	X	X		
	6		8	X	X	X	X	X	
4	7		4	X	X	X	X	X	
5	8		4	X	X	X	X	X	X
6	9		4	X	X	X	X	X	X
7	None								
8	10		4	X	X	X	X	X	X

to you, you should go through the exercises for about 20 minutes, twice per day. If you cannot find time for two practices per day, one is acceptable but not as good as twice per day. If you cannot, or will not, practice regularly, then you probably will not receive the major benefits of the training. Questions?

Migraine Patient: How does relaxing my muscles affect my headache?

Therapist: Learning to relax specific muscles over time leads to a lower overall state of arousal. This in turn starts to relax that part of your nervous system causing your headache problem.

A variety of relaxation approaches have been used with headache sufferers ranging from simple, passive meditation as described by Benson (1975) in the book *The Relaxation Response*, to more active, involved forms embodying portions of Jacobson's (1938) progressive relaxation procedure. The procedure we use in our work with patients draws heavily from Bernstein and Borkovec's (1973) adaptation of Jacobson's procedure. We have evolved a fairly standard protocol which involves administration of 10 individual sessions spaced over an 8-week period. Spacing of procedures as well as content of each session are summarized in Table 13.4.

Having explained the procedure to the patient, it is now time to review specifics of what is involved. The procedure begins with sequential tension and relaxation cycles of 14 separate muscle groupings in 18 separate steps:

1. Right hand and lower arm (by having the patient make a fist and simultaneously tense the lower arm)
2. Left hand and lower arm
3. Both hands and lower arms
4. Right upper arm (by having the patient bring his/her hand to the shoulder and tense the bicep)
5. Left upper arm
6. Both upper arms
7. Right lower leg and foot (by having the patient point his/her toe and tensing the calf muscles)
8. Left lower leg and foot
9. Both lower legs and feet
10. Both thighs (by pressing the knees and thighs tightly together)
11. Abdomen (draw the abdominal muscles in tightly)
12. Chest (by having the patient take a deep breath and holding it)
13. Shoulders and lower neck (by having the patient "hunch" his/her shoulders or draw his/her shoulders towards the ears)
14. Back of the neck (have the patient press

head backwards against a headrest or chair)

15. Lips (by pressing them together very tightly but not clenching the teeth)
16. Eyes (by closing the eyes tightly)
17. Lower forehead (by having the patient frown and draw the eyebrows together)
18. Upper forehead (by having the patient wrinkle the forehead area)

Before actually administering treatment it is helpful to have the patient engage in a few practice tension-release cycles. Typical problems that occur at this time are incomplete tensing, overzealous tensing, or tensing adjacent muscles as well as the target group at the same time. The patient needs to learn to tense just the muscle being targeted at the moment and then to relax it completely when the tension cycle is completed. You might have the patient hold his or her arm straight out while tense and then let it drop when relaxed with you catching it to illustrate this point. Before proceeding, ask if the patient has ever experienced pain or strain in any particular muscle group; if so, omit this muscle group from the training sequence. Instruct the patient to tense the muscle group anywhere from 5 to 10 seconds, and during this to attend specifically to the sensations of tension in that particular muscle group and area of the body. Instruct the patient to notice the particular sensations when the muscle tension is stopped by comparing it to the tension state. Thus, a critical component involves learning to discriminate various tension states.

When you instruct the patient to begin a tension cycle, instructions like the following are used:

> Now I want you to tense the muscles in your
> _____ . Go ahead, make it tight—
> make it tight, feel the tension, feel the tightness, pay attention to the tightness. Now, I want you to relax your muscles, let them completely relax, notice the relaxed feeling you have in your muscles, notice that they are beginning to feel a little heavy and a little bit warm.

Some therapists feel it is helpful to continue this "relaxation banter" during the 20 to 30 seconds in between tension cycles by drawing the patient's attention to feelings of relaxation radiating through the body, feelings of warmth, feeling of heaviness, etc. The therapist continues in this manner until every muscle group has been tensed and relaxed.

At this point it often is helpful to have the patient scan through every muscle group in the instructed order to see whether any group contains residual tension. This can be accomplished by you verbally reviewing each muscle group and having the subject signal if the group is still tense by raising a finger. If so, have the patient readminister a tension and release cycle to that muscle grouping.

Once completed, we have the patient engage in a deepening exercise. Verbatim instructions include:

> Now I want you to relax all the muscles of your body; just let them become more and more relaxed. I'm going to help you to achieve a deeper state of relaxation by counting from one to five. As I count you will feel yourself becoming more and more deeply relaxed; . . . farther and farther down into a deep restful state of deep relaxation. One . . . you are becoming more deeply relaxed. Two . . . down, down into a very relaxed state. Three . . . Four . . . more and more relaxed . . . Five. Deeply relaxed.

Once the deepening suggestions have been administered, then instruct the person to breathe slowly, deeply, and evenly through the nose and concentrate on breathing with each inhalation and exhalation. Finally, tell the patient to begin to say the word "relax" with each exhalation. Allow 1 to 2 minutes for this focus on breathing and repeat the instructions at least one additional time. Verbatim instructions include:

> I want you to remain in your very relaxed state . . . I want you to begin to attend just to your breathing. Breathe through your nose; slowly, deeply, and evenly. Notice the cool air as you breath in . . . and the warm moist air as you exhale . . . Just continue to attend to your breathing . . . Now each

time you exhale, mentally repeat the word relax: inhale, exhale, relax . . . inhale, exhale, relax . . . Continue this for a couple of minutes.

Now it is time to alert the patient, and this should be done in a gradual manner. Verbatim instructions include:

Now I am going to help you return to your state of alertness. In a little while, I will begin counting backwards from five to one. You will gradually become more alert. When I reach two, I want you to open your eyes. When I get to one, you will be entirely aroused up in your normal state of alertness. Ready now? Five . . . Four . . . You're becoming more and more alert. You feel very refreshed . . . Three . . . Two . . . Now your eyes are open and you begin to feel very alert. Returning completely to your normal state . . . One.

Discuss with the patient how this particular session was experienced, noting any particular problems or adjustments that you will need to make for the next session. Remind the patient to practice at home; and, if you like, you may ask the patient to make a rating on each relaxation practice session which indicates how deeply relaxed they became (say on a scale from 1 to 10).

In subsequent sessions, the number of tension and release cycles is gradually reduced and additional procedures are added in order to make relaxation a more portable, readily used coping procedure for dampening physiological arousal. In Session 2, the only new twist is to teach the patient how to imagine a peaceful/tranquil situation to serve as an additional aid to relaxation. If the patient believes it will be helpful to have an audio tape to assist in the relaxation training, a tape of the muscle tension cycle should be made at this session. This session is selected for audiotaping rather than the initial session because it is likely that this session will move a little more smoothly and won't be interrupted by questions and elaborations.

Ask the patient to describe an event or situation that occurs frequently and that is very positive or relaxing for him or her. The therapist might suggest a situation of his or her own if the patient has trouble. Most patients end up selecting a vacation activity or scene, such as relaxing on the banks of a favorite lake or sunning themselves on the beach at oceanside. Have the patient provide as much detail as possible about the relaxing situation, noting whether he or she is standing, sitting, or lying, how he or she is dressed, if anyone else is present, the location of the sun, etc. At the end of the tension and release cycle and after the deepening exercise has been provided, then verbally instruct the patient to imagine this particular situation by calling attention to various details he or she has previously provided. Once the image is vivid in the patient's mind, have him or her continue imagining for 3 to 5 minutes. At the end of this time, alert the patient and end the session.

In Sessions 3 and 4, an additional focus is added to the relaxation training, consisting of something we call discrimination training, which is designed to help the patient become more aware of the tension in his or her body and to be able to detect tension early enough to counteract it and prevent headache. Using the hand and lower arm for a demonstration, first have the patient engage in a complete tension and release cycle. Next, have the patient tense the hand and arm only one half as much as before, noting the sensations when relaxing it. Next, have the patient tense the muscle by one half again as much, which is actually one fourth of the level of tension. If the patient is able to do this, then continue with the complete cycle of tension and release exercises, informing the patient that the discrimination training will be introduced during practice with the neck and facial muscles, the site of headache pain. When you get to the neck and eye exercises, add the discrimination training steps as follows. First, the patient engages in a complete tension and release cycle, which is followed by a cycle that generates one half of the tension and is subsequently released, followed by a final cycle that has the patient tense by one fourth the level. Remind the patient to pay special attention to the sensations of tension and how they differ from cycle to cycle.

In Sessions 5 and 6, the patient is taught to reduce the number of muscle contractions to a total of eight muscle groupings. These consist of: (a) both hands and lower arms, (b) both legs and thighs, (c) abdomen, (d) chest, (e) shoulders, (f) back of neck, (g) eyes, and (h) forehead. (Have the patient select only one of the two tension-producing cycles.) For the lower arms, have the patient hold both arms out, flex slightly at the elbow, and simultaneously tense the hands, lower arms, and upper arms. Inform the patient that reducing the number of muscle groups is a step towards shortening the procedure and making it "more portable" and more readily usable. Go through the various muscle groupings with the patient to make certain he or she understands how the condensed tensing is done. The interval between tension and release cycles should be approximately 30 seconds now. In Session 5, otherwise continue the procedure as done previously.

At Session 6, the idea of "relaxation by recall" is introduced, which is just another procedure to help the patient become relaxed readily and quickly in most situations. In relaxation by recall, the patient attempts to become relaxed without going through the tension-release cycles. Before starting, remind the patient of the system you have developed to signal when a particular muscle is not sufficiently relaxed. Begin by having the patient focus attention on the muscles in the arms, being very careful to identify the feelings or sensations of tension or tightness that might be present; have the patient especially focus on any feelings of tension. Then ask the patient to attempt to recall what it was like when he or she released the tension from that particular muscle group. Allow 30 to 40 seconds for this (which may be accompanied by therapist banter). At the end of this interval, ask the patient to signal if the muscles are not deeply relaxed. If not, attempt one additional time for the patient to become relaxed through suggestion only. If the patient is not deeply relaxed at this point, then have the

patient actually complete a tension-release cycle. If the patient indicates that he or she is relaxed without the tension cycle or following the tension-release cycle, proceed to the next muscle group. Proceed through all eight muscle groupings, followed by the deepening by counting exercise, attention to breathing, and subvocalizing the word relax with exhalations periodically. The only exception is the chest, which the patient should tense by the actual breathing exercise. If the patient is moderately or completely successful with this procedure, have the patient utilize relaxation by recall during home practice. If the patient was chiefly unsuccessful with this procedure, have the patient continue the eight actual muscle tension-release cycles.

In Sessions 7, 8, and 9, the muscle groups are reduced from eight to four: arms, chest, neck, and face (especially eyes and forehead). For the arms, use both arms together with fists closed and the arms flexed slightly at the elbow. For the chest, use the deep breath, which is held. For the neck, have the patient slightly hunch the shoulders while drawing in and pressing backwards on the neck. For the face, have the patient close the eyes tightly while drawing up the rest of the face. Have the patient go through complete tension and relaxation cycles for these four muscle groups, followed by the deepening by counting and the attention to breathing. Next, alert the patient and then see if he or she can relax these four groups entirely by recall. Introduce actual tensing cycles as needed. At the end of Session 8, while the patient is continuing to remain relaxed, introduce the notion of "cue-controlled relaxation" by having the patient take a deep breath and think of the word "relax." Have the patient repeat this several times. Inquire if the patient is becoming relaxed to just this word. The sequence for cue-controlled relaxation is take a deep breath, consciously exhale, and say to oneself, "relax." Instruct the patient to begin using this cue-controlled relaxation procedure at various times throughout the day, noting that it is a quick, and hopefully effective and transportable, response.

At Session 10, have the patient go through

the four muscle groups by relaxation by recall only, and review all prior procedures: complete tension cycles, discrimination training, eight muscle groups, relaxation through recall, four muscle groups, cue-controlled relaxation, and relaxation as a coping strategy throughout the day.

Clinical Considerations

Training should initially be done in a relatively quiet, distraction-free environment while the patient is sitting in a chair that lends support to all major muscle groups. At the start of each session, the patient should loosen any tight or restrictive clothing and remove his or her glasses (possibly take out contact lenses), and the lighting should be adjusted to his or her preference. The trainer should use a calm, soothing tone of voice. We typically conduct all relaxation training live rather than by audio tape, because of the limited research supporting the latter (Paul & Tremble, 1970). By conducting training live, the therapist can spot problem areas and can correct them when need be. This also allows the therapist to make other necessary adjustments. There is nothing magical about the particular muscle group sequence nor the comments made by the therapist between tension-release cycles to facilitate relaxation, but the training should be done in a consistent order.

Some patients may be leery of hypnosis and liken relaxation training to hypnosis. We tell them that it does have some similarities, but that it really is not hypnosis per se, and assure them that no hypnotic suggestions will be administered. Occasionally, a patient may experience "relaxation-induced anxiety" (Heide & Borkovec, 1983). A very small portion of patients (in our experience no more than 1 to 2%) experience a sudden increase in anxiety during the relaxation induction that ranges from mild to a minor panic attack. It is important at these times for the therapist to remain calm and not panic, to reassure the patient that everything is all right, and to have the patient sit up for a few minutes and even walk around the room if necessary before resuming training. It is important that aversive thoughts and sensations that accompany the panic attack not become conditioned to the consultation room, the therapist, or the treatment situation in general. Doing the above should help lessen the chance of this happening. A third problem is muscle spasm, which is handled by stopping the relaxation induction, having the patient relax or massage the affected muscle until the spasm has decreased, resuming the relaxation training after warning the patient not to tense so hard, and avoiding the spasmed muscle until the next session.

We have a preference for augmenting relaxation practice with audio tapes made during an actual session. The value of home practice tapes seems to be that they control the pacing and duration of the home practice sessions. (Left to their own devices, patients may rush through the exercises and report taking as few as 8 minutes to complete a session.) Some patients worry about getting the sequence of exercises right (the tape eliminates this concern), and some patients claim it's just not the same when they try to do it by themselves. Patients who find audio tapes helpful initially need to be gradually "weaned" from the audio tape. Through Session 6, we allow the patients to use the audio tapes on a daily basis, but suggest that they begin to alternate practice with and without the tape beginning at Session 7. This alternating pattern is gradually increased until by Session 10 the patients are no longer using the audio tapes.

Biofeedback Treatment Procedures

The following are verbatim instructions to be used when administering EMG biofeedback:

Therapist: Your treatment consists of something called biofeedback training. The main idea involved is to help you learn how to control certain physiological responses. In your particular case, we want you to learn how to relax the muscles of your forehead, scalp, and face.

It has been shown in numerous clinics

and laboratories that teaching people to control the forehead muscles, and especially how to really relax these muscles, can have a very beneficial effect on tension headache like yours. As explained earlier, your headache is caused by your muscles becoming tight. People like yourself are generally not even aware their muscles are becoming tense until it's too late and they have a headache (which is a signal that the muscles have been too tense, too long). With biofeedback you'll become more aware of when your muscles are just starting to become tense so you can relax them and stop your headaches.

There are three basic parts to biofeedback: First, we need an electronic gadget to detect very small changes in a particular response, changes so small that you ordinarily cannot detect them. In this case it is very small changes in muscle tension in your forehead. These sensors detect the levels of muscle tension. [Show forehead electrodes to the patient.] It will be necessary for me to clean the skin of your forehead very well so that we get a good contact.

Second, we need to be able to convert these changes to a signal you can easily understand. We do this electronically, also.

Finally, we feed or present this information back to you (hence, biofeedback). For this purpose we will use this speaker. We have several different kinds of auditory feedback and will let you try different ones to see which works best for you. For example, the pitch of the tone may go up or down as you become more tense or more relaxed. Or there may be a series of clicks, with faster clicks meaning increasing tension and slower clicks meaning relaxation.

There are two important parts of learning to control a response: first, you can use the biofeedback situation as your own laboratory in which you can discover what strategies or tactics or maneuvers work for you. Thus, we encourage you to experiment, to try new ideas or images that you think might work for you.

Second, and very important, is to *let the response occur*, to be somewhat passive. If you try to force it, to make your forehead less tense, you may become *more tense* as

you try. So remember to relax and *let your forehead* become more relaxed.

Questions?

Patient: Can I be shocked by the sensors?

Therapist: No, they are perfectly safe.

They work much like a thermometer. A thermometer puts no heat into a person's body; it only reads the temperature of the object it comes into contact with. These sensors work in an analogous way. They measure the tiny amount of electrical activity that is generated when muscles contract, but the electrical activity flows only one way. The sensors do not pass any electrical current into your body.

The following instructions are for autogenic feedback.

Therapist: Your treatment consists of something called biofeedback training. The main idea involved is to help you to learn how to control certain physiological responses. In this particular case, we want you to learn how to warm your fingers and hands.

It was first discovered at the Menninger Clinic, a famous psychiatric center in Kansas, that patients with vascular headaches, especially migraine, who could learn to warm their hands fairly rapidly and who practiced this hand warming regularly, had a marked decrease in headache intensity and frequency. The basic treatment effect has been replicated in many different laboratories and clinics.

It is not entirely clear why handwarming is helpful, but we think it involves the following. Blood flow to your hands (which is what makes them warm) and to your head is controlled by the same part of your nervous system. As the activity level in this part of your nervous system slows down, the blood vessels in your fingers open up and allow more heat-enriched blood to flow into them. It is the relaxing of the nervous system which occurs as you warm your hands that leads to improvement in your headache.

There are three basic parts to biofeedback: First, we need an electronic gadget to detect very small changes in a particular response, changes so small that you ordinarily cannot detect them. In this case it is very small changes in temperature. This little sensor detects the temperature changes. [Show thermistor to patient.]

Second, we need to be able to convert these changes to a signal you can easily process. We do this electronically, also.

Finally, we feed or present this information back to you (hence, biofeedback). For this purpose we will use this electronic meter. Thus, as the temperature goes up, the pen on the meter will move to the right.

There are two important parts of learning to control a response: First, you can use the biofeedback situation as a laboratory in which you can discover what strategies or tactics or maneuvers work for you. Thus, we encourage you to experiment, to try ideas or images that you think might work for you.

Second, and very important, is to *let the response occur*, to be somewhat passive. If you try to force it, to make your hands warmer, typically they will become cooler. So remember to relax and let your hands become warm.

Once you have learned how to warm your hands, we will want you to practice warming them on a regular daily basis and also as a way of possibly aborting the headache.

Questions?

Patient: Will it work if I place my hand in a bowl of warm water?

Therapist: That's a good question. Researchers have actually tested that and the answer is, no, it doesn't work. It isn't hand warming per se that causes the effect; warmth in the hands is just an indication that nervous system activity is decreasing. Warmth produced by external means doesn't lead to the effect. The warming has to occur because of internal changes.

In our research, each biofeedback session encompasses a number of phases, including an adaptation period, an in-session baseline, a first "self-control" baseline, biofeedback training itself, and a second self-control assessment. We know that when an individual is first attached to the monitoring equipment, his or her physiological activity will fluctuate for a period of time (Lichstein,

Sallis, Hill, & Young, 1981). The clinician will want to wait a few minutes for the patient to become habituated. It is then helpful to take a "resting baseline" to use as a comparison for judging progress. Two "self-control" assessments are taken by us, but the therapist may want to omit one of these in the interest of time. The reason for collecting "self-control" data is to assess how much the patient is able to control the response when instructed to do so, but in the absence of any tangible feedback. During these readings you would instruct the patient as follows:

I want you to do what you can to relax your muscles (or to raise your hand temperature) as much as you can, but without having the feedback signal to aid you. When you leave the therapy session, you will not have the biofeedback unit with you; and this will allow me to gauge how well you will be able to do this on your own, as well as how much you have learned during the treatment session.

It is our impression that feedback sessions should run approximately 20 to 40 minutes, adjusting the duration to fit the patient. When the patient begins to feel he or she is gaining some control over the target response, then the patient is urged to start using biofeedback as a coping response (when muscles become slightly tense, at the first sign of a headache, or when some change in hand temperature is noticed). In research the number of treatment sessions has varied substantially from a low of 7 to highs of 20 or more. Our research has involved anywhere from 10 to 16 sessions, with sessions being held twice per week at first. Number of days between sessions is gradually increased over time to facilitate transfer of skills to the natural environment.

One question that immediately surfaces is how does the clinician decide how many sessions to administer to a given patient? We can think of two rules to guide this decision. First, one can continue treatment until the patient believes maximum benefit has been gained from the procedure (until headaches have either markedly decreased or the patient has continued the procedures for a certain period of time with no change or further improvement). Second, the therapist might continue until the patient evidences sufficient self-control abilities. Several researchers have advocated this "training to criterion" notion. Unfortunately, there are no universally accepted criteria at present. Most of the studies that have shown a treatment effect with EMG biofeedback have produced mean decreases on the order of 50% or greater for forehead muscle tension level. It is not possible to provide an absolute level here, because this varies as a function of the biofeedback unit used. As regards thermal biofeedback, Fahrion (1978) advocates that patients be trained until they can regularly warm the hands in the presence of feedback to 95.5°F, while Sargent, Solbach, Coyne, Spohn, and Segerson (in press) advocate training patients until they can reliably produce a 1°F temperature rise within 1 minute from a resting/stable baseline. Validity data to support these claims are lacking, and they are provided here only as potential guides to the therapist.

At the Menninger Foundation, the institution where autogenic feedback originated, autogenic phrases are introduced in the first session, during which all forms of feedback are withheld from the patient (Sargent, Green, & Walters, 1973). The patient is instructed as follows:

> At today's session, I'm going to be in a room with you during the actual biofeedback, reading you a list of what we call autogenic phrases. These phrases are designed to help you achieve an overall physiological state of relaxation and are designed specifically to help you warm your hands. Many patients use methods other than autogenic phrases to try to increase their hand temperature. For instance, some people imagine that their hands are over a fire, or imagine blood flowing to their fingertips, etc. For today, let's try the autogenic phrases and see how they work. I will be watching the monitor today and will be giving feedback on how you're doing. During our next session, you'll be looking at the monitor yourself. The reason I'll be providing you with feedback is be-

TABLE 13.5. AUTOGENIC PHRASES

1. I feel quite quiet.
2. I am beginning to feel quite relaxed.
3. My feet feel heavy and relaxed.
4. My ankles, my knees, and my hips feel heavy, relaxed, and comfortable.
5. My solar plexus, and the whole central portion of my body, feel relaxed and quiet.
6. My hands, my arms, and my shoulders, feel heavy, relaxed, and comfortable.
7. My neck, my jaws, and my forehead feel relaxed. They feel comfortable and smooth.
8. My whole body feels quiet, heavy, comfortable, and relaxed.
9. I am quite relaxed.
10. My arms and hands are heavy and warm.
11. I feel quite quiet.
12. My whole body is relaxed, and my hands are warm, relaxed and warm.
13. My hands are warm.
14. Warmth is flowing into my hands, they are warm, warm.
15. Warm.

Note. From "Preliminary report on the use of autogenic feedback training in the treatment of migraine and tension headaches" by J.D. Sargent, E.E. Green, and E.D. Walters, *Psychosomatic Medicine*, 35, p. 131. Reprinted by permission.

cause people get so concerned over whether or not their hand temperature has increased that they are unable to become relaxed, and warm their hands. Hopefully, that won't happen today. [The trainer then reads the phrases in Table 13.5 in verbatim fashion. The top set of phrases is designed to elicit a state of total body relaxation and passive concentration while the bottom set of phrases is designed to facilitate warming in the hands.]

Clinical Considerations

The practitioner will be confronted by an overwhelming number of biofeedback devices from which to choose. Factors to consider are cost, ease of use, reliability and accuracy of equipment, and whether a permanent record of the physiological activity is desired (Andrasik & Blanchard, 1983). Nearly all of the commercially available temperature trainers are reliable, accurate, and inexpensive, but few make available a permanent trace. There is an additional factor to consider when purchasing EMG biofeedback equipment. The electromyogram signal has an estimated frequency range (or something referred to as band pass) of approximately 1 to 1,000 Hz. Our laboratory polygraph has a band pass of 3 to 300 Hz. Most commercial or self-contained EMG biofeedback devices have a much more restricted band pass, typically only from 100 to 200 Hz. These devices, therefore, eliminate much of the EMG signal, and a large amount of relevant muscle activity does occur below 100 Hz.

Another consideration concerns feedback modality. Most EMG biofeedback devices are equipped to provide auditory as well as visual feedback, but researchers and clinicians have shown a near unanimous preference for auditory feedback alone. A scant amount of research suggests individuals perform better at EMG biofeedback when their eyes are closed, and keeping the eyes closed also has the beneficial effect of minimizing signal artifacts due to eye movement. Conversely, in the area of thermal biofeedback, clinicians and researchers seem universally to prefer a visual feedback modality. We routinely provide patients various types of feedback displays and allow them to select the one or combination they prefer. Another choice concerns binary (on, off) versus continuous or analog display. In providing binary biofeedback, a criterion level is specified and the feedback stimulus is turned on or off whenever the response meets or exceeds the criterion. We prefer an analog signal because it insures that feedback is continuously available to patients.

There is no consensus regarding the optimal length of a feedback session. A length of 20 minutes probably serves as a minimum; patients can become fatigued when feedback sessions go much beyond 40 minutes. We conducted an investigation to determine if frequent breaks were helpful during provision of feedback (Andrasik, Pallmeyer, Blanchard, & Attanasio, 1984). Migraine patients receiving continuous biofeedback evidenced modest degrees of acquisition, while the group receiving frequent rest periods (60 seconds of thermal biofeedback followed by 10 seconds of rest) actually deteriorated. Comments from patients assigned to the interrupted condition indicated they found the frequent rest breaks to be highly disruptive and annoying. Interestingly, individuals assigned to the continuous condition indicated they rarely maintained a constant attention to the tone, but rather took "mental breaks" on an as-needed basis. It may be that rest breaks are facilitative, but they should not be provided as frequently as every minute. Perhaps an administration schedule of something like 5 minutes of biofeedback with a 30- to 60-second rest break might be helpful for patients who fatigue easily. We use this type of training schedule in research with young children.

Another important consideration is how the therapist interacts with the patient during biofeedback. Research suggests that therapists possessing a "warm, friendly, supportive manner" are the most desirable (Taub, 1977), as is true with all therapy. A related consideration concerns whether the therapist is present during feedback training and, if so, how much the therapist should interact with the patient. The only available investigation (Borgeat, Hade, Larouche, & Bedwani, 1980) revealed that very active coaching by a therapist (coaching, encouraging, providing information about overall progress, and looking with the patient for causes of poor performance) actually interfered with progress during EMG biofeedback. If the therapist is present during provision of feedback, then he or she needs to be certain not to be too intrusive and to reserve most comments until biofeedback proper is concluded.

Preparation and selection of sensor placement needs consideration. In EMG recordings it is important to prepare the skin surface carefully by lightly abrading the skin (to remove dead skin cells, makeup, and surface oils) and then cleansing with an alcohol solution. This is necessary to minimize the resistance between electrodes. Surface preparation is less critical when applying a thermal probe; one needs only to be sure that the surface is relatively clean. The thermal sensor is usually attached either with paper tape or a velcro band. Either way, it is important that the fastening device not be applied too tightly, as this may act as a tourniquet and cut off the blood supply. It is wise to run the cable from the thermal probe down the individual's finger and attach it to the base of the finger or the hand to control for "stem effects" (Taub & School, 1978). The EMG sensors (three in number) are typically placed across the forehead when administering biofeedback to tension headache sufferers (Basmajian & Blumenstein, 1980). The two active electrodes are centered over each eye approximately 1 inch above each eyebrow. The remaining or ground electrode is placed midway between these two (directly above the bridge of the nose). Originally it was thought that this type of placement recorded muscle activity fairly restrictively from the frontalis muscles. Basmajian (1976) has pointed out, however, that when electrodes are placed in this manner they actually pick up electrical signals down to the first rib. This fortuitous electrode placement practice ends up being highly desirable, as tension headache sufferers often experience pain in the upper shoulders, neck, and back of the head as well.

Some investigators have argued that EMG placements should vary as a function of site or origin of headache pain. Again, there is no strong empirical evidence supporting this viewpoint. The most reasonable course would be to start with the conventional frontal recording site and, if met with minimal success, to change to a new recording site if pain is experienced predominantly in places other than the forehead area. If the practitioner has equipment that will allow monitoring from more than one site, then feedback could be alternated or sampled at various sites throughout treatment. One last question concerns where to place the thermal probe. We typically use the ventral surface of the index finger of either hand, although others have used the little finger or the web dorsum. We are unaware of any data suggesting that one site is any better than another.

With either modality, the patient is encouraged early on to experiment with a variety of strategies for controlling the feedback signal. Although the goal is to lower EMG activity and to raise hand temperature, attention is devoted early on to discovering what factors cause the signal to go in the nontherapeutic direction so that the patient can prevent or minimize these occurrences in the future. Various somatic (primarily breathing and positioning of arms, shoulders, etc.) and imaginal (thermally based imagery, relaxing imagery, etc.) strategies are typically suggested to patients. They are told, though, that the strategy they ultimately select may be quite idiosyncratic, so they should explore and seek to find what works best for them. Patients are encouraged to test the responsiveness of the biofeedback display, for example, by deliberately tensing their forehead. A not uncommon response in thermal biofeedback is for the patient initially to experience a marked degree of temperature cooling when efforts are made to warm the hand. One can almost predict that this will occur with very achievement-oriented individuals. In thermal biofeedback, passive forms of relaxation, or what some term passive volition, appear to work best. Failures occasioned by trying too hard are used to illustrate to patients the effects that emotional processes, and their approach to problem-solving in particular, can have upon their physiological functioning.

A few additional problems routinely come up when administering biofeedback to patients. Gaining control of a physiological response is difficult and can generate frustration in patients. Early failure experiences may cause patients to avoid or ignore the feedback display and to engage in negative or counterproductive self-statements. To minimize these occurrences, we inform patients of the difficulty of the task and of tendencies we have observed for patients to self-derogate after failure experiences. This permits patients to attribute failure experiences to the difficulty of the task, rather than to personal inadequacies (Lynn & Freedman, 1979). Judicious control of the feedback display, such as arranging feedback so that small changes in the therapeutic direction are presented to the patient as large-magnitude changes, is helpful in the initial sessions.

Patients frequently encounter "learning plateaus" and feel as if they are stuck at a certain level of performance. Patients are informed early on that these plateaus will occur and not to become distressed by them. When a learning plateau occurs, in addition to giving support to the patient, you might have the patient engage in some bidirectional control (alternately increasing and decreasing the response). It is quite easy for individuals to raise their EMG level, and this may serve to counteract any frustration resulting from minimal progress. It is not uncommon for a migraine patient to have relatively warm hands (in the low 90's) at the start of a biofeedback training session. Of course, the higher the starting temperature, the more difficult it is for the individual to show further increases in hand temperature. You might point out that just because his or her temperature is high during the session does not mean that it will be high outside of the session or in stress-producing situations. This is also an instance where training in bidirectional control might be useful.

A new feature we have recently added to biofeedback is "discrimination training." This was instituted in response to a case study by Gainer (1978). After extensive training with thermal biofeedback, his patient demonstrated a pronounced ability to raise her hand temperature upon request, but this was of no value in controlling her migraines. Gainer speculated that this patient, although evidencing heightened self-control abilities, could not discriminate or did not know when to apply her hand warming skills. Comparisons between the patient's perceived changes in hand temperature and her actual changes revealed poor correspondence, confirming Gainer's hunch. In subsequent sessions, training was instituted to rectify this situation. At each discrimination-training session, the patient was presented 60 training trials of either 15- or 30-second duration, separated

by a 5-second break. The patient was instructed to increase her hand temperature during each discrimination-training trial while, most importantly, focusing on the sensations in her hand. During the break, the patient was informed of the magnitude and direction of change relative to the preceding trial. Following training, the patient revealed markedly improved abilities to discriminate hand temperature changes. By having the patient implement hand warming when changes were first detected, migraine attacks disappeared completely, and medication was no longer needed. An 8-month follow-up revealed a high level of maintenance of treatment gains.

Discrimination training is done at our clinic by periodically turning off the feedback display, having the patient attempt alternately to raise, lower, or keep the response the same, asking the patient to "guess" the physiological value, and then providing feedback as to accuracy. We believe this procedure helps enable patients to apply self-regulation skills at the first sign of an attack and have begun to use it on a regular basis. Again, there is no controlled research documenting the utility of discrimination training.

Another issue concerns home practice and application of relaxation skills as a coping response. Clinicians have universally accepted that patients need to engage in post-therapy practice two times per day for a period of 20 minutes each. Whether this amount of practice is critical is again unknown. One investigation (Libo & Arnold, 1983) found support for the importance of home practice, but the results did not conform to a "dose-response" relationship. Rather, the relationship was essentially "all-or-none"; virtually any level of practice was better than no practice for maintaining treatment gains. Those who had ceased home practice revealed the poorest response, while those who practiced achieved an enhanced response. Successful patients reported they practiced relaxation when needed, rather than according to a set schedule.

We view home practice as an important step to coping with the problems of everyday living that can lead to stress buildup and headache. Early in treatment, when patients are struggling to acquire skills, we believe it is best for the patient to set aside specific periods during the day for practice. Initially, we review a patient's schedule to help identify a time and place most conducive to practice. Subsequently, patients are instructed to vary the time and location of practice, performing some at work if convenient. We offer patients home biofeedback trainers to use outside of treatment initially. As with audio tapes during relaxation training, we have patients use these trainers during every home practice initially, then begin to alternate practice with and without the trainer, and then increase the number of times the trainer is not used so that by the end of treatment patients will no longer be dependent on them.

Once the patient feels accomplished at relaxation, he or she is then instructed to begin to use relaxation skills as a means for coping with tension and headache-related stress and distress. Patients are informed that, although a single dose of stress can lead to a headache if large enough, headache is most often caused by a build-up of stress from the day-to-day, small-scale ups and downs we all experience. The goal now is to begin to handle each up and down on the spot to prevent the effects from accumulating throughout the day. At this point, patients are instructed to distribute practice throughout the day; instead of two 20-minute practices the patient is encouraged to practice eight times for 5 minutes, then ten times for 4 minutes, etc. Conspicuous display of prompts in the home and work environment can help remind patients to engage in frequent, brief relaxation practices (affix a symbol or the word "relax" to an item frequently seen during the day, such as the telephone, desk, wristwatch, appointment book, etc.). Contingency management may be necessary for patients who don't find the promise of future benefits to be sufficiently compelling to sustain current practice. Treatment of a 10-year-old female migraineur is a case in point.

Despite consultations from several medical specialists and administration of various medications, the young girl's headaches had remained on a steadily deteriorating course for the past 5 years (five to seven severe headache episodes per month with most accompanied by nausea and vomiting). Initial assessment revealed two situations were most reliably associated with headache: being "keyed up" and experiencing "academic pressures." Thermal biofeedback augmented by various relaxation procedures was initiated, and the patient quickly mastered the ability to raise her hand temperature. This by itself had no appreciable effect on her headaches, however, as the child experienced considerable difficulty applying her newly acquired self-regulation skills in the situations most needed. For example, periods of extended, vigorous play with friends and relatives regularly precipitated headache. She acknowledged this relationship, but was unwilling to moderate her play behavior because she found it so immediately enjoyable. School was stressful because of her high standards for performance and her manner of exam preparation. The patient and her best friend studied together and quizzed each other when preparing for examinations. These sessions would often end with the patient becoming quite upset and engaging in a number of negative self-statements.

A contingency contract was established with the mother wherein the patient was monetarily reinforced first for regular home practice, next for periodically interrupting her intense play to complete a brief biofeedback practice to prevent her from becoming overly "keyed up," and finally for persisting at biofeedback when experiencing headache as an attempt to abort the headache.

School-related stresses were dealt with in two ways: (a) by inviting her friend to therapy, modeling alternative ways for them to discuss examinations and other academic matters in a less stressful manner, and teaching the friend to "coach" the patient in the application of hand-warming when needed; and (b) by assisting the patient in analyzing and changing her self-critical and unrealistic performance demands by cognitive reappraisal and self-statement training (use of positive, coping self-statements).

At the last contact the patient was described as being more in control of her headaches, less reactive and better able to handle emotional upsets, and no longer viewed by her family as "sick." Although not completely free of headache, her headaches were much less frequent and when present they were of significantly reduced duration and intensity, as judged by diary records completed by the patient and her parents. Nausea and vomiting, frequent accompaniments of headache in the past, were no longer present. Her medication had been completely eliminated, too. Inspection of school attendance records revealed no further absences as a result of headache.

Children, as this case illustrates, present a particular challenge. The interested reader is referred to Attanasio et al. (in press) for a more expanded discussion of problems that are likely and adaptations that are necessary when utilizing biofeedback with children.

This case illustrates one final point—that relaxation and biofeedback often are not applied in a vacuum. Cognitive and other behavioral coping strategies (see Holzman, Turk, & Kerns, chapter 3 of this volume) often end up being useful during treatment. More than one biofeedback patient has stated midway during treatment, "Can we turn the machine off today; I'd like to talk about something that's bothering me." One unique advantage of biofeedback and relaxation is that they afford patients who are not psychologically minded, or who initially are uncomfortable divulging personal information, an acceptable "physical" treatment alternative. Over time, many of these patients become more aware of and more receptive to dealing with their psychological concerns.

REFERENCES

Ad Hoc Committee on Classification of Headache. (1962). Classification of headache. *Journal of the American Medical Association*, *179*, 717–718.
Ala-Hurula, V., Myllyla, V., & Hokkanen, E. (1982). Ergotamine abuse: Results of ergotamine discontinuation, with special reference to the plasma concentration. *Cephalalgia*, *2*, 189–195.
Andrasik, F. (in press). Tension headache. In M. Hersen & C.J. Last (Eds.), *Behavior therapy casebook*. NY: Springer.
Andrasik, F., & Blanchard, E.B. (1983). Application of biofeedback to therapy. In C.E. Walker (Ed.), *Handbook of clinical psychology: Theory, research and practice* (pp. 1123–1164). Homewood, IL: Dorsey.
Andrasik, F., Blanchard, E.B., Ahles, T., Pallmeyer, T., & Barron, K.D. (1981). Assessing the reactive as well as the sensory component of headache pain. *Headache*, *21*, 218–221.
Andrasik, F., Blanchard, E.B., Arena, J.G., Teders, S.J., Teevan, R.C., & Rodichok, L.D. (1982). Psychological functioning in headache sufferers. *Psychosomatic Medicine*, *44*, 171–182.
Andrasik, F., Pallmeyer, T.P., Blanchard, E.B., & Attanasio, V. (1984). Continuous versus interrupted schedules of thermal biofeedback: An exploratory analysis with clinical subjects. *Biofeedback and Self-Regulation*, *9*, 291–298.
Attanasio, V., Andrasik, F., Burke, E.J., Blake, D.D., Kabela, E., & McCarran, M.S. (in press). Clinical issues in utilizing biofeedback with children. *Clinical Biofeedback and Health*.
Bakal, D.A. (1982). *The psychobiology of chronic headache*. NY: Springer Publishing Co.
Basmajian, J.V. (1976). Facts versus myths in EMG biofeedback. *Biofeedback and Self-Regulation*, *1*, 369–371.
Basmajian, J.V., & Blumenstein, R. (1980). *Electrode placement in EMG biofeedback*. Baltimore, MD: Williams & Wilkins.
Benson, H. (1975). *The relaxation response*. NY: William Morrow.
Bernstein, D.A., & Borkovec, T.D. (1973). *Progressive relaxation training*. Champaign, IL: Research Press.
Blanchard, E.B., & Andrasik, F. (1982). Psychological assessment and treatment of headache: Recent developments and emerging issues. *Journal of Consulting and Clinical Psychology*, *50*, 859–879.
Blanchard, E.B., Andrasik, F., Jurish, S.E., & Teders, S.J. (1982). The treatment of cluster headache with relaxation and thermal biofeedback. *Biofeedback and Self-Regulation*, *7*, 185–191.
Blanchard, E.B., Andrasik, F., Neff, D.F., Jurish, S.E., & O'Keefe, D.M. (1981). Social validation of the headache diary. *Behavior Therapy*, *12*, 711–715.
Blanchard, E.B., O'Keefe, D., Neff, D., Jurish, S., & Andrasik, F. (1981). Interdisciplinary agreement in the diagnosis of headache types. *Journal of Behavioral Assessment*, *3*, 5–9.

Blanchard, E.B., Andrasik, F., Neff, D.F., Teders, S.J., Pallmeyer, T.P., Arena, J.B., Jurish, S.E., Saunders, N.L., Ahles, T.A., & Rodichok, L.D. (1982). Sequential comparisons of relaxation training and biofeedback in the treatment of three kinds of chronic headache or, the machines may be necessary some of the time. *Behaviour Research and Therapy, 20,* 1–13.

Borgeat, F., Hade, B., Larouche, L.N., & Bedwani, C.N. (1980). Effects of therapist active presence on EMG biofeedback training of headache patients. *Biofeedback and Self-Regulation, 5,* 275–282.

Budzynski, T., Stoyva, J., & Adler, C. (1970). Feedback-induced relaxation: Application to tension headache. *Journal of Behavior Therapy and Experimental Psychiatry, 1,* 205–211.

Budzynski, T.H., Stoyva, J.M., Adler, C.S., & Mullaney, D.J. (1973). EMG biofeedback and tension headache: A controlled outcome study. *Psychosomatic Medicine, 6,* 509–514.

Cox, D., & Thomas, D. (1981). Relationship between headaches and depression. *Headache, 21,* 216–263.

Daly, E.J., Donn, P.A., Galliher, M.J., & Zimmerman, J.S. (1983). Biofeedback applications to migraine and tension headache: A double-blinded outcome study. *Biofeedback and Self-Regulation, 8,* 135–152.

Davis, R.A., Wetzel, R.D., Kashiwagi, M.D., & McClure, J.N. (1976). Personality, depression and headache. *Headache, 16,* 246–251.

Diamond, S. (1983). Depression and headache. *Headache, 23,* 123–126.

Diamond, S., & Dalessio, D.J. (1982). *The practicing physician's approach to headache* (3rd ed.). Baltimore, MD: Williams & Wilkins.

Fahrion, S.L. (1977). Autogenic biofeedback treatment for migraine. *Mayo Clinic Proceedings, 52,* 776–784.

Gainer, J.C. (1978). Temperature discrimination training in the biofeedback treatment of migraine headache. *Journal of Behavior Therapy and Experimental Psychiatry, 9,* 185–188.

Haynes, S.N. (1980). Muscle contraction headache: A psychophysiological perspective of etiology and treatment. In S.N. Haynes & L.R. Gannon (Eds.), *Psychosomatic disorders: A psychophysiological approach to etiology and treatment.* NY: Gardner.

Heide, F.J., & Borkovec, P.D. (1983). Relaxation-induced anxiety: Paradoxical anxiety enhancement due to relaxation training. *Journal of Consulting and Clinical Psychology, 51,* 171–182.

Holroyd, K.A., & Andrasik, F. (1982). A cognitive-behavioral approach to recurrent tension and migraine headache. In P.C. Kendall (Ed.), *Advances in cognitive-behavioral research and therapy* (Vol. 1, pp. 275–320). NY: Academic.

Jacobson, E. (1938). *Progressive relaxation.* Chicago: University of Chicago Press.

Jay, G.W., Renelli, D., & Mead, T. (1984). The effects of propranolol and amitriptyline on vascular and EMG biofeedback training. *Headache, 24,* 59–69.

Kudrow, L. (1976). Hormones, pregnancy and migraine. In O. Appenzeller (Ed.), *Pathogenesis and treatment of headache.* NY: Spectrum Publications.

Kudrow, L. (1980). *Cluster headache: Mechanisms and management.* NY: Oxford University Press.

Kudrow, L. (1982). Paradoxical effects of frequent analgesic use. In M. Critchley, A.P. Friedman, S. Gorini, & F. Sicuteri (Eds.), *Advances in neurology: Headache: Physiopathological and clinical concepts* (Vol. 33). NY: Raven Press.

Kudrow, L. (1983). Pathogenesis of vascular headache. In W.H. Rickles, J.H. Sandweiss, D. Jacobs, & R.N. Grove (Eds.), *Biofeedback and family practice medicine* (pp. 41–59). NY: Plenum.

Lance, J.W. (1978). *Mechanism and management of headache* (3rd ed.). Boston: Butterworth.

Lance, J.W., Curran, D.A., & Anthony, M. (1965). Investigations into the mechanism and treatment of chronic headache. *Medical Journal of Australia, 2,* 904–914.

Leviton, A. (1978). Epidemiology of headache. In V.S. Schoenberg (Ed.), *Advances in neurology* (Vol. 19, pp. 341–352). NY: Raven Press.

Libo, L.M., & Arnold, G.E. (1983). Relaxation practice after biofeedback therapy: A long-term follow-up study of utilization and effectiveness. *Biofeedback and Self-Regulation, 8,* 217–227.

Lichstein, K.L., Sallis, J.F., Hill, D., & Young, M.C. (1981). Psychophysiological adaptation: An investigation of multiple parameters. *Journal of Behavioral Assessment, 3,* 111–121.

Luborsky, L., Docherty, J.P., & Penick, S. (1973). Onset conditions for psychosomatic symptoms: A comparative review of immediate observation with retrospective research. *Psychosomatic Medicine, 35,* 187–204.

Lynn, S.J., & Freedman, R.R. (1979). Transfer and evaluation of biofeedback treatment. In A. Goldstein & F. Kanfer (Eds.), *Maximizing treatment gains: Transfer enhancement in psychotherapy.* NY: Academic Press.

Olesen, J., Lauritzen, M., Tfelt-Hansen, P., Henriksen, L., & Larson, B. (1982). Spreading cerebral oligemia in classical- and normal cerebral blood flow in common migraine. *Headache, 22,* 242–248.

Packard, R.C. (1979). What does the headache patient want? *Headache, 19,* 370–374.

Paul, G.L., & Trimble, R.W. (1970). Recorded versus "live" relaxation training and hypnotic suggestion: Comparative effectiveness for reducing physiological arousal and inhibiting stress response. *Behavior Therapy, 1,* 285–302.

Price, D.D., McGrath, P.A., Rafii, A., & Buckingham, B. (1983). The validation of visual analog scale as ratio scale measures for chronic and experimental pain. *Pain, 17*, 45–56.

Raskin, N.H., & Appenzeller, O. (1980). *Headache.* Philadelphia: Saunders.

Sargent, J.D., Green, E.E., & Walters, E.D. (1972). The use of autogenic training in a pilot study of migraine and tension headaches. *Headache, 12*, 120–124.

Sargent, J.D., Green, E.E., & Walters, E.D. (1973). Preliminary report on the use of autogenic feedback training in the treatment of migraine and tension headaches. *Psychosomatic Medicine, 35*, 129–135.

Sargent, J.D., Walters, E.D., & Green, E.E. (1973). Psychosomatic self-regulation of migraine headache. *Seminars in Psychiatry, 5*, 415–428.

Sargent, J., Solbach, P., Coyne, L., Spohn, H., & Segerson, J. (in press). Results of a controlled, experimental, outcome study of nondrug treatments for the control of migraine headaches. *Journal of Behavioral Medicine.*

Schultz, J.H., & Luthe, W. (1969). *Autogenic training* (Vol. 1): NY: Grune & Stratton.

Sicuteri, F., (1982). Natural opioids in migraine. In M. Critchley, A. Friedman, S. Gorini, & F. Sicuteri (Eds.), *Advances in neurology: Headache: Physiopathological and clinical concepts* (Vol. 33). NY: Raven Press.

Solbach, P., Sargent, J., & Coyne, L. (1984). Menstrual migraine headache: Results of a controlled, experimental, outcome study of nondrug treatments. *Headache, 24*, 75–78.

Sovak, N., Kunzel, M., Sternbach, R.A., & Dalessio, D.J. (1981). Mechanism of the biofeedback therapy of migraine: Volitional manipulation of the psychophysiological background. *Headache, 21*, 89–92.

Stoyva, J., & Budzynski, T. (1974). Cultivated low arousal—An antistress response? In L.V. DiCara (Ed.), *Limbic and autonomic nervous systems research* (pp. 369–394). NY: Plenum.

Taub, E. (1977). Self-regulation of human tissue temperature. In G.E. Schwartz & J. Beatty (Eds.), *Biofeedback: Theory and research.* NY: Academic.

Taub, E., & School, P.J. (1978). Some methodological considerations in thermal biofeedback training. *Behavioral Research Methods and Instrumentation, 10*, 617–622.

Thompson, J.K., Haber, J.D., & Tearnan, B.H. (1981). Generalization of frontalis electromyographic feedback to adjacent muscle groups: A critical review. *Psychosomatic Medicine, 43*, 19–24.

Ziegler, D.K., Rhodes, R.J., & Hassanein, R.S. (1978). Association of psychological measurements of anxiety and depression with headache history in a nonclinical population. *Research Clinical Studies in Headache.* Basel: Karger.

MEDICAL LIBRARY
W. C. B.
DOWNSVIEW REHAB. CENTRE

14 THE PROCESS OF PSYCHOLOGICAL CONSULTATION IN PAIN MANAGEMENT*

Roy Cameron
Larry F. Shepel

Psychological factors play an important role in determining how pain is experienced and expressed (Melzack & Wall, 1982; Turk, Meichenbaum, & Genest, 1983). As the evidence supporting this proposition mounts, psychologists are becoming involved increasingly in the assessment and treatment of pain patients. As this consultation role develops, working relationships are evolving between psychologists and members of other health professions including physicians, surgeons, nurses, and physiotherapists. Consultation across professional boundaries can be awkward, because the process involves individuals who usually have strikingly different theoretical backgrounds, diverse approaches to problems, and idiosyncratic technical vocabularies. Psychological consultation is complicated by the fact that the patient may

misunderstand and resent the consultation. If things are to run smoothly, the consultation process needs to be considered carefully.

Consultation involves a blend of science and art. The scientific side tends to be emphasized, and this is as it should be. Consultants are, above all, experts who are conversant with pertinent scientific literature, so that their assessment and treatment procedures are updated and refined as research findings emerge. Anyone working in a clinical setting, however, knows that there is an art to developing effective consultation. We have had patients refuse to see us (not to mention threaten us with legal action or physical assault) because we had blundered badly in the way we had arranged the consultation. No matter how expert consultants may be, they cannot do much for patients who are not prepared to cooperate. It is obviously important to do everything possible to arrange the consultation so that patients will be at ease and cooperative.

This chapter represents our attempt to pre-

*The authors are grateful to Myles Genest, Arnold Holzman, Donald Meichenbaum, Kenneth Prkachin, Barr Taylor, Dennis Turk, Carl Von Baeyer, and Cynthia Zeeve for their helpful comments on an earlier draft of this chapter.

sent our thoughts regarding the art of consultation. We don't want to pretend to be virtuoso consultants prescribing definitive guidelines for consultation. Our reflections are based solely on 8 years of learning, much of it by trial and error, as we've worked as consultants in a university hospital setting. Glitches still arise. It is our hope that the suggestions we offer from our experience will stimulate clinicians to think systematically about the consultation process, and how it might be improved, in their individual situations.

INFORMING REFERRAL AGENTS ABOUT PSYCHOLOGICAL SERVICES

Most physicians responsible for managing pain patients have not had much exposure to psychologists or to contemporary clinical psychology. They are unlikely to make referrals unless they have some understanding of the services provided by psychologists and also some reasonable basis for believing that these services are of value. If we are to establish productive consultation, potential referral agents must have basic information.

What information should they have, and how can they get it? At the most fundamental level, we believe that it is important for potential referral agents to have at least rudimentary information about psychological assessment and treatment procedures. If they are going to refer patients, they should have enough information about commonly used procedures so that they can answer patients' questions reasonably without seeming evasive. Moreover, they should have a general understanding of both the empirical support for the procedures used by the psychologist and the limitations of these methods. This information provides a basis for establishing realistic expectations regarding the utility of the services offered. It is beyond the scope of the present chapter to provide an overview of this material here. Succinct summaries of psychological assessment and treatment procedures, written specifically for a medical audience,

are available elsewhere (Cameron & Shepel, 1983; Cameron, Shepel, & Bowen, 1983).

There are a number of ways to inform medical colleagues about the nature of psychological consultation. The most straightforward approach, of course, is to speak directly with clinicians who inquire about making referrals. This personal contact is indispensable, but it is inefficient to rely upon it as the sole means of communication. Conversations between busy clinicians tend to be rushed, cryptic, and easily forgotten. Continuing education sessions and hospital rounds provide excellent opportunities to inform other professions about psychological services. Papers outlining psychological assessment and treatment procedures, such as those noted above (Cameron & Shepel, 1983; Cameron et al., 1983), may be passed on to interested clinicians. Psychologists who work extensively with pain patients, and get referrals from many different sources, may find it worthwhile to prepare a brief handout summarizing important information for referral agents.

The medium for dissemination of information needs to be tailored to individual circumstances. A busy family physician who is only peripherally interested in pain problems will not likely read a long paper on pain. A surgeon who specializes in chronic pain may not be satisfied with anything less. The point to be emphasized is that all referring agents need to have a reasonable understanding of psychological assessment and treatment procedures if consultation is to proceed smoothly.

SELECTING PATIENTS FOR REFERRAL

In most acute care medical settings, it is clearly both impractical and unnecessary to conduct formal psychological assessments with all pain patients. Referral agents usually screen patients, requesting psychological consultation on a selective basis. What criteria should be used to determine whether psychological consultation is warranted? In the absence of empirically established criteria, we suggest that referral might be considered with patients who manifest any of the following:

1. Evidence of notable psychological distress (e.g., depression, anxiety, irritability);
2. Evidence of a stressful personal situation (e.g., *chronic tensions* such as marked vocational or marital dissatisfaction, or a *major life change* such as bereavement or occupational change);
3. Complaints that are anatomically implausible or that appear disproportionate to organic findings;
4. Social isolation;
5. Evidence of drug abuse (alcohol, analgesics, psychotropic medications); and/or
6. A problem that is chronic or becoming so.

Patients who meet one or more of these criteria warrant careful consideration from a psychological point of view, and a formal psychological assessment might be considered.

THE REFERRAL PROCESS

Psychological consultation is of little or no value unless the patient cooperates with the psychologist. If patients are comfortable and confident about a psychological assessment, they are likely to be candid and forthcoming in their description of difficulties. On the other hand, if they are apprehensive and wary, they are likely to be guarded and reticent about problems. In extreme cases, defensive patients may decline flatly to participate in a psychological assessment.

It is understandable that pain patients might balk at the suggestion that they see a psychologist. They typically believe, generally quite correctly, that their problems have a physical basis. Hence, the relevance of a psychological consultation may not be evident to the patient. The meaning of the referral also may be unclear. The patient may infer that the physician making the referral believes the problem to be somehow less than real, or believes the patient to be seriously maladjusted psychologically. Patients who interpret the referral this way are likely to be guarded with the psychologist. Their defensiveness may be expressed in the form of hostility, reticence, or a Pollyanna presentation,

with the patient doing everything possible to project an image of robust psychological health. Such patients often deny even the most mundane difficulties in a way that undermines confidence in the veracity of their accounts. Hence, defensiveness is likely to result in the psychologist developing incomplete or distorted views of patients and their circumstances, thereby diminishing the value of the consultation.

The referral process may influence the attitude of the patient toward the psychological assessment and hence the success of the consultation. A particularly embarrassing example will illustrate how badly referrals can be botched. A man, scheduled to see one of us (Cameron will identify himself here to absolve Shepel of any responsibility!) at 9 a.m., arrived early. The man was pacing the hall, livid with anger, when the psychologist arrived. He had a lot to say, in a voice loud enough to be heard in all the offices and waiting rooms throughout the large area housing Psychology and Psychiatry. Among other things, he shouted that if it weren't for his bad back, he'd throw us all "out the goddam window." It was a nasty scene.

It turned out that the man had reason to be upset. We later confirmed his report that he had not been told that the "doctor" he had been asked to see was a psychologist. He lived hundreds of miles away. As he was unemployed, he could not afford to stay in town overnight, so he had driven most of the night in order to arrive in time for his early morning appointment. We had not checked with him to verify that the appointment time we booked through his doctor would be convenient for him. Driving seriously aggravated his back pain, so he was extremely uncomfortable and irritable when he arrived. He had been in our hospital for a couple of weeks for an extensive work-up, but due to a miscommunication a psychological assessment was not booked during his hospitalization. Instead, he was scheduled to return for an outpatient appointment a few days after discharge. Thus, he had had to make a special trip, which was taxing both physically and financially. Although his reaction was certainly extreme, the man's anger and his refusal to work with a psychologist were understandable. If we had handled things properly, we might have been able to conduct an assessment and perhaps have found a way to work constructively with this dolorous man.

Based on our clinical experience, we have come to believe that the following guidelines for making referrals may be useful. Clinicians making referrals to psychologists (or other nonmedical consultants) are likely to reassure their patients if they arrange the referral with these guidelines in mind.

Clearly Identify Nonmedical Consultants

Tell the patient directly that the consultant is a psychologist (or social worker, etc.). An awkward situation arises when the patient first becomes aware of the nature of the consultation upon arrival. The person is likely to be at least surprised and quite possibly upset and defensive. At this point the referring clinician is not at hand to provide reassurance, and the consultant's attempts to be reassuring are weakened by the fact that the patient has no basis for having confidence in a stranger.

Acknowledge that the Problem is Legitimate

Patients may become defensive if they infer from the referral that they are suspected of being malingerers or hypochondriacs. They may be reassured by an unequivocal statement indicating that the physician has no doubt that the pain is real. This reassurance is easy for physicians to give, and for patients to receive, if a demonstrable organic basis for the problem has been established

The credibility of the verbal reassurance also is likely to be high if the psychological consultation is arranged concurrently with ongoing physical investigations. When the psychological assessment comes only after physical tests have been completed and proven negative, the context of the referral may prompt the patient to conclude that

physical causes have been ruled out and that the problem is now being "dismissed" as psychological.

Potential problems arise when complaints appear to be disproportionate to organic findings. Even in this situation it may be helpful for the physician to acknowledge that the patient's distress is real. These people do appear to be in pain, although the source is unclear. Clinicians referring such patients might consider saying something along these lines to provide reassurance that the problem is being taken seriously:

> You're obviously living with a great deal of pain. We've checked you over thoroughly, and we haven't found anything to worry about. This isn't at all unusual, even with people who have severe pain. Since you are having so much pain, I don't just want to let you go with the expectation that you will improve naturally. I want to make sure that we do everything possible to get you back on track as quickly as possible. There are a number of things that you can do to help yourself. I'd like you to see X, a physiotherapist who can show you some exercises that I think will be very helpful, Y, an occupational therapist who will teach you how to move in ways that will help you avoid aggravating the problem, and Z, a psychologist who specializes in helping people with pain find ways to reduce discomfort.

Provide a Positive Rationale for the Referral

Wary patients may misperceive the psychologist as an adversary who is going to raise questions about the legitimacy of their pain problems or about their emotional stability. If so, it may be difficult for the psychologist to win the patient's confidence and cooperation. It is important that the referring clinician introduce the psychologist as an ally who is going to look for practical solutions to problems, so that the patient does not mistakenly believe that the psychologist is charged with passing judgment on the patient or the problem.

The rationale should be honest, positive, reflect respect and concern, and make sense to the patient. For instance, a surgeon considering surgery might say:

> I'd like you to see Dr. Z, a psychologist, before we decide what to do. Dr. Z has been very helpful to many of my patients, and I'd like to make sure that we are as thorough as possible so that we don't overlook anything that might be helpful to you. If we can avoid surgery, I'd like to do that. If we do decide to go ahead and operate, I want to make sure that we do everything we can to help you get back on track and Dr. Z is often helpful with this.

If surgery is not an option, the psychologist may be introduced as someone who frequently is able to help patients find ways to ease discomfort and reestablish normal activities. If the physician is able to provide specific examples of some common psychological interventions (e.g., training in muscular relaxation to counteract feelings of tension and irritability) and emphasize the desirability of nonmedical treatments, this may be helpful.

Inform Other Staff of the Rationale

The referring clinician is not necessarily the only staff member who influences the patient's perception of the psychological referral. Apprehensive patients may ask other clinical and clerical staff members about the reason for the consultation. If all staff members offer a similar reassuring rationale, this is likely to set the patient at ease. However, if staff members are uncomfortable and evasive because they do not understand the rationale, or if they give conflicting explanations to a skeptical patient, the patient may become even more defensive. It is helpful if all staff having contact with pain patients are prepared to answer patients' questions in an informed, straightforward, matter-of-fact way.

If it is feasible, there may be an advantage in having the same psychologist(s) assigned to a ward on an ongoing basis. This makes it possible for the psychologist to establish a positive personal reputation among nursing staff and veteran patients. A surprising number of patients have reported spontaneously that they were reassured about the referral when nurses or "old" patients vouched for the psychologist they were scheduled to see.

Avoid Making Cynical Comments about the Referral

Clinicians sometimes make cynical comments about patients while arranging a psychological consultation. This cynicism is understandable given the exasperation we all experience working with certain patients. Moreover, cynical comments are often intentionally funny and may reflect a kind of gallows humor rather than a mean spirit. Cynical attitudes, however, are contagious. Pervasive cynicism among staff members may be perceived by, and influence, patients. There have been a few occasions when we have discovered that patients had overheard the referring clinician make pejorative comments while arranging a psychological consultation (e.g., "What a crock! Get one of the spooks to have a look at her."). Patients who sense that the referring agent is cynical about the consultation are almost certain to arrive in a defensive, resentful state of mind. This makes it difficult to establish the rapport, trust, and cooperation required to carry out a useful psychological assessment.

If the Referral is Routine, Let Patients Know This

In some clinics all patients see a psychologist as a matter of routine. If so, the patient may be reassured by knowing this. Naturally, if psychological referrals are *not* routine, patients should not be misled into believing that they are. Such deception is not only ethically dubious, but also easily detected through conversations with other patients or staff members. Hence, well-intentioned attempts to reassure patients by duping them into believing that a referral is routine may backfire and undermine trust in the referring clinician. To maintain a sense of trust, statements about the referral being routine should be qualified carefully as appropriate (e.g., "I regularly refer people who have longstanding problems like yours to make sure that we are thorough and don't overlook anything that might help.").

Personalize the Referral

Personalized conversation can help explain the referral, while at the same time helping to establish a comfortable, friendly, warm tone. Discussion of the referral can be personalized in at least four ways. First, the referring clinician can speak hypothetically about his or her own probable reactions to the sort of problem the patient has been experiencing. Second, allusion can be made to any specific personal difficulties the patient may have mentioned. Third, the psychologist can be described in a personal way. Apprehension may be alleviated if, for instance, the psychologist is described as a down-to-earth, practical, friendly sort of person. Fourth, it may be useful to describe briefly or to allude to instances in which the psychologist was able to help people with difficulties similar to those of the current patient. If it is convenient, or if a patient is especially wary, arrangements might be made for the patient to speak with previous patients who benefited from working with the psychologist.

This sort of personalization can be done quite simply and briefly. For instance, the referring physician might say something like this:

> Problems like yours are not easy to live with. I know that if I had to put up with the pain and disability you've had to live with for as long as you have, it would certainly affect me and my family in ways that would create lots of stresses and strains. Although we haven't talked about this much, I've heard you mention that you often feel tense and grouchy and that your kids get on your nerves when you're not feeling well. This is normal for anyone in pain; virtually all my patients who have problems like yours experience these things. In fact, it's so common that I routinely refer anyone who's had pain

for any length of time to see Dr. Smith. She's a psychologist who specializes in working with pain patients. She's really enthusiastic, and practical and easy to get along with. Everyone I've ever sent to her has liked her as a person, and she's been really helpful to quite a few of my patients.

Obviously the buildup needs to be realistic, but there's no reason not to be as enthusiastic as possible. Patients pick up our optimism and enthusiasm, and these attitudes counteract apprehension.

Note that the Referral Does Not Imply a Transfer

Patients will be resentful if they suspect that they are being "dumped" by being referred to a psychologist. They may be reassured if they understand clearly that the physician or surgeon responsible for their overall management will (a) follow through with any further tests or consultations necessary to ensure a thorough physical work-up and (b) continue to be available for consultation, monitoring, and supervision. The physician can emphasize that a comprehensive team approach that brings together a wide range of expertise is used to ensure that the evaluation is thorough.

INTAKE

The intake process, as well as the referral process, deserves consideration. For instance, in booking appointments it is important to set aside enough time to complete a thorough assessment without being rushed. The appointment is likely to be much longer than most clinical appointments, and patients should anticipate this. We typically discuss the time requirements with patients in advance and make sure that the appointment times are convenient. Scheduling sometimes has presented serious problems in the past. For instance, the man described earlier was given an early morning appointment that was extremely inconvenient, and this helped set in motion a train of events that resulted in the consultation being aborted. At other times patients being picked up by relatives at a prearranged time have become perfunctory in their involvement in the assessment as they began to worry about keeping someone waiting.

Once the psychologist actually meets the patient, the first objective is to establish rapport and a sense of confidence and alliance. The way in which this sort of ambience is created will vary from patient to patient and from psychologist to psychologist: Friendly spontaneity is the key ingredient we try to assure.

Before plunging ahead with an assessment, we want to make certain that the patient understands how the psychological assessment is relevant to the investigation and solution of the pain problem. We usually ask the patient to describe the rationale for the assessment that was provided by the referring clinician. The rationale, as the patient understands it, is then fleshed out or clarified if necessary. We note that it is completely normal for people who experience persistent pain to experience psychological distress and interpersonal difficulties as a result of the pain. We may enumerate some of the common problems (e.g., irritability, sleep difficulties, a sense of discouragement) that are experienced to some degree by almost all pain patients. We may underscore this point by mentioning that, indeed, these difficulties are so pervasive that most of our clinical time is spent working with pain patients. We may add that we find it very rewarding work because there are good, practical ways to relieve many of the common difficulties experienced by pain patients. In short, we try to convey in an enthusiastic way a sense that we may well have something practical to offer.

Humor can be useful during this initial rapport-building phase. For instance, in a low key, humorous way we may acknowledge that many patients are uneasy about seeing a psychologist. We have a backlog of funny anecdotes told to us by previous patients about their initial reactions when they were asked to see "the shrink". We often tell one or two of these stories if the current patient seems un-

easy. It is implicitly clear from the anecdote that we had gone on to establish warm, amicable relationships with these earlier apprehensive patients, and this, as well as the humor, may help to build rapport with the current patient.

Finally, during this rapport-development phase, we talk explicitly about the consultation procedure and about confidentiality issues to reassure patients that they will not lose control of the process. We mention, for instance, that we will discuss our findings and recommendations with them. We let them know that we will not try to force any treatment on them. If we think we might have something useful to offer, we'll let them know what we've got in mind and they will be able to make a decision about whether or not they want to give it a try. With respect to confidentiality, we tell patients that we will treat the information they provide with strict confidence: There will be only two copies of our report, one of which will stay in our file, with the other copy going to the referring agent. No copy will be placed in the general medical chart. No copies will be released without the specific written permission of the patient. With patients who are seriously concerned about confidentiality (e.g., those with compensation claims pending often fall into this category), we discuss fully our approach to confidentiality (see below).

As we move from the rapport-building phase to the assessment proper, we usually ask the patient to describe the problem and its history. This tends to put patients at ease because this material is usually well rehearsed and not emotionally charged. It also helps to establish a sense that we are going to focus on the patient's presenting problem and not conduct an interview geared toward a purely psychological workup. A patient once remarked that "I was afraid you were going to ask me all sorts of irrelevant questions looking for signs of mental illness. I was relieved when you focused on problems I identified. You seemed to be practical and straightforward, and that meant a lot." We want to do everything we can to encourage this sort of attitude. If patients trust us enough to report problems, with the expectation that we are prepared to try to help them find solutions, the consultation is likely to be successful.

ASSESSMENT

Since this chapter is concerned with consultation issues, not assessment per se, we will not discuss assessment procedures here. A number of detailed reviews of assessment procedures are available (e.g., Cameron & Shepel, 1983; Fordyce, 1976; Turk et al., 1983). We will limit our focus to links between the assessment and the consultation process.

The Assessment Question

Effective consultation requires that the referral agent and the psychologist have a shared understanding of the purpose of the assessment. The person who initiated the referral must be asking a question that the psychologist can address, and the psychologist must address the question that the referring clinician has asked. What, then, is the right question?

The most appropriate question to be addressed, in our view, is "What might be done to help this patient experience less distress and disability?" Posing the assessment question this way promotes a good working relationship with the patient, since it means that the psychologist is establishing an alliance with the patient to search for practical solutions to problems that are identified. Moreover, the referring clinician is likely to get information that is useful for formulating a comprehensive treatment plan.

Although the referral question we framed may seem self-evident, psychologists often are called upon to address other questions, some of which seem inappropriate. For instance, we sometimes have been asked to determine whether a given patient's problem is "functional." This question is problematic because there is no reason to believe that psychological and physical difficulties are mutually exclusive. Hence, evidence that a patient has

psychological difficulties can in no way be used to rule out an organic basis for the problem. We have seen patients who have had obvious psychological difficulties, who nonetheless were found eventually to have equally impressive physical problems as well. In a striking case of this type, we were asked to see a woman whose expressions of pain seemed extraordinarily histrionic, and who appeared on the basis of both interview impressions and psychological test data to have flagrant psychological problems. Nevertheless, the surgeon responsible for her management followed through with a thorough work-up and discovered an elusive but life-threatening condition that undoubtedly was causing his patient great pain.

Psychological assessment sometimes is requested to confirm other diagnostic labels as well. For example, we have been asked to evaluate "hysterical predisposition" or "hypochondriacal tendencies." This sort of labeling is of dubious value: The meaning of the label is usually unclear, and the label provides no information about what might be done to help the patient. Moreover, since such labels tend to have pejorative connotations, they may engender negative perceptions of the patient and pessimism regarding the prognosis. None of this is likely to be helpful to the patient.

Psychological assessment sometimes is requested to determine the probability that a given patient will respond favorably to a treatment (e.g., surgery) under consideration. This sort of prediction would be valuable if it could be achieved with accuracy and confidence. The available data suggest, however, that we must be very cautious about attempting such prediction. A number of studies have examined treatment outcomes in relation to pretreatment scores on the Minnesota Multiphasic Personality Inventory (MMPI). High pretreatment scores on certain MMPI scales have been found to be associated with poor response to surgical procedures (Blumetti & Modesti, 1976; Pheasant, Gilbert, Golforb, & Herron, 1979; Wiltse & Rocchio, 1975), conservative treatment

(McCreary, Turner, & Dawson, 1979), and anesthesiologic and psychiatric interventions (Strassberg, Reimherr, Ward, Russell, & Cole, 1981). However, some investigators failed to find a significant relationship between pretreatment MMPI scores and response to surgical (Waring, Weisz, & Bailey, 1976) and rehabilitative treatment (Cummings, Evanski, Debenedetti, Anderson, & Waugh, 1979). Moreover, when pretreatment MMPI scores are correlated with response to treatment, the correlation is sometimes so modest as to be of limited value clinically (Pheasant et al., 1979).

Although some clinicians seem to believe that they can make accurate judgements and predictions based on clinical impressions, the empirical evidence suggests that subjective clinical prediction is much more fallible than is commonly recognized (e.g., Chapman & Chapman, 1969; Meehl, 1955; Nisbett & Ross, 1980). In the absence of evidence that treatment outcome for individual patients can be predicted accurately and consistently across patient samples and clinical settings, undertaking an assessment to predict treatment response appears risky.

REVIEWING FINDINGS AND RECOMMENDATIONS WITH PATIENTS

We make a point of discussing our findings, impressions, and recommendations with patients during the final phase of the assessment process. This is helpful in a number of ways. First, it provides an incentive for us to think and talk about the problem in practical, constructive, nontechnical terms. Second, it gives the patient an opportunity to correct misperceptions and to provide relevant information we may have overlooked. We explicitly encourage patients to let us know what they think of our formulation so that we can correct erroneous impressions or straighten out misunderstandings. Third, it enables us to assess the patient's perceptions of our assessment and recommendations. Fourth, this open approach tends to build confidence and

trust. And, finally, it makes it possible for us to take responsibility for presenting the assessment to the patient. This is usually preferable, from the point of view of everyone concerned, to simply passing on a report to the referring agent, leaving it to the latter to discuss with the patient a psychological report that he or she may not fully understand or feel comfortable discussing.

As we talk about our findings with the patient, we emphasize that we do not have the "big picture." We note that we will pass on a report to the referring agent. Once all consultants have reported to the referring agent, it will be up to the latter to "put all the pieces together" and decide what should be done. Patients may become confused by piecemeal, unintegrated information from consultants, and it is important for them to know who has ultimate responsibility for pulling things together and formulating a management plan.

To minimize defensiveness, we try to link our feedback to the patient's self-report as much as possible. For example, if a patient has a clinically significant elevation on scale 2 (Depression) of the MMPI, we might say, "There were no surprises on the test. You mentioned during our interview that you sometimes feel blue and discouraged, and your responses during the test reflected that. The test helps us gauge how serious problems like this are. Your responses suggested that your spirits do get pretty low at times and that we might want to work on this to see if we can find ways to help you get charged up and improve your mood." If there is a discrepancy between test results and self-report during interview, we typically go over pertinent test responses individually and discuss problems acknowledged on the test that did not surface during the interview. For example, we might say, "in responding to the test, you indicated that you often . . . and sometimes . . . . I'm glad we caught this, because I didn't pick it up during the interview, and we can often do something about this." Organizing feedback around the patient's own words and avoiding labels and technical language (e.g., clinical names of MMPI scales) tend to make the process relatively comfortable and to promote clear communication.

REPORTING FINDINGS AND RECOMMENDATIONS

We have developed a few simple guidelines that we use for reporting findings. First, we have found it useful to provide an "interim report" to the referring agent prior to finalizing our formulation. Second, we try to separate observation from inference. Third, we try to evolve recommendations that are practical given the patient's circumstances.

Interim Reporting

We find it useful to make an "interim report" to the referring agent as soon as possible after seeing the patient. Typically, this report is verbal. Our goal is to offer a tentative formulation and, perhaps, tentative recommendations. The preliminary, tentative tone of the report helps to establish a collaborative relationship with the referral agent, who finds it easy to contribute to the formulation process. If, in contrast, a formulation is phrased dogmatically, or with a sense of finality, the referring agent, who may for good reason disagree with the psychological formulation, is placed in the position of having to challenge or ignore the report. We explicitly solicit the referring agent's reactions to our tentative formulation. This makes it possible to work toward a formulation that takes into account information that may have been unavailable or overlooked during the psychological assessment but is deemed important by the referring agent.

The referring agent's reactions to the interim report also provide information about his or her impressions of the patient. It is important to bear these in mind in formulating the case to ensure that the formulation is credible to the referring agent. For instance, a patient initially may be somewhat abrasive, but then settle down and become pleasant as rapport is established. If the referring agent has spent little time with the patient and not yet established a comfortable relationship, he

or she may find the patient irritating, with few redeeming qualities. If the psychologist's report describes the patient as a pleasant person, without noting the initial abrasiveness and irritation, the referring agent may be inclined to discount the psychologist's perceptions.

In the interim report we note the additional information we want to collect to refine our formulation. For instance, we often want to know how family members perceive the patient and the problem. Sometimes the referring agent is able to provide valuable information directly (e.g., a family physician may know the family very well). In other cases, the referring agent can help expedite the information-gathering process (e.g., by letting the psychologist know that a family from out of town has an appointment to speak with the surgeon and that it might be possible for the psychologist to arrange an interview during the same visit).

As part of the interim report, we indicate how the patient perceives our formulation and recommendations. It is particularly important to let the referring agent know about any reservations the patient may have about either the formulation or the recommendations. Failure to do this may result in an awkward situation if the referring agent begins to discuss our report with the patient without recognizing that the patient is not in full agreement.

We have contrived an illustrative segment of an interim report that is concerned with the hypothetical patient's mood.

Sample Segment of Interim Report

> While Mr. X. denied depression on interview, he did acknowledge biological concomitants of depression: loss of appetite and weight, sleep disturbance (both sleep onset insomnia and early morning wakening), and loss of interest in sexual activity. Moreover, there was a clinically significant elevation on the Depression scale of the MMPI and a striking lack of animation during the interview. Thus, although he denied depression per se, Mr. X. appeared to be remarkably

subdued and he acknowledged difficulties often associated with depression.

Mr. X.'s account suggested that the problems just described are secondary to his back injury and not related to endogenous depression. He denied either a personal or family history of emotional difficulties. The difficulties he described (sleep disturbance, etc.) reportedly developed several weeks after his injury as he began to realize that his back problem was not going to be relieved quickly. He has not worked for 4 months, but he is not eligible for compensation since his injury did not occur at work. He has been living on savings, which are now almost exhausted. He has had to restrict leisure activities (hunting, fishing, snowmobiling, etc.). He said that he is, quite understandably, "worried" and "discouraged" by all this.

Mr. X. indicated that he is perplexed about the nature of his problem, the treatment plan, and the prognosis. He has seen a number of specialists and consultants both before and since his admission here. He has received what he perceives to be fragmentary, and sometimes vague and contradictory, information from these people. He would appreciate an opportunity to discuss findings and plans with someone who is in a position to provide an integrated, comprehensive overview. Although he is rather reserved and shy, he has many questions, and I think that it would be useful to draw him out and discuss things thoroughly.

If the "depressive" complaints Mr. X. reported are indeed secondary to his injury, these problems may dissipate to the extent that the pain problem can be resolved. Assuming that Mr. X. will continue to experience some discomfort and disability, training in pain management skills may be useful. Also, treatment for the secondary problems, notably sleep disturbance, might be considered. Normally, I would encourage Mr. X. to consult a local psychologist, psychiatrist, or social worker for these services. However, this is not feasible since he lives in an isolated community where there are no mental health professionals available. I am prepared to offer him self-administered treatments (e.g., stimulus control strategies and relaxation training for sleep disturbance)

and to see him periodically to check on his progress. He seems to be interested in this, but he is still hoping that you will be able to resolve his problem surgically. If antidepressant medication is considered at some point, it will be important to bear in mind that Mr. X. does not see himself as depressed. The rationale for prescribing the medication should take this into account: It might be noted that pain patients with his constellation of problems sometimes benefit from medications commonly used to treat depression.

Normally the interim report is made verbally, so the tone tends to be less formal, and the communication process is more interactive than this written example would suggest.

Separating Observation and Inference

We try to describe concretely the observations that we regard as key to the formulation of the case. For example, with the hypothetical interim report above, the observations that prompted us to regard the man as depressed, despite his denial, are noted. We attempt to separate observation and inference for two reasons.

First, by making the process of observation and inference explicit, our formulation may be disputed. It may be that our observations are incomplete, or that some other formulation may be derived from the observations assembled. Conversely, if the person reading the report has had a different impression of the patient, linking the formulation to observation may convince the reader that the person who prepared the report had a more complete understanding of the problem and that the unexpected formulation therefore deserves serious consideration. In either case, describing observations and deriving the formulation from the observations provides a basis for discussing the case as objectively as possible. This tends to avert standoffs, with the consultant and the referring agent having different perceptions that are difficult to reconcile because the formulation process has been implicit rather than explicit.

Second, the report may serve an educational function if important observations are noted and the formulation process is made explicit. Most pain patients are not seen by psychologists. There may be some advantage to training medical colleagues how to think like psychologists, so that they can approach the psychological aspects of their patients' problems in a systematic way. A report that help them learn what information psychologists regard as pertinent, and how this information is used to develop a treatment plan, may be useful for this purpose.

Formulating Practical Recommendations

An assessment undertaken for the purpose of identifying potential solutions to problems is likely to culminate in a set of recommendations. To be practical, recommendations should be specific. For instance, it is more helpful to recommend a specific form of behavioral treatment to deal with a particular problem than it is to recommend unspecified "psychotherapy." It is important to avoid recommendations that are unacceptable to the patient or that are impractical because the services recommended are not available to the patient (e.g., people in outlying communities may not have access to psychological services).

If the rationale for the recommended treatment will affect its acceptability to the patient, this should be noted with the recommendation (e.g., a patient might balk at being treated for depression, but be willing to take antidepressant medication, honestly identified as such, if it is offered with the explanation that problems similar to the patient's are sometimes relieved by this medication even though the drug is most often used for its anti-depressant effects).

If psychologists recommend some form of psychological treatment, it is also helpful for them to offer to serve as a liaison in helping to arrange appropriate treatment (e.g., by contacting the most appropriate psychologist in the patient's home town).

CONFIDENTIALITY

Psychological reports often contain highly sensitive personal information. Care needs to be taken to protect the patient's privacy. On a number of occasions, patients have complained to us that the psychological report had been released against their wishes. Consultants need to do everything possible to ensure that the confidentiality of reports is not violated.

We tried to find a simple solution for this problem at University Hospital. As we made inquiries, it became evident that clinicians who received authorized requests for information typically turned these over to clerical staff for action. Although the psychological report was stamped "CONFIDENTIAL," it was often copied and sent out with medical and surgical reports. Staff interpreted "Confidential" to mean that the report could be sent to others, as long as the person requesting materials was "legitimate" and would in turn treat the information as "confidential." If this principle applied throughout the system, confidential materials could range far afield indeed. It simply did not occur to some staff members that this practice of circulating confidential reports might violate the patient's right to privacy. The essential problem seemed to be a lack of awareness about how the psychological report should be treated.

Given this formulation of the problem, we decided to stamp instructions for protecting privacy on the report itself. We replaced the "CONFIDENTIAL" stamp with one which reads "FOR CONFIDENTIAL use of the listed referring agent ONLY. NOT TO BE COPIED OR RELEASED. Anyone requesting information should be referred to the Division of Psychology, University Hospital."

To further protect patient privacy, we stopped placing psychological reports of medical and surgical patients in the general medical record. Now the only copy of the report that leaves our office goes to the referring agent. A memo is entered in the medical record noting that the patient was seen in our department and directing requests for information to our department. By not placing the psychological report in the main medical record, we protect the patient's privacy directly, as many people who do not need to see the psychological report have access to these records. Moreover, when we tell referring agents about this arrangement, it impresses upon them that we take the issue of confidentiality very seriously; in addition, it implies that if a report is released, there will be no possibility of responsibility being diffused.

A third measure for preserving the confidentiality of reports involves requiring that authorizations to release information indicate specifically and explicitly that the psychological report is to be released. It is not uncommon, in our experience at least, to receive a photocopy of a "blanket" release form signed by a patient. It is not clear whether or not the patient intended to authorize release of the psychological report by signing the form. We return general release forms with a note indicating that we require specific authorization before we can send out a report.

These measures seem to have reduced problems with breaches of confidentiality. In the 12 months following introduction of these measures, we had no complaints about unauthorized releases of information. In retrospect, we were able to recall specifically eight complaints during the previous 12 months. We have published a more extended discussion of our approach and its effects elsewhere (Cameron & Shepel, 1981).

It may be worth noting that by asking our referring agents to direct requests for information to us, we create opportunities to provide revised reports tailored to the needs of the new requesting agent. For example, if a patient was referred originally by a surgeon, we might have collected information not deemed relevant to the surgeon's management of the case and hence not included in our formal report. If the surgeon's patient eventually seeks psychiatric treatment, the psychiatrist may request a copy of the psychological report. If the request for the report comes to the psychologist, he or she is able to write an expanded report based on the origi-

nal notes. Conversely, sensitive personal information included in a report may be removed before the report is forwarded to a compensation board, etc., when this information is irrelevant to such an agency's needs and purposes. This opportunity to "rewrite" reports not only helps to protect the patients' privacy (as in the second case), but also serves them better clinically (as in the first case). The time required to dictate a letter revising the original report is minimal, as the basic case formulation has been completed.

We should, perhaps, note that we carefully discussed our new policies with everyone affected in advance. We spoke, for instance, with referring agents, heads of clinical departments, nurses, medical records personnel, and the Workers' Compensation Board. We encountered no difficulty. However, making changes like this abruptly and unilaterally, without prior consultation, could meet with some resistance.

CONSULTATION ISSUES IN TREATMENT

Psychological consultants can contribute to patient management in a number of ways. Most obviously, they can provide direct treatment to patients. In addition, they may provide consultation to physicians, nurses, physiotherapists, and others who are providing treatments. These two roles will be discussed separately.

Providing Psychological Treatment

The psychological assessment sets the stage for treatment. Indeed, in a real sense, treatment begins during the assessment. As we collect information, we want to try to develop a highly differentiated conceptualization of the problem. We assume that "pain" is a complex experience which may involve any or all of the following:

1. Unpleasant physical sensations over which patients have no voluntary control (e.g., burning, numbness);

2. Unpleasant physical sensations over which they can exert some control (e.g., discomfort related to sustained contraction of voluntary muscles, hyperventilation);
3. Pain-related cognitions (e.g., labeling the pain "unbearable");
4. Pain-related emotions (e.g., irritability, depression);
5. Pain-related behaviors (e.g., lying down, complaining of pain); and/or
6. Secondary problems arising from the pain (e.g., sleep difficulties).

Our assumption is that, although some of these elements may not be under voluntary control, the patient can learn to control many facets of the pain experience.

This microscopic analysis is often novel for the patient. Because so many ingredients of the pain experience are potentially under some degree of voluntary control, the detailed analysis lays the groundwork for developing a rationale for psychological intervention. During the course of the assessment, we encourage the patient to notice aspects of the experience that are amenable to control. As we move toward the end of the assessment, we describe change strategies that patients might want to use to deal with specific problems they have identified. We let them know that treatment along the lines we have described is available, and we encourage them to try it.

The credibility of the procedures may be enhanced if the rationale is not merely presented abstractly, but linked to vivid metaphors and simple demonstrations. For instance, in introducing attention diversion as a general strategy, we often ask the patient to imagine watching TV. The person is to think of one TV channel as the pain channel. If the channel selector is switched to a different channel, the "pain signal" is still there, but is not received. Attention diversion is likened to this sort of "switching process." At this point the patient may be asked to notice the sensations in his thighs and buttocks as he sits: He likely becomes aware of real sensations that weren't previously registering because he wasn't "tuned in." We may go on to suggest that pain somehow tends to capture our attention, as attested to by the common experience of "worrying" an aching tooth with our tongues. We continue our story by indicating that people can learn to reduce their experience of pain and discomfort by learning to turn their attention away from pain, and we describe some striking examples of this. Finally, we may draw on the patient's or our own experiences blocking out pain (e.g., serious injuries occurring during competitive athletic activities may have been unnoticed completely as long as attention was focused on the activity).

The process of engaging the patient's interest is difficult to describe. We attend as carefully as we can to this issue, however. If we are perfunctory, abstract, or unenthusiastic about describing our treatment approach, or if we fail to help patients see it as plausible and pertinent to their experience, patients may go through the motions without really becoming involved in our treatments. This virtually guarantees failure.

An actual demonstration of technique effectiveness can be very persuasive. For example, patients who reported feeling "strung out" and exhausted because they could not get to sleep have sometimes fallen into a sound sleep during a leisurely relaxation induction. They subsequently have little doubt that the relaxation procedure can help them relax and perhaps even get to sleep. Other patients who have gone through relaxation training have been delighted when we provided EMG feedback that demonstrated unequivocally that indeed they did have the capacity to relax themselves voluntarily.

Patient expectations about treatment outcome need to be clarified. Most patients who have had longstanding, intractable problems will continue to experience discomfort even if treatment is successful. The goal of treatment often is to train coping skills that allow the person to live more comfortably with the problem, rather than to eradicate the problem totally. Qualifying the treatment goal this way may actually enhance the credibility of many of our procedures. Patients may, for instance, dismiss relaxation training as a curative treatment, but have little difficulty accepting it as valuable for learning to cope with the problem.

It is perhaps worth noting that the goal of treatment need not be limited to management of pain and associated problems. There is an inherently negative focus to such treatment. Patients who want to improve their relationships, productivity, or sense of self-esteem, or to pursue some other positive objective, should be encouraged to do so. It may be very therapeutic to shift the focus to the development of behavior patterns and habits of mind that enhance the quality of life and foster confidence and self-esteem. There is a tendency for pain to fall into the background, though not necessarily decrease, when attention and strivings are reoriented this way. In a sense, this orientation is consistent with the operant approach to pain management (Fordyce, 1976), with its emphasis on the importance of staff disregarding pain behaviors as much as possible and focusing instead on the development of "well behaviors." Our discussion of treatment issues reflects our cognitive-behavioral orientation. It is obviously not intended to be an exhaustive overview. More comprehensive reviews of cognitive-behavior techniques and other approaches are available in other chapters of this volume and elsewhere (e.g., Roy & Tunks, 1982; Turk et al., 1983).

Providing Consultation to Caregivers

Most care received by pain patients comes from surgeons, physicians, nurses, physiotherapists, and other professionals who are not psychologists. Physical ministrations have psychological as well as physical sequelae (Frank, 1974; Shapiro & Morris, 1978). The psychologist can play a valuable role if he or she is able to help members of other disciplines recognize how they can avoid psychological pitfalls and actively promote the psy-

chological well-being of individual patients as they go about their work.

The operant approach to rehabilitation, described in detail by Fordyce (1976), has widespread applicability. Care-givers may not recognize that they themselves may exacerbate patient complaints and disabilities by selectively attending to such behaviors, thereby inadvertently reinforcing them. From an operant point of view, it seems prudent instead to emphasize indications of achievement and improvement. Indeed, it is possible and often quite easy to carefully structure a rehabilitation program in a way that virtually guarantees and calls attention to improved functioning (see Fordyce, 1976, for details).

As we talk with patients, we listen for, and inquire about, things doctors (nurses, psychologists, etc.) have said or done that were particularly helpful or especially distressing. Patients not infrequently will single out some specific experience that they claim had an important effect on them, for better or worse. We then look for opportunities to provide feedback, in tactful ways that respect the patient's privacy if that is an issue.

One theme that has emerged is that patients have expressed gratitude for reassuring information that helps them interpret their experiences in benign ways. For instance, we talked postoperatively with the patient of a psychologically gifted surgeon. This woman reported that she still seemed to have much of her original pain, as well as the expected postoperative pain. She said that she was relieved that the surgeon had told her *before* the operation to expect this, as he thought she had a severely irritated nerve that would take some time to get back to normal after surgical decompression. Moreover, after the operation he had come in to say that he had found what he had been expecting. He evidently went on to describe very graphically that, instead of being white, the compressed tissue was "the color of a plum skin." The surgeon's conversations left her with a clear sense that the likely cause of her problem had been found and with a benign, plausible interpretation for her continuing pain. All of this was especially reassuring to her because an earlier surgeon had performed surgery that resulted in no improvement, then allegedly told her that there was nothing wrong with her.

Some communications create problems. Using unnecessarily technical language and discussing important matters at inappropriate times represent common complaints. One experience that comes to mind illustrates both points. A man, who initially was quite guarded during a postoperative interview, finally implied that he was thinking of suing for malpractice. According to his report, a resident had come in when he was still recovering from the anesthetic, and told him that "a nerve decompressed during surgery." He interpreted this to mean that things had gone wrong and that he had been injured. Instead, the resident had been trying to reassure him that the decompression procedure that had been planned had in fact been accomplished successfully.

Reports like these have led us to believe that pain patients often have difficulty interpreting their problems. To what do they attribute chronic pain? To what do they attribute pain that develops or lingers postoperatively? It is important for caregivers to elicit patients' understanding of the information they have been given and to correct misinterpretations.

Often it is not possible to provide definitive answers. Nonetheless, obvious misperceptions can be ruled out for the patient. For example, a man was admitted to a surgical ward although he was scheduled for conservative treatment. He became sullen and withdrawn. It turned out that he thought he was to have surgery, although this was never contemplated or mentioned to him. He interpreted the "cancellation" of the operation as evidence that he was beyond help and on a degenerative course. Clearing up this misunderstanding had a salutary effect on the man's morale.

Patients often have attributional problems when pain recurs when they resume normal activities after a period of disability. Does the pain mean they should refrain from activity because they are aggravating a mechanical problem? Several patients have reported that their surgeons told them that, because they had not been using certain muscles during their period of disability, they should expect these muscles to be out of condition and to become painful with significant activity. This advance warning helped them dismiss the pain as normal and continue building up their activity levels gradually.

It is not clear how many patients are disabled by overreacting to normal muscular pain during recovery, but we have seen some dramatic examples of this. The most memorable was a woman who was not doing well several months after surgery and who was therefore sent for a psychological assessment. She had been involved heavily in competitive sports prior to her back problem, and the recognition she had received for her athletic achievements had been an important source of self-esteem. She found that exercise was painful after surgery and interpreted this as meaning that she could no longer be active without risking damage to her back. She dropped out of athletic activities and became quite isolated and depressed. After consultation with the surgeon, the psychologist encouraged her to entertain the possibility that the pain was related to being out of condition. A plan was developed that would allow her to work back into shape. Within a period of several weeks she was fully active. Treatment was terminated when she bowled several games in one day without pain. A 2-year follow-up review indicated that she continued to be fully active with no pain.

The general point to be made here is that the manner in which caregivers interact with patients can influence patients' attitudes, moods, and behaviors. A psychologist who is able to shed light on these processes can make a significant contribution to the pain management team. Calling attention to particularly helpful conversations or other maneuvers that have had salutary psychological consequences is an effective way to encourage these behaviors.

THE LARGER PICTURE

We have discussed consultation issues in fairly specific terms. Somehow the big picture can get lost in all of this detail. We have enjoyed thoroughly the consultation work we have done. It has been intellectually stimulating, emotionally satisfying, and a great deal of fun. No doubt we can attribute this in part to the fact that we have been fortunate enough to work with interesting, open-minded, curious, capable colleagues.

It is not all a matter of good luck, however. All of us on the pain management service have made a point of getting to know each other personally. We don't just send reports to each other. We talk face to face about patients and ideas. We exchange papers of general interest. We've watched each other work with patients. We're not bureaucratic. We use and enjoy humor. In short, we've invested a great deal in creating a work environment and interaction patterns that suit us. We have a sense that the cultivation of a comfortable, stimulating ambience, where people are concerned with challenging and affirming each other, is the real key to successful consultation.

REFERENCES

Blumetti, A.E., & Modesti, L.M. (1976). Psychological predictors of success or failure of surgical intervention for intractable back pain. In J.J. Bonica & D. Albe-Fessard (Eds.), *Advances in pain research and therapy* (Vol. 1, pp. 323–325). New York: Raven Press.

Cameron, R., & Shepel, L. (1981). Strategies for preserving the confidentiality of psychological reports. *Canadian Psychology, 22,* 191–193.

Cameron, R., & Shepel, L.F. (1983). Psychological assessment. In W.H. Kirkaldy-Willis (Ed.), *Managing low back pain* (pp. 63–73). New York: Churchill Livingstone.

Cameron, R., Shepel, L.F., & Bowen, R.C. (1983). Psychological treatment of back pain and associated problems. In W.H. Kirkaldy-Willis (Ed.), *Managing low back pain* (pp. 229–239). New York: Churchill Livingstone.

Chapman, L.J., & Chapman, J.P. (1969). Illusory correlation as an obstacle to the use of valid psychodiagnostic signs. *Journal of Abnormal Psychology, 74,* 271–280.

Cummings, C., Evanski, P.M., Debenedetti, M.J., Anderson, E.E., & Waugh, T.R. (1979). Use of the MMPI to predict outcome of treatment for chronic pain. In J.J. Bonica & V. Ventafridda (Eds.), *Advances in pain research and therapy* (Vol. 2, pp. 667–670). New York: Raven Press.

Fordyce, W.E. (1976). *Behavioral methods for chronic pain and illness.* St. Louis, MO: C.V. Mosby.

Frank, J.D. (1974). *Persuasion and healing* (rev. ed.). New York: Schocken.

McCreary, C., Turner, J., & Dawson, E. (1979). The MMPI as a predictor of response to conservative treatment for low back pain. *Journal of Clinical Psychology, 35,* 278–284.

Meehl, P. (1955). *Clinical vs. statistical prediction.* Minneapolis: University of Minnesota Press.

Melzack, R., & Wall, P.D. *The challenge of pain.* Hammondsworth, England: Penguin, 1982.

Nisbett, R., & Ross, L. (1980). *Human inference: Strategies and shortcomings of social judgment.* Englewood Cliffs, NJ: Prentice-Hall.

Pheasant, H.C., Gilbert, D., Goldfarb, J., & Herron, L. (1979). The MMPI as a predictor of outcome in low-back surgery. *Spine, 4,* 78–84.

Roy, R., & Tunks, E., Eds. (1982). *Chronic pain: Psychosocial factors in rehabilitation.* Baltimore, MD: Williams and Wilkins.

Shapiro, A.K., & Morris, L.A. (1978). Placebo effects in medical and psychological therapies. In S.L. Garfield & A.E. Bergin (Eds.), *Handbook of psychotherapy and behavior change* (2nd ed., pp. 369–410). New York: John Wiley.

Strassberg, D.S., Reimherr, F., Ward, M., Russell, S., & Cole, A. (1981). The MMPI and chronic pain. *Journal of Consulting and Clinical Psychology, 49,* 220.

Turk, D.C., Meichenbaum, D., & Genest, M. (1983). *Pain and behavioral medicine: A cognitive behavioral perspective.* New York: Guilford.

Waring, E.M., Weisz, G.M., & Bailey, S.I. (1976). Predictive factors in the treatment of low back pain by surgical intervention. In J.J. Bonica & D. Albe-Fessard (Eds.), *Advances in pain research and therapy* (Vol. 1, pp. 939–942). New York: Raven Press.

Wiltse, L.L., & Rocchio, P.D. (1975). Preoperative psychological tests as predictors of success of chemonucleolysis in the treatment of the low-back syndrome. *Journal of Bone and Joint Surgery, 57-A,* 478–483.

15 COMMONALITIES AMONG PSYCHOLOGICAL APPROACHES IN THE TREATMENT OF CHRONIC PAIN: SPECIFYING THE META-CONSTRUCTS

Dennis C. Turk
Arnold D. Holzman

The regulation of pain and suffering has been a preoccupation since the beginning of time. There are references to strategies to ameliorate pain in the Egyptian papyri, the Koran, and the Bible. Philosophers, religious leaders, health care providers, and layman alike have speculated as to the nature and cause of pain while seeking effective means of relief. The therapeutic armamentarium has consisted of a dizzying array of modalities. Consider the following melange: surgery, dorsal column stimulation, hot packs, cold packs, traction, massage, cupping, trephinning, palliative radiotherapy, nerve blocks, steroid injections, manipulations of the spine, transcutaneous nerve stimulation, muscle relaxants, anti-inflammatory medication. This list includes just some of the treatment modalities administered by the many different kinds of health care professionals who work with patients with chronic pain. Throughout history, almost every organic and inorganic substance has been ingested and nearly every part of the nervous system has been severed, all in the quest to eliminate pain. Many other approaches have been employed outside of the purview of medical practitioners, for example, copper bracelets, faith healing, distraction, "rational repudiation" through logical means, and the use of "patent" medicine, to name only a few.

We can note two general points about the lists that we have enumerated. First, at least some patients appear to derive benefit from each of the diversity of strategies, no matter how esoteric, whereas other patients, no matter what is tried, find no relief. We might be tempted to conclude that those who receive relief from modalities that do not have a scientific basis must have had "psychogenic pain," in other words, their pain was not real. This conclusion illustrates the frustration of the health care provider that occurs by assuming that one can separate psychological factors from physical ones. In reality, it may be more appropriate to view pain from a multidimensional perspective, with an interaction between physical and psychological contributors to the pain experience. This is basically the view that has been advocated by Melzack and his colleagues in the gate control theory (Melzack & Casey, 1968; Melzack & Wall, 1965). There is increasing evidence that pain extends beyond the sole contribution of sensory phenomena to include cognitive, affective, and behavioral factors (e.g., Liebeskind & Paul, 1977; Weisenberg, 1977).

Second, despite increasing knowledge, pain and pain control remain poorly understood and treatment procedures remain inadequate. Physicians have frequently noted that procedures designed to cut or block the pain pathways for patients with ostensibly the same pain syndromes have proven to be differentially effective, with frequent recurrences of pain in those patients who at first appeared to be responsive.

Commentators on the current state of understanding have concluded that, despite the magnitude of the problem and the abundance of literature on the topic, amazingly little is known about the etiology and, consequently, the most effective treatment for many pain syndromes (e.g., Flor & Turk, 1984; Greene, 1980). Nachemson (1979) summarized the current situation regarding back pain in the following way:

> Having been engaged in this field for nearly 25 years and having been clinically engaged in back problems for nearly the same period of time, and as a member and scientific adviser to several international back associations, I can only state that for the majority of our patients, the true cause of low back pain is unknown. (p. 143) . . . since the cause is unknown there is only symptomatic treatment available. (p. 145)

Similarly, Greene (1980) described the situation for another pain syndrome, temporomandibular myofascial pain dysfunction syndrome in this way:

> Rarely in the history of dentistry have so many labored for so long, only to end with extreme disagreement. After more than half a century, the myofascial pain-dysfunction (MPD) syndrome continues to be one of the most controversial areas in dentistry. (p. 284)

Frustration with the inadequacies of conventional theories and treatment modalities has resulted in a search for alternative treatments. Some have looked to the Orient, seeking panaceas in acupuncture, yoga, and various herbal preparations. Others, having more faith in Western technologies, have embraced biofeedback and different types of physical exercise apparatus. As would be expected, each of these approaches has provided some relief for some patients with some syndromes; but there are many for whom adequate control of pain remains elusive.

Interestingly, the success of the treatment modality is often unrelated to the rationale for the treatment. For example, thermal and frontalis EMG biofeedback have been reported to be successful for treating migraine and tension headaches, respectively. Yet, the association between reduction in psychophysiological activity and reports of reduced pain has not been consistently demonstrated (Turk, Meichenbaum, & Berman, 1979).

Thus, Melzack and Casey (1968) suggest:

> The surgical and pharmacological attacks on pain might well profit by redirecting thinking toward the neglected and almost forgotten contribution of motivational and cognitive processes. Pain can be treated not only by trying to cut down sensory input by anesthesthetic blocks, surgical intervention, and the like but also by influencing the motivational-affective and cognitive factors as well. (p. 435)

In this book, we have brought together a set of contributors who have described some of the most recent advances and innovations in the use of psychological modalities to treat chronic pain, including: operant conditioning, cognitive-behavior modification, social skills training, support, hypnosis, family therapy, and biofeedback. In addition, chapters were included that described the use of psychological modalities with several specific populations, namely, children, cancer patients, and headache patients.

As with many of the treatment modalities there is some support for the efficacy of each of these approaches. We are struck with the similarity of the conclusions despite the diversity of approaches. The question remains how to explain these results. In the remainder of this chapter, we will consider what "meta-constructs" or common features are present among the approaches described in the preceding chapters. It is important to realize that the amount of emphasis and the degree of incorporation of these constructs will vary, yet we believe that they are sufficiently frequent to warrant consideration as "common features," or what some in the psychotherapy literature have called the "nonspecifics" of therapy.

COMMON FEATURES AMONG PSYCHOLOGICAL APPROACHES

Reconceptualization

Examination of each of the chapters reveals that, regardless of the specific modalities employed, each provides a conceptualization of the cause of the patient's pain that is consistent with the modality(ies) incorporated in the treatment regimen. That is, the practitioner provides a rationale of the patient's pain that makes it appear amenable to the treatment offered. Some rationales (e.g., operant conditioning, biofeedback) are stated explicitly at treatment onset, whereas others are more implicitly conveyed during treatment (e.g., family therapy, group therapy). For example, the operant conditioning therapist (Fordyce, 1976; Roberts, chapter 2 of this volume) provides a learning or conditioning model to explain the development and maintenance of chronic pain. The therapist with this orientation explains that behaviors that are initially appropriate during acute

pain may become reinforced over time. These same behaviors that are adaptive for acute conditions are maladaptive in chronic pain and lead to greater incapacity and suffering. On the other hand the group therapist may communicate the treatment rationale more subtly by allowing patients to learn to cope more successfully by providing the group as a vehicle for in vivo learning and modeling of appropriate behaviors (Gentry and Owens, chapter 7 of this volume).

The vast majority of patients have already evolved their own idiosyncratic views that are likely to be based on a somatic rather than a psychological causation. Therefore, the reconceptualization process appears to be especially important when a psychologically oriented treatment is to be offered. Patients are likely to be skeptical, if not hostile, toward an approach that is incompatible with their perspective (Cameron, 1978; Cameron & Shepel, chapter 14 of this volume). They are likely to be concerned that a psychologically oriented treatment is being prescribed because their pain is not being taken seriously and is not being viewed as "real." We would speculate that failure to present an acceptable explanation, regardless of how effective the treatment approach, is doomed from the outset.

The cognitive-behavioral approach (Turk, Meichenbaum, & Genest, 1983; and chapter 3 of this volume) places the greatest amount of emphasis on the importance of the role of the reconceptualization process. According to adherents of this approach, a critical component of treatment is preparing the client for the treatment modalities to be employed, so that patient and therapist expectations are the same. Regardless of the treatment being offered, the patient must come to believe that the modalities offered match the problem and that treatment is likely to be successful.

Turk, Holzman, and Kerns (in press) have suggested that the reconceptualization process serves five crucial functions:

1. It provides a more benign view of the problem than the patient's own view;

2. It translates patients' symptoms into difficulties that can be pinpointed as specific, addressable problems rather than problems that are vague, undifferentiated, overwhelming, and uncontrollable;

3. It recasts problems in forms that are amenable to solutions and thus the reconceptualization should foster hope, positive anticipation, as well as expectancy for success;

4. It prepares patients for interventions contained within the treatment regimen that are directly linked to the conceptualization that is proposed;

5. It creates a positive expectancy that the treatment being offered is appropriate for the problem. (pp. 25–26)

Optimism and Combating Demoralization

Each treatment approach, whether implicitly or explicitly stated, provides a message of hope and optimism. When patients have experienced unremitting pain for long periods of time, they are usually demoralized. They have received multiple interventions, yet they still have pain. Health care providers seem impotent, and the patients may feel that there is little hope of a satisfactory resolution to their problem. Their experience of pain is unrelenting and beyond anyone's control.

All of the treatment approaches described in this book convey a sense of hope. The message is that "We understand your situation and your pain and we have ways of helping you." A sense of optimism is presented along with the description of the intervention. This sense of optimism permeates the entire treatment process.

Cognitive-behavioral approaches (Holzman, Turk, & Kerns, chapter 3 of this volume) emphasize the need to alter patients' beliefs that pain is an all encompassing state over which they can exert little control. The treatment rationale must confront the sense of helplessness and hopelessness experienced by the patient. The cognitive-behavioral practitioner attempts to combat demoralization by educating patients so as to translate their view

of pain from an overwhelming, continuous assault to a view of their problems as potentially manageable and under their control. In short, the practitioner of this approach attempts to help the patient view himself as competent and resourceful and his efforts at coping with the pain as likely to be successful.

Biofeedback practitioners and those who espouse the operant perspective combat demoralization by providing feedback concerning success. In biofeedback, the patient is directly provided continuous information about his or her control over physiological functioning. Threshold levels and target physiological responses can be selected so that the patient is likely to perceive maximal reinforcement, thereby ensuring that he or she remains in treatment.

In operant conditioning, patients are provided with specific behavioral regimens (i.e., "up-time," physical exercise). These regimens are designed so that the patient is likely to gain positive reinforcement, thereby facilitating "shaping" of improved functioning and maintaining motivation for treatment. Social reinforcement is employed through the treatment setting milieu. Charts to record activity levels are employed to demonstrate improvements in activity throughout the treatment regimen, to provide self-reinforcement, and to be used by the treatment team as the basis for praise and evaluation of treatment progress.

Individualization of Treatment

Despite the fact that the different treatment approaches described include specific techniques, each of them individualizes the intervention to meet the needs of the particular patient. Thus, the nature of the physical exercise regimen will vary according to the age, sex, and physical status of individual patients. Barber (chapter 10 of this volume) describes the use of different hypnotic strategies depending upon the patient's idiosyncratic style and needs. Cognitive-behavioral and operant-conditioning practitioners individualize the nature of goals and homework assignments.

The flexibility of these approaches is important, as they should not be viewed as being rigidly applied. Thus, both the specific goals of treatment and the nature and content of the modalities employed are tailored to meet the needs of the individual patient. The treatments are not presented in a rigid or lock-step manner, as might be assumed from reading descriptions of various approaches in some texts.

Active Patient Participation and Responsibility

Unlike somatic treatments, where emphasis is based on the skills of the health care provider, psychologically based treatments rely heavily on the skills and active participation of the patients in their own treatment. Thus, most of the interventions described in this book depend upon the patient practicing specific skills (e.g., relaxation) or performing activities *outside* of the therapeutic milieu. Things are not done to a passive patient, as is the case with surgery and conventional medical treatments. Rather, the efficacy of the treatment is largely a function of the actions of the patient.

Each of the psychologically oriented treatments relies heavily on the patient's assuming responsibility for much of the treatment. Some programs have fairly rigid exclusion criteria, with the lack of motivation being an important consideration (e.g., Anderson, Cole, Gullickson, Hudgens, & Roberts, 1977). It is imperative that patients understand their own responsibility and are willing to accept this in treatment. This requirement contrasts with that of more somatic treatments where the patient relinquishes most responsibility to the health care provider.

The active acceptance of responsibility by the patient is particularly important for those treatment approaches that rely on outpatient treatment. Assuming the patient is seen for therapy, whether hypnosis, group therapy, biofeedback, or traditional supportive therapy, this leaves the patient on his or her own to adhere to and to practice the various skills covered during treatment sessions, and to engage in specific tasks or assignments if prescribed (e.g., physical exercise). Even inpatient programs will discharge patients who will then return to their natural environment. Patients will be expected to continue practicing and using skills and information developed during the inpatient hospitalization.

In sum, all of the psychological modalities incorporate a collaborative relationship between the practitioner and the patient. Practitioners work with patients, not on them.

Skills Acquisition

Psychological interventions share a concern with the acquisition of new skills or strengthening of existing skills. Biofeedback emphasizes patients' learning how to control physiological functioning; hypnosis incorporates attention diversion and focusing skills; family therapy emphasizes communication skills; cognitive-behavioral approaches incorporate problem-solving and stress-management skills; eclectic programs (Newman & Seres, chapter 5 of this volume) include, among other procedures, acquisition of information on body mechanics and assertiveness. Thus, in a sense, each treatment includes a skills-acquisition component.

This skills-acquisition component can be contrasted with somatic treatments, where, with the exception of physical therapy, the patient is not expected to learn anything. Again, the contrast of an active versus passive patient can be noted.

Self-Efficacy

In laboratory studies of pain tolerance, subjects who believed they had control over a noxious stimulus, who knew what to expect, or who confronted a predictable aversive stimulus, demonstrated increased tolerance for nociceptive stimulation compared to subjects with minimal perceived control, who did not know what to expect, or who were confronted with an unpredictable stimulus (e.g., Averill, 1973; Bowers, 1968; Johnson, 1973).

Several clinical studies have reported that the success of biofeedback treatments for various pain syndromes seemed to be unrelated to actual psychophysiological changes following treatment. Rather, success following biofeedback seemed to be associated with increased perceptions of self-control (e.g., Flor, Haag, Turk, & Koehler, 1983; Holroyd & Andrasik, 1978; Nouwen & Solinger, 1979).

Somatic treatments place heavy emphasis on what Bandura (1977) has labeled "outcome efficacy"—the expectancy that the treatment will be beneficial for the patient's problem. In contrast, psychological treatments focus on both outcome efficacy and what Bandura (1977) has labeled "self-efficacy"—the belief that the patient can himself perform the requisite behavioral strategies (e.g., relaxation, control of muscular activity, stress management, assertion) when the situation warrants. The distinction between outcome efficacy and self-efficacy is important, because a patient may believe that the specific treatment would be effective for others with similar problems (high outcome efficacy) but doubt that he will be able to acquire or use the specific techniques incorporated within the treatment (low self-efficacy) (Turk & Meichenbaum, in press).

Self-Attribution of Change

The psychologically oriented treatments encourage the patient to attribute goal accomplishments to himself, or herself; that is, self-reinforcement is implicitly conveyed by all of these approaches. The operant-conditioning therapist positively reinforces the patients' performance of "well-behaviors" (i.e., activity); the cognitive-behavior therapist emphasizes the accomplishments that the patients bring about; the biofeedback therapist weans patients from the psychophysiological apparatus and encourages them to practice the skills that they have learned in their natural environment. In a sense, the message is not what a fine job the therapist has done but rather how well the patient has learned to take charge of his life and his pain.

It is our belief that the seven interrelated constructs just discussed are inherent in all of the psychologically oriented treatments described in this book. Much greater attention has been given to the specifics of various treatment modalities, the size, composition, and placement of electrodes in biofeedback, the nature of the imagery employed in cognitive behavior modification, details of the exercise charts employed by operant-conditioning practitioners, and the method of trance induction employed in hypnotherapy. These factors are important, but it is our opinion that excessive emphasis on the specifics to the exclusion of the seven meta-constructs outlined will likely mitigate successful utilization of various treatment modalities. Treating chronic pain is a complex process that requires a set of many skills in addition to specific details related to any one treatment modality.

SOME DIFFERENCES AMONG PSYCHOLOGICAL APPROACHES

We have identified a set of meta-constructs that appear to be inherent in all psychological approaches. There are, however, a number of factors that differentiate these approaches beyond the characteristics of the specific techniques and modalities employed.

Role of Assessment in Treatment

Examination of each of the chapters included reveals that the relationship between assessment and treatment varies greatly. Most of the chapters rely on the use of interviews and the standardized questionnaires (e.g., Minnesota Multiphasic Personality Inventory [MMPI]). The cognitive-behavioral approaches with both adults (Holzman, Turk, & Kerns, chapter 3 of this volume) and children (Varni, Jay, Masek, & Thompson, chapter 11 of this volume) place greater emphasis on comprehensive and multimodal assessment. Cleeland and Tearnan (chapter 12 of this volume) also describe the importance of comprehensive assessment in developing specific treatment regimens for cancer patients.

Assessment can be used for at least three purposes — for screening, as a basis for prescription, and for evaluation of treatment progress and efficacy (Turk & Kerns, 1985). Assessment can serve solely as a screening function to rule out those individuals for whom the treatment is deemed inappropriate. Different practitioners have different criteria for deciding who is likely to benefit from the particular approach and who is inappropriate. It is incumbent upon practitioners to consider such questions as: "Who is a likely candidate for biofeedback versus hypnosis?", "Are there some patients who are not likely to benefit from group therapy?", and "What criteria should I employ to decide whether a patient should be treated on an inpatient rather than an outpatient basis?" Assessment can be employed to provide relevant information to assist in such decision making.

A second function of assessment is for deciding upon the focus, or which components of treatment to emphasize. Practitioners can use a range of assessment techniques to assist them in deciding whether the spouse should be included, whether depression needs to be treated, what specific goals should be addressed, and so forth.

The third function of assessment relates to evaluation. How does the practitioner determine the success of his or her intervention? And how does he or she develop information as to the nature of patients, specifically what demographic, physiological, and psychological characteristics distinguish the best candidates? Evaluation need not wait until the end of treatment, rather it can be viewed as an ongoing process. Goals may need to be altered, treatment modalities may need to be added or modified. The practitioner needs to be aware that assessment and treatment are in actuality inextricably linked. A number of texts are available that focus on instruments

and procedures available for use in assessing patients with chronic pain (e.g., Jacox, 1977; Melzack, 1983; Turk et al., 1983).

Family Involvement

The degree of emphasis on the involvement of the family varies from therapies with minimal attention and involvement to family therapy where the family is the major focus of attention. It is interesting to consider how little attention is typically given to families when the treatment of chronic pain is discussed (Flor & Turk, 1985). Families are rarely discussed, and usually they are viewed as possibly contributing to the problem by positively reinforcing pain behaviors and punishing reinforcing well behaviors (Roberts, chapter 2 of this volume).

Chronic pain takes place within the family context. All aspects of the family's life are affected — roles, financial, activity. We have observed in our pain program that spouses of chronic pain patients report being up to four times more depressed than the patients (!) and suffering from a variety of other psychological and psychophysiological problems. The impact of chronic pain on family members is a neglected area. The role of the family in treatment is thus far a poorly researched area and an area that may be found to be of great importance (Roy, chapter 8 of this volume).

Specificity of Treatment Goals

The development of specific treatment goals also varies. The cognitive-behavioral and operant approaches place great emphasis on specific, individualized goals. In contrast, group approaches (Gentry and Owens, chapter 7 of this volume), eclectic approaches (Newman and Seres, chapter 5 of this volume), and hypnotic approaches (Barber, chapter 10 of this volume) make little mention of goals.

The goals of treatment vary from alleviation of pain, as is often the case with biofeedback employed with headache patients

(Andrasik, chapter 13 of this volume) and with hypnosis, to learning to live more effectively despite pain as emphasized in the eclectic approach and in operant conditioning, to coping more effectively with pain as in the case of cancer patients and patients treated within the cognitive-behavioral perspective.

The attention to medication reduction also varies, from the operant and cognitive-behavioral approaches always addressing medication when indicated to the group therapy, family therapy, and hypnotic approaches giving little direct attention to medication reduction. As Cleeland and Tearnan (chapter 12 of this volume) note, the importance of medication reduction varies to some extent based on the specific population treated.

Philosophies differ on these specific dimensions, and there are no clearcut guidelines to help the practitioner decide how much to emphasize them. To some extent they will depend upon the particular patient being treated.

Attention to Dysphoric Mood

Depression has been documented as a frequent concomitant of chronic pain (e.g., Romano & Turner, 1985; Roy, Thomas, & Mates, 1984). Some reports have indicated the incidence of depression among chronic pain patients to be as high as 100%, although the majority of studies suggest that around 50% of chronic pain patients are significantly depressed (e.g., Kamlinger, Swanson, & Maruta, 1983; Lindsay & Wychoff, 1981). Several explanations for the incidence of depression have been offered. Perhaps the most prevalent view is that depression is an understandable secondary reaction to a chronic, incapacitating medical condition, and as the condition persists, dysphoric mood increases. There are some data to suggest that depression following a medical problem may, in a recursive manner, lead to increased physiological problems subsequent to the initial physical one (Aneshensel, Frerichs, & Huba, 1984).

Although the secondary reaction model makes intuitive sense, it is inadequate because it does not account for the fact that at least 50% of chronic pain patients do not demonstrate significant depression. Thus, it seems likely that other factors must be involved in determining why some patients become depressed and others do not.

From a psychoanalytic perspective, Blumer & Heilbronn (1982) have speculated that chronic pain reflects an underlying depressive state in a "pain-prone" personality. According to this model, those pain patients who appear depressed after the onset of the medical problem were actually depressed prior to the manifestation of their pain syndrome and, in fact, pain is only the surface symptom of a primary affective disorder. At the present time, there is little empirical support for this model, and the conceptualization has been seriously challenged (France, Krishnan, Houpt, & Maltbie, 1984; Turk & Salovey, 1984).

An alternative possibility is that patients who become depressed following the onset of pain had some emotional difficulties prior to pain and the medical problem simply served to exacerbate preexisting problems. This explanation is difficult to verify, as it relies on retrospective reporting that may be biased. Following the development of symptoms, it is all too easy to search for prior causal factors as explanations.

Recently, Turk and his colleagues (Kerns & Turk, 1984; Turk, Kerns, & Rudy, 1984; Turk & Salovey, 1984) have proposed an explanation consistent with contemporary cognitive (Beck, 1967; Rehm, 1977; Seligman, 1975) and behavioral formulations (Lewinsohn, 1974) of depression. According to this cognitive-behavioral conceptualization, depression among chronic pain patients is both a function of negative cognitions (e.g., perceptions of helplessness and limited self-control), as well as of reduction in response-contingent reinforcement associated with declines in activity and instrumental behavior. Those patients who become depressed following pain onset are the ones who appraise their situation as beyond their control, and they perceive their pain as drastically interfering with all aspects of their life and the degree of satisfaction they experience. One important factor that appears to contribute as a buffer against the development of depression is social support, especially by the spouse (Kerns & Turk, 1984).

The treatment modalities described in previous chapters frequently acknowledge the problem of dysphoric mood, but they vary greatly as to whether they directly or indirectly attend to it. For example, Merskey (chapter 4 of this volume) provides a detailed discussion of dysphoric mood among pain patients and notes the use of antidepressant medication, as do Newman and Seres (chapter 5 of this volume). In contrast, several of the other chapters indirectly address depression by trying to increase physical activity and by positively reinforcing other well behaviors (e.g., operant conditioning, Roberts, chapter 2 of this volume), by increasing perceptions of self-control and self-efficacy (e.g., biofeedback, Belar & Kibrick, chapter 9 of this volume), or by assisting patients to alter their appraisals of their situation (e.g., cognitive-behavioral intervention, Holzman et al., chapter 3 of this volume).

The effect of different treatment approaches on dysphoric mood, as well as on reports of pain and activity, should be examined. Is it necessary for treatments to directly address problems of dysphoric mood, or will improvements in activity, perceptions of control, and reduction in perceived intensity of pain indirectly result from alleviation of emotional distress? Research needs to address the sequence of therapeutic progress and not only the outcome. Follow-up studies to examine the order of change as well as the association of mood and other dependent measures also need to be conducted.

CONCLUDING COMMENTS

We need to note that many of the specific treatment modalities described in this book can be incorporated with each other as well as with existing somatic treatment interventions. That is, psychological approaches need not be viewed exclusively as alternatives to conventional medical and surgical regimens. As demonstrated in the chapters by Cleeland and Tearnan and by Belar and Kibrick in this volume, the strategies described are readily incorporated into ongoing treatment programs.

All of the psychological treatments attempt to encourage sufficient intrinsic and extrinsic motivation so that gains made during treatment are generalized beyond the therapeutic setting and are maintained over extended periods of time. Many patients will continue to experience pain (hopefully, at least, at some reduced level of intensity), despite the best efforts of health care providers. The important issue is how to help patients accept this while at the same time encouraging them to continue to adhere to the therapeutic regimens (e.g., physical exercise, relaxation, attention diversion, open communication). We may expect that the naturally reinforcing properties of successful treatment outcome should lead to continued adherence to strategies learned during treatment. Nevertheless, we know from other areas that successful treatment outcome is often not enough to ensure continued adherence (e.g., Marlatt & Gordon, 1980). Adherence is a major problem for all medical treatments and attention to this topic is greatly needed. No psychologically oriented treatment modality, no matter how powerful, is likely to have long-lasting benefits if the patients do not continue to make use of what has been learned during treatment.

Psychological approaches should not be viewed as panaceas; rather, the techniques and approaches should be viewed as tools to enhance the practitioner's therapeutic arsenal. Used appropriately, these approaches can be valuable in helping to alleviate suffering for the millions of chronic pain patients who are experiencing unremitting pain. In our opinion the most pressing questions that need to be addressed by all investigators in this area are: *"What patients, with what set of characteristics (demographic, psychological, somatic), are most likely to benefit from what set of treatment modalities?* We might hope for the day that we can be sufficiently knowledgeable to prescribe treatment modalities based on empirical evidence and not solely on the practitioner's clinical experience.

REFERENCES

Anderson, T.P., Cole, T.M., Gullickson, G., Hudgens, A., & Roberts, A.H. (1977). Behavior modification of chronic pain: A treatment program by a multidisciplinary team. *Journal of Clinical Orthopedics, 129,* 96–100.

Aneshensel, C., Frerichs, R.J., & Huba, G.J. (1984). Depression and physical illness: A multiwave, nonrecursive causal model. *Journal of Health and Social Behavior, 25,* 350–371.

Averill, J.R. (1973). Personal control over aversive stimuli and its relationship to stress. *Psychological Bulletin, 80,* 286–303.

Bandura, A. (1977). Self-efficacy: Toward a unifying theory of behavioral change. *Psychological Review, 84,* 191–215.

Beck, A.T. (1967). *Depression.* New York: Harper & Row.

Blumer, D., & Heilbronn, M. (1982). Chronic pain as a variant of depressive disease: The pain-prone disorder. *Journal of Nervous and Mental Disease, 170,* 381–406.

Bowers, K.S. (1968). Pain, anxiety, and perceived control. *Journal of Consulting and Clinical Psychology, 32,* 596–602.

Cameron, R. (1978). The clinical implementation of behavior change techniques: A cognitively oriented conceptualization of therapeutic "compliance" and "resistance." In J.P. Foreyt and D.P. Rathjen (Eds.), *Cognitive behavior therapy: Research and application* (pp. 233–250). New York: Plenum Press.

Flor, H., Haag, G., Turk, D.C., & Koehler, G. (1983). Efficacy of EMG biofeedback, pseudotherapy, and conventional medical treatments for chronic rheumatic pain. *Pain, 17,* 21–32.

Flor, H., & Turk, D.C. (1984). Etiological theories and treatment for chronic back pain: I. Somatic factors. *Pain, 19,* 105–121.

Flor, H., & Turk, D.C. (1985). Chronic illness in an adult family member: Chronic pain as a prototype. In D.C. Turk and R.D. Kerns (Eds.), *Health, illness, and families: A life-span perspective.* New York: Wiley-Interscience.

Fordyce, W.E. (1976). *Behavioral methods for chronic pain and illness.* St Louis, MO: C.V. Mosby.

France, R.D., Krishnan, R.R., Houpt, J.L., &

Maltbie, A.A. (1984). Differentiation of depression from chronic pain with the dexamethasone suppression test and DSM-III. *American Journal of Psychiatry, 141,* 1577–1579.

Greene, C.S. (1980). Myofascial pain-dysfunction syndrome: Nonsurgical treatment. In B. Sarnat & D.M. Laskin (Eds.), *The temporomandibular joint: A biological basis for clinical practice* (pp. 315–334). Springfield, IL: Charles C. Thomas.

Holroyd, K.A., & Andrasik, F. (1978). Coping and self-control of chronic tension headache. *Journal of Consulting and Clinical Psychology, 46,* 1036–1045.

Jacox, A.K. (Ed.) (1977). *Pain: A source book for nurses and other health professionals.* Boston: Little, Brown.

Johnson, J.E. (1973). Effects of accurate expectations about sensation on the sensory and distress components of pain. *Journal of Personality and Social Psychology, 27,* 261–275.

Kamlinger, K.G., Swanson, D.W., & Maruta, T. (1983). Are patients with chronic pain depressed? *American Journal of Psychiatry, 140,* 747–749.

Kerns, R.D., & Turk, D.C. (1984). Depression and chronic pain: The mediating role of the spouse. *Journal of Marriage and the Family, 46,* 845–852.

Lewinsohn, P.M. (1974). Clinical and theoretical aspects of depression. In K.S. Calhoun, H.E. Adams, & Mitchell, K.M. (Eds.), *Innovative treatment methods for psychopathology* (pp. 201–217). New York: John Wiley & Sons.

Liebeskind, J.C., & Paul, L.A. (1977). Psychological and physiological mechanisms of pain. *Annual Review of Psychology, 28,* 41–60.

Lindsay, P.G., & Wyckoff, M. (1981). The depression-pain syndrome and its response to antidepressants. *Psychosomatics, 22,* 571–577.

Marlatt, G.A., & Gordon, J.R. (1980). Determinants of relapse: Implications for the maintenance of behavior change. In P.O. Davidson & S.M. Davidson (Eds.), Behavioral medicine: *Changing health life styles* (pp. 107–131). New York: Brunner/Mazel.

Melzack, R. (Ed.) (1983). *Pain measurement and assessment.* New York: Raven Press.

Melzack, R., & Casey, K.L. (1968). Sensory, motivational and central control determinants of pain: A new conceptual model. In D. Kenshalo (Ed.), *The skin senses* (pp. 168–187). Springfield, IL: Charles C. Thomas.

Melzack, R., & Wall, P.D. (1965). Pain mechanisms: A new theory. *Science, 150,* 971–979.

Nachemson, A. (1979). A critical look at the conservative treatment of low back pain. *Scandinavian Journal of Rehabilitation Medicine, 11,* 143–149.

Nouwen, A., & Solinger, J.W. (1979). The effectiveness of EMG biofeedback training in low back pain. *Biofeedback and Self-Regulation, 4,* 103–111.

Romano, J.M., & Turner, J.A. (1985). Chronic pain and depression: A review. *Psychological Bulletin, 97,* 18–34.

Rehm, L.P. (1977). A self-control model of depression. *Behavior Therapy, 8,* 787–804.

Roy, R., Thomas, M., & Mates, M. (1984). Chronic pain and depression: A review. *Comprehensive Psychiatry, 25,* 96–105.

Seligman, M.E.P. (1975). *Helplessness: On depression, development and death.* San Francisco: Freeman.

Turk, D.C., Meichenbaum, D.M., & Berman, W.H. (1979). Application of biofeedback for the regulation of pain: A critical review. *Psychological Bulletin, 86,* 1322–1338.

Turk, D.C., Holzman, A.D., & Kerns, R.D. (in press). Treatment of chronic pain: Emphasis on self management. In K.A. Holroyd & T. Creer (Eds.), *Handbook of self-management in health psychology and behavioral medicine.* Orlando, FL: Academic Press.

Turk, D.C., & Kerns, R.D. (1985). Assessment in health psychology: A cognitive-behavioral perspective. In P. Karoly (Ed.), *Measurement strategies in health psychology.* New York: Wiley-Interscience.

Turk, D.C., Kerns, R.D., & Rudy, T.E. (1984, August). *Identifying the links between chronic illness and depression.* Paper presented at the annual meetings of the American Psychological Association, Toronto, Canada.

Turk, D.C., & Meichenbaum, D. (in press). Behavioral approaches in pain management. In G. Burrows, D. Elton, & G. Stanley (Eds.), *Handbook of chronic pain management.* Amsterdam: Elsevier Science.

Turk, D.C., Meichenbaum, D., & Genest, M. (1983). *Pain and behavioral medicine: A cognitive-behavioral perspective.* New York: Guilford.

Turk, D.C., & Salovey, P. (1984). "Chronic pain as a variant of depressive disease": A critical reappraisal. *Journal of Nervous and Mental Disease, 172,* 1–7.

Weisenberg, M. (1977). Pain and pain control. *Psychological Bulletin, 84,* 1008–1044.

AUTHOR INDEX

SUBJECT INDEX

ABOUT THE EDITORS
AND CONTRIBUTORS

Arnold D. Holzman, PhD is an Assistant Clinical Professor of Psychology in Psychiatry at the Yale University School of Medicine. He is the former Director of the Pain Management Program at the West Haven Veterans Administration Medical Center and is currently in practice in New Haven, Connecticut. He is an attending psychologist at the West Haven Veterans Administration Medical Center and a consultant at the Newington Children's Hospital, Newington, Connecticut. Dr. Holzman has presented workshops and papers at various conferences, universities and medical settings, and has consulted to pain management programs throughout the United States. Dr. Holzman has published numerous scientific articles and chapters in professional journals and books.

Dennis C. Turk, PhD is internationally known for his work in the assessment and treatment of chronic pain and is considered to be the authority on the cognitive-behavioral treatment of pain. From 1977 to 1985 he was on the faculty of the Department of Psychology, Yale University. He is currently Director of the Center for Pain Evaluation and Treatment, University of Pittsburgh School of Medicine. Dr. Turk is a founding member of both the International Association for the Study of Pain and the American Pain Society. Dr. Turk has presented papers and workshops at numerous conferences and hospitals throughout the United States and Canada.

Dr. Turk has published over 50 papers in books and scientific journals, has prepared a tape series on the treatment of chronic pain, and has recently published two books, *Pain and Behavioral Medicine* with Donald Meichenbaum and Myles Genest, and *Health, Illness and Families* with Robert Kerns.

Frank Andrasik, PhD is an Associate Professor of Psychology and Associate Director of the Center for Stress and Anxiety Disorders at the State University of New York at Albany. His teaching and research interests center chiefly on pain and stress management with children and adults.

Joseph Barber, PhD is Assistant Clinical Professor, Department of Psychiatry, UCLA, and maintains a private practice in psychology in Los Angeles. He is the co-editor (with Cheri Adrian) of *Psychological Approaches to the Management of Pain*, is Abstracts Editor of *The American Journal of Clinical Hypnosis*, and has published widely in professional journals.

Cynthia D. Belar, PhD is Chief Psychologist in the Department of Psychiatry, Kaiser-Permanente Medical Center, Los Angeles, California, where she also serves as Clinical Director of Behavioral Medicine.

Roy Cameron, PhD received his doctorate from the University of Waterloo. He has been a faculty member in the Department of Psychology at the University of Saskatchewan, and is currently Associate Professor and Chairman, Department of Health Studies, University of Waterloo.

Charles S. Cleeland, PhD is a Professor of Neurology (Neuropsychology), and Director of the Pain Research Group and the Biofeedback Clinic at the University of Wisconsin Medical School. His research includes studies of pain in cancer and other disease and of behavioral intervention in neurologic disease.

Al S. Fedoravicius, PhD received his PhD in Clinical Psychology from the University of Waterloo in 1971. He has been a faculty member at Xavier University in Ohio and at the University of Cincinnati Medical School, where he was the Director of the Psychosomatics Unit and the Chronic Illness Behavior Program. Currently, he is the Coordinator of the Behavioral Medicine Program at the Albuquerque VA Medical Center, and is an adjunct faculty member in the departments of Psychology and Psychiatry at the University of New Mexico.

W. Doyle Gentry, PhD is currently in private practice with Psychological Associates of Lynchburg, Virginia. He is Clinical Professor of Behavioral Medicine and Psychiatry, University of Virginia, and is Founding Editor-in-Chief, *Journal of Behavioral Medicine.*

Susan M. Jay, PhD is Director of Research and Education, Psychosocial Program, Division of Hematology-Oncology, Children's Hospital of Los Angeles, and Assistant Professor of Pediatrics, University of Southern California, Los Angeles.

Stephen A. Kibrick, PhD is a clinical psychologist in the Behavioral Medicine unit of the Department of Psychiatry, Kaiser-Permanente Medical Center, Los Angeles, California, where he has served as Director of the Stress Management/Biofeedback program since 1977.

Ben J. Klein, MA is a graduate student in the Department of Psychology at the University of New Mexico, where he received his MA degree in 1984. He is currently (1985–1986) an intern at the University of Washington School of Medicine.

Bruce J. Masek, PhD is Assistant Professor of Psychology, Department of Psychiatry, Harvard Medical School and the Children's Hospital, Boston.

Harold Merskey, DM is Professor of Psychiatry, University of Western Ontario and Director of Education and Research at London Psychiatric Hospital, London, Canada. He was educated at the Universities of Oxford and London, England, and was Physician in Psychological Medicine at The National Hospitals for Nervous Diseases, Queen Square and Maida Vale, London, England.

Richard I. Newman, PhD is Assistant Clinical Professor of Psychiatry at the University of Oregon Health Sciences Center and Co-Director of the Northwest Pain Center. He is the current President of the Western U.S.A. Pain Society.

Daniel Owens, PhD is currently in private practice with Psychological Associates of Lynchburg, Virginia. He received his doctorate in Clinical Psychology from Ohio State University in 1980.

Alan H. Roberts, PhD was formerly a professor at the University of Minnesota where he founded and directed the Pain Clinic and the Pain Treatment Program from 1969 until 1979. He is currently the Director of the Behavioral Medicine Program at Scripps Clinic and Research Foundation in La Jolla, California.

Ranjan Roy, Adv. Dip. SW was educated at St. Stephen's College, Delhi, India; London School of Economics in the U.K.; and School of Social Work, University of Toronto, Canada. He is an Associate Professor in Social Work, as well as Psychiatry, at the University of Manitoba, Canada.

Joel Seres, MD is a Board Certified neurosurgeon who established the Northwest Pain Center in 1972. He is an Associate Clinical Professor of Neurosurgery at the Oregon

Health Sciences University and Director of the Northwest Pain Center. He is currently President-Elect of the American Academy of Algology, a physician group specializing in pain management.

Larry F. Shepel, PhD received his doctorate from the University of Saskatchewan. He is currently Head of the Division of Psychology at University Hospital, Saskatoon, and an Associate Professor in the Department of Psychology, University of Saskatchewan.

Blake A. Tearnan, PhD is an academic staff psychologist for the Department of Neurology, University of Wisconsin Medical School.

Karen L. Thompson, MA is a doctoral graduate student, Department of Psychology, University of Southern California, Los Angeles.

James W. Varni, PhD is Co-Director, Behavioral Pediatrics Program, Orthopaedic Hospital, and Clinical Associate Professor of Psychology, Pediatrics and Psychiatry, University of Southern California, Los Angeles.

Pergamon General Psychology Series

Editors: Arnold P. Goldstein, Syracuse University
Leonard Krasner, SUNY at Stony Brook